CENTRAL NERVOUS SYSTEM EFFECTS OF HYPOTHALAMIC HORMONES AND OTHER PEPTIDES

Central Nervous System Effects of Hypothalamic Hormones and Other Peptides

Edited by

Robert Collu, M.D.
Pediatric Research Center
Sainte-Justine Hospital
Montreal, Quebec, Canada

André Barbeau, M.D.
Clinical Research Institute
of Montreal
Montreal, Quebec, Canada

Jacques R. Ducharme, M.D.
Pediatric Research Center
Sainte-Justine Hospital
Montreal, Quebec, Canada

Jean-Guy Rochefort, Ph.D.
Abbott Laboratories Limited
Montreal, Quebec, Canada

Raven Press ▪ New York

Raven Press, 1140 Avenue of the Americas, New York, New York 10036

Made in the United States of America

Library of Congress Cataloging in Publication Data
Main entry under title:

Central nervous system effects of hypothalamic hormones
and other peptides.

Includes bibliographical references and index.
1. Neuroendocrinology. 2. Central nervous system.
3. Hypothalamic hormones. 4. Endorphins, I. Collu,
Robert. [DNLM: 1. Peptides—Pharmacodynamics.
2. Pituitary hormone releasing hormones—Pharmacodynamics. 3. Central nervous system—Drug effects.
QU68 C396]
QP356.4.C45   612'.8'04   77-94310
ISBN 0-89004-347-7

Foreword

The discovery of hypophysiotropic hypothalamic hormones has been one of the major advances in neuroendocrinology made in the last decade. The importance of this discovery was recognized by the awarding of the 1977 Nobel Prize in Physiology and Medicine to Dr. R. Guillemin and to Dr. A. V. Schally, who were the first to establish the structures of TRH, LH-RH, and somatostatin.

A great deal of research from several laboratories and clinics around the world indicates that these peptides may also exert actions outside the anterior pituitary. This book contains the most up-to-date evidence for the participation of these peptides in the modulation of central nervous system activities. The significance of the presence in the brain and in the anterior pituitary of peptides with opioid-like activities is also reviewed in this volume.

The International Society of Neuroendocrinology was pleased to co-sponsor the Symposium (held in Montreal in May 1978) on which this volume is based, and hopes that this book will help stimulate future advances in the field of neuroendocrinology.

Luciano Martini, M.D.

Preface

The period between 1945 and 1960 was the golden age of steroids; now is the golden age of peptides. The elucidation of the amino acid sequence of the two chains of insulin and the synthesis of vasopressin and oxytocin in the early 1950s ushered in this new era. Since then, mainly due to technical refinements that allow for the determination of the composition and amino acid sequence of peptides from minute amounts of material, we have witnessed the growth and maturation of "peptidology."

Particularly exciting to scientists involved in such diverse fields as psychiatry, endocrinology, and neurology have been recent demonstrations that the brain manufactures several peptides, and that these peptides may influence brain functions. A review of this evidence is presented in this volume. Data are presented indicating that hypothalamic-releasing and release-inhibiting factors, endorphins, vasoactive intestinal peptide, neurotensin, substance P, bombesin, and even anterior pituitary hormones may be found in significant amounts in various areas of the brain, possibly synthesized *in situ* by peptidergic neurons, and that these substances may have powerful effects on central nervous system functions. Pioneer work in this field demonstrated that ACTH fragments—recently shown to be present in the hypothalamus and mesencephalon several weeks after hypophysectomy—can influence memory. Data by several workers on the localization of TRH, LH-RH, and SRIF in several extrahypothalamic areas have given solid anatomical support to physiologists and their data on central nervous system effects of these compounds.

Psychiatrists and neurologists have benefited from experimental work with psychoactive brain peptides, and new concepts and modalities of therapy are being developed for old diseases such as Parkinson's disease and schizophrenia.

With the new concept of APUD cells, the entire body appears now as an orchestra of endocrine instruments in which the brain retains its role of conductor but in a completely new role of master gland. It is indeed the era of Neuroendocrinology, a heretofore mainly experimental subspecialty that is now considered to be a major clinical discipline. We present this book as an expression of confidence in a bright new science, in new ideas, and in new hopes.

Robert Collu
André Barbeau
Jacques-Raymond Ducharme
Guy Rochefort

Contents

Contributors

F. Aichner
Clinic of Neurology
University of Innsbrück
Innsbrück, Austria

Elisabeth Arnauld
Division of Neurology
Montreal General Hospital
Montreal, Quebec, H36 1A4 Canada

André Barbeau
Département de Neurobiologie
Institut de Recherches Cliniques de
  Montréal
Montréal, Québec, H2W 1R7 Canada

Gordon Bautz
Department of Pharmacology
Hoffmann-La Roche Inc.
Nutley, New Jersey 07110

M. Beaulieu
Medical Research Council Group in
  Molecular Endocrinology
Centre Hospitalier de l'Université
  Laval
Québec, Québec, Canada

S. Benjannet
Protein and Pituitary Hormone
  Laboratory
Clinical Research Institute of
  Montreal
Montreal, Quebec, Canada

R. Benoit
Division of Neurology
McGill University
Montreal, Quebec, Canada

Garth Bissette
Department of Psychiatry
Biological Sciences Research Center
University of North Carolina
Chapel Hill, North Carolina 27514

Howard W. Blume
Division of Neurology
Montreal General Hospital
Montreal, Quebec, H36 1A4 Canada

J. R. Boissier
Centre de Recherches Roussel-
  UCLAF
Romainville, France

Paul Brazeau
Division of Neurology
McGill University
Montreal, Quebec, Canada

Michael J. Brownstein
Laboratory of Clinical Science
National Institute of Mental Health
Bethesda, Maryland 20014

John F. Bruni
Department of Physiology
Neuroendocrine Research Laboratory
Michigan State University
East Lansing, Michigan 48824

M. A. Carino
Department of Pharmacology
School of Medicine
University of Washington
Seattle, Washington 98195

M. G. Caron
Medical Research Council Group in
  Molecular Endocrinology
Centre Hospitalier de l'Université
  Laval
Québec, Québec, Canada

G. Charpenet
Centre de Recherche Pédiatrique
Hôpital Sainte-Justine
Montréal, Québec, H3T 1C5 Canada

Steven R. Childers
Johns Hopkins University
School of Medicine
Baltimore, Maryland 21205

Michel Chrétien
*Protein and Pituitary Hormone
Laboratory
Clinical Research Institute of
Montreal
Montreal, Quebec, H2W 1R7 Canada*

Robert Collu
*Centre de Recherche Pédiatrique
Hôpital Sainte-Justine
Montréal, Québec, H3T 1C5 Canada*

David H. Coy
*Endocrine and Polypeptide
Laboratories
Veterans Administration Hospital
New Orleans, Louisiana 70146*

P. Crine
*Protein and Pituitary Hormone
Laboratory
Clinical Research Institute of
Montreal
Montreal, Quebec, H2W 1R7 Canada*

Lionel Cusan
*Laboratory of Molecular En-
docrinology
Le Centre Hospitalier de l'Université
Laval
Québec, Québec, Canada*

F. Denizeau
*Centre de Recherches Roussel-
UCLAF
Romainville, France*

T. Di Paolo
*Medical Research Council Group in
Molecular Endocrinology
Centre Hospitalier de l'Université
Laval
Québec, Québec, Canada*

Carol A. Dudley
*Physiology Department
Southwestern Medical School
University of Texas Health Sciences
Center
Dallas, Texas 75235*

Jacques R. Ducharme
*Centre de Recherche Pédiatrique
Hôpital Sainte-Justine
Montréal, Québec, Canada*

André Dupont
*Laboratory of Molecular En-
docrinology
Le Centre Hospitalier de l'Université
Laval
Québec, Québec, Canada*

J. Epelbaum
*Division of Neurology
McGill University
Montreal, Quebec, Canada*

C. Euvrard
*Centre de Recherches Roussel-
UCLAF
Romainville, France*

Louise Ferland
*Medical Research Council Group in
Molecular Endocrinology
Centre Hospitalier de l'Université
Laval
Québec, Québec, Canada*

Henry G. Friesen
*Department of Physiology
University of Manitoba
Winnipeg, Manitoba, Canada*

Joseph Gardner
*Endocrine and Polypeptide
Laboratories
Veterans Administration Hospital
New Orleans, Louisiana 70112*

F. Gerstenbrand
*Clinic of Neurology
University of Innsbrück
Innsbrück, Austria*

Roger Guillemin
*Laboratories for Neuroendocrinology
The Salk Institute
La Jolla, California 92112*

Victor Havlicek
*Department of Physiology
University of Manitoba
Winnipeg, Manitoba, R3E OW3
Canada*

A. Horita
Department of Pharmacology
School of Medicine
University of Washington
Seattle, Washington 98195

W. Dale Horst
Department of Pharmacology
Hoffmann-La Roche Inc.
Nutley, New Jersey 07110

Ivor M. D. Jackson
Tufts University School of Medicine
New England Medical Center
    Hospital
Boston, Massachusetts 02111

Abba J. Kastin
Endocrinology Section of the Medical
    Service
Veterans Administration Hospital
New Orleans, Louisiana 70146

G. L. Kovács
Department of Pathophysiology
University Medical School
Szeged, Hungary

C. Kozma
Clinic of Neurology
University of Innsbrück
Innsbrück, Austria

Fernand Labrie
Medical Research Council Group in
    Molecular Endocrinology
Centre Hospitalier de l'Université
    Laval
Québec, Québec, Canada

T. R. Lahann
Department of Pharmacology
School of Medicine
University of Washington
Seattle, Washington 98195

H. Lai
Department of Pharmacology
School of Medicine
University of Washington
Seattle, Washington 98195

Yvon Lamour
Division of Neurology
Montreal General Hospital
Montreal, Quebec, H36 1A4 Canada

André Lemay
Department of Obstetric and Gyne-
    cology
Hôpital St-François d'Assise
Québec, Québec, Canada

Morris A. Lipton
Department of Psychiatry
Biological Sciences Research Center
University of North Carolina
Chapel Hill, North Carolina 27514

Martin Lis
Protein and Pituitary Hormone
    Laboratory
Clinical Research Institute of
    Montreal
Montreal, Quebec, H2W 1R7
    Canada

Peter T. Loosen
Department of Psychiatry
Biological Sciences Research Center
University of North Carolina
Chapel Hill, North Carolina 27514

Luciano Martini
Istituto di Farmacologia
Milan, Italy

Joseph Meites
Department of Physiology
Neuroendocrine Research Laboratory
Michigan State University
East Lansing, Michigan 48824

Robert L. Moss
Physiology Department
Southwestern Medical School
University of Texas Health Sciences
    Center
Dallas, Texas 75235

Charles B. Nemeroff
Department of Psychiatry
Biological Sciences Research Center
University of North Carolina
Chapel Hill, North Carolina 27514

Richard D. Olson
Department of Psychology
University of New Orleans
New Orleans, Louisiana 70122

Alan J. Osbahr III
Department of Psychiatry
Biological Sciences Research Center
University of North Carolina
Chapel Hill, North Carolina 27514

Jaak Panksepp
Department of Psychology
Bowling Green State University
Bowling Green, Ohio 43403

Escipion Pedroza
Department of Medicine
Veterans Administration Hospital
New Orleans, Louisiana 70112

Georges Pelletier
Medical Research Council Group in
  Molecular Endocrinology
Le Centre Hospitalier de
  l'Université Laval
Québec, Québec, G1V 462 Canada

Quentin J. Pittman
Division of Neurology
Montreal General Hospital
Montreal, Quebec, H36 1A4 Canada

W. Poewe
Clinic of Neurology
University of Innsbrück
Innsbrück, Austria

Arthur J. Prange, Jr.
Department of Psychiatry
Biological Sciences Research Center
University of North Carolina
Chapel Hill, North Carolina 27514

V. Raymond
Medical Research Council Group in
  Molecular Endocrinology
Le Centre Hospitalier de
  l'Université Laval
Québec, Québec, Canada

J. P. Raynaud
Centre de Recherches Roussel-
  UCLAF
Romainville, France

Ram B. Rastogi
Division of Pharmacology
Bio-Research Laboratories
Connlab Holdings Limited
Montreal, Quebec, Canada

Seymour Reichlin
Tufts University School of Medicine
New England Medical Center
  Hospital
Boston, Massachusetts 02111

Leo P. Renaud
Division of Neurology
Montreal General Hospital
Montreal, Quebec, H36 1A4 Canada

Peter Riskind
Physiology Department
Southwestern Medical School
University of Texas Health Sciences
  Center
Dallas, Texas 75235

Catherine Rivier
Laboratories for Neuroendocrinology
The Salk Institute
La Jolla, California 92112

Jean Rivier
Laboratories for Neuroendocrinology
The Salk Institute
La Jolla, California 92112

Jean-Guy Rochefort
Abbott Laboratories Ltd.
Montreal, Quebec, Canada

Curt A. Sandman
Department of Psychology
Ohio State University
Columbus, Ohio 43210

Andrew V. Schally
Endocrine and Polypeptide
  Laboratories
Veterans Administration Hospital
New Orleans, Louisiana 70146

Nabil S. Seidah
Protein and Pituitary Hormone
  Laboratory
Clinical Research Institute of
  Montreal
Montreal, Quebec, H2W 1R7
  Canada

Janos Seprodi
Department of Medicine
Veterans Administration Hospital
New Orleans, Louisiana 70112

Solomon H. Snyder
Johns Hopkins University
School of Medicine
Baltimore, Maryland 21205

Nena Spirt
Department of Pharmacology
Hoffmann-La Roche Inc.
Nutley, New Jersey 07110

Yvette Taché
Centre de Recherche Pédiatrique
Hôpital Sainte-Justine
Montréal, Québec, H3T 1C5 Canada

G. Telegdy
Department of Pathophysiology
University Medical School
Szeged, Hungary

Robert D. Utiger
Departments of Psychiatry, Pharma-
*   cology, and Medicine*
University of Pennsylvania
School of Medicine
Philadelphia, Pennsylvania 19104

Wylie Vale
Peptide Biology Laboratory
The Salk Institute
La Jolla, California 92112

Dean A. Van Vugt
Department of Physiology
Neuroendocrine Research Laboratory
Michigan State University
East Lansing, Michigan 48824

Tj. B. van Wimersma Greidanus
Rudolf Magnus Institute for
*   Pharmacology*
Utrecht, The Netherlands

R. Veilleux
Medical Research Council Group in
*   Molecular Endocrinology*
Centre Hospitalier de l'Université
*   Laval*
Québec, Québec, Canada

Jesus A. Vilchez-Martinez
Department of Medicine
Veterans Administration Hospital
New Orleans, Louisiana 70112

Ian C. Wilson
Division of Research
North Carolina Department of Mental
*   Health*
Raleigh, North Carolina 27611

Andrew Winokur
Departments of Psychiatry, Pharma-
*   cology, and Medicine*
University of Pennsylvania
School of Medicine
Philadelphia, Pennsylvania 19104

Thyrotropin-Releasing Hormone

Central Nervous System Effects of Hypothalamic
Hormones and Other Peptides, edited by Collu et al.
Raven Press, New York © 1979.

Distribution and Biosynthesis of TRH in the Nervous System

Ivor M. D. Jackson and Seymour Reichlin

Division of Endocrinology, Department of Medicine, Tufts University School of Medicine,
New England Medical Center Hospital, Boston, Massachusetts 02111

It is well substantiated that the anterior pituitary gland of mammalian species is regulated by the hypothalamus through the synthesis and secretion of releasing factors, or hormones, by peptidergic neurons (16,184). The isolation and synthesis of three of these hypothalamic hypophysiotropic hormones—thyrotropin-releasing hormone (TRH), luteinizing hormone-releasing hormone (LH-RH), and growth hormone-release inhibiting hormone (somatostatin)—have provided powerful tools for the investigation of pituitary function and permitted the development of specific radioimmunoassays for the measurement of these substances at exceedingly low concentrations (191,231). A wholly unanticipated outcome of these methodologic developments was the finding that most of neural TRH (and somatostatin) is located outside the hypothalamus (91,92). Further, these hormones are present in inframammalian species (92) although the functional significance of this phylogenetic distribution remains to be determined (93). Even more surprising was the discovery that both TRH (103,152) and somatostatin (3,170) are found in anatomic locations not heretofore considered part of the nervous system.

It is believed that the hypothalamic peptidergic neurons producing the hypophysiotropic hormones are in turn regulated by neurotransmitters, especially of the monoaminergic type, and that the peptidergic neuron acts as a "neuroendocrine transducer," converting neuronal information from the brain into chemical information (237). Subsequently it was recognized that the chemical products of the peptidergic neurons may themselves function as neurotransmitters (131). Still to be determined is the question of whether the same kind of hormonal feedback and/or neurotransmitter control characteristic of the hypothalamus is also operative at extrahypothalamic sites. The development of techniques to purify hypophysiotropic hormones (e.g., affinity chromatography and cellular localization with immunohistochemistry) have made important methodologic contributions to determining the physiologic importance of these hormones.

The finding of extrahypothalamic brain sources of hypophysiotropic hormones provides some support for the "ependymal tanycyte hypothesis," which proposes that a portion of the releasing hormones reaches the portal vessels by trans-median eminence transport; it is postulated that the releasing hormones are secreted into the ventricular system, taken up by the lumenal processes of the tanycytes of the median eminence (ME), and then actively transported for release at the capillary end of the cell (122).

DISTRIBUTION OF THYROTROPIN-RELEASING HORMONE IN MAMMALS

Hypothalamus

It has been recognized since the early 1950s that the hypothalamus exerts an important influence on the regulation of the pituitary-thyroid axis (for reviews see refs. 183,186). Finally in 1969, following rigorous chemical analysis of large numbers of ovine and porcine hypothalamic fragments, the chemical structure of TRH was elucidated in the laboratories of Guillemin and Schally and was shown to be a tripeptide amide (P-glu-His-Pro-NH$_2$) of molecular weight 362 (18,30).

The availability of chemically pure synthetic TRH permitted the development of a radioimmunoassay for TRH by several groups including those of Utiger (6), Wilber (150), Porter (166), and ourselves (100). The conjugation of TRH to a large carrier-weight protein such as bovine serum albumin (6) or bovine thyroglobulin (101) permits the generation of antibody to TRH in rabbits with a high degree of sensitivity and specificity. The levels of immunoreactive (IR)-TRH in the rat hypothalamus reported from different laboratories ranged from 2.7 to 15.7 ng (9,101,102,165). We found considerable variation in the amount of IR-TRH in different groups of rat hypothalami in different experiments. These variations may relate to the size of tissue block in different experiments but might also reflect seasonal or other differences. Bassiri and Utiger (9) also reported variations in the levels of IR-TRH in the hypothalamus when experiments were performed at different time intervals.

We found immunoreactive TRH readily detectable in porcine hypothalami (500 pg/mg tissue wet weight), hamster hypothalami (480 pg/mg tissue wet weight), and human stalk median eminence (SME), with values up to 300 pg/mg tissue (101). Recent studies by Okon and Koch (162), Guansing and Murk (77), and Kubek et al. (125) demonstrated substantial quantities of TRH throughout the hypothalamus and SME of humans.

Ablation of the "thyrotrophic" area of the hypothalamus induces hypothyroidism in the rat, but the TRH levels in the hypothalamus of such lesioned animals were as much as 35% of the values found in the controls (104) (Table 1). The persistence of significant TRH levels in the hypothalamus following lesion explains the fact that depression of base-line thyroid

TABLE 1. *Effect of a lesion of the "thyrotropic area" of the hypothalamus on the hypothalamic and brain content of TRH*

	Lesion[a]	Control[a]	Significance
Hypothalamus	3.6 ± 0.3[b]	9.4 ± 0.5	$p < 0.001$
Extrahypothalamic brain	17.0 ± 0.9	18.9 ± 0.7	$p > 0.1$

From ref. 104.

[a] Six lesioned and seven control rats were studied.

[b] Results are expressed as nanograms per whole tissue (mean $\pm$ SEM).

function after such a procedure is never as severe as that occurring after hypophysectomy. Studies by Browstein et al. (28), utilizing a technique which allows discrete nuclei to be dissected from the brain of the rat, showed that TRH, although present in highest concentrations within nuclei of the "thyrotrophic area," was also found in the hypothalamus outside this region. Their data are in keeping with our findings in lesioned animals as well as our report (102) of a gradient of TRH from dorsal hypothalamus (49 pg/mg tissue) to SME (3,570 pg/mg tissue) (Table 2).

TRH has been reported to show immunofluorescent staining of nerve terminals in the medial part of the external layer of the median eminence (84), but no immunopositive TRH perikarya were observed. Although there are a number of reports from different laboratories of immunopositive staining for LH-RH and somatostatin in the hypothalamic region (see refs. 91–93 for review), there have been no other reports of the immunohistochemical distribution of TRH in the hypothalamus or elsewhere in the central nervous system (CNS).

TABLE 2. *TRH distribution in rat brain*

Brain area	TRH (pg/mg tissue)	
	Mean	Range
Extrahypothalamic brain		
Brainstem	5	4–5
Cerebellum	2	1–3
Diencephalon	6	3–12
Olfactory lobe	6	5–8
Cerebral cortex	2	1–3
Hypothalamic-pituitary complex		
Dorsal hypothalamus	49	41–61
Ventral hypothalamus	64	23–106
Stalk median eminence	3,570	920–7,600
Posterior pituitary	155	150–160
Anterior pituitary	10	8–11

From ref. 102.

It may be that TRH is broken down in the preparation of the section, or its special subcellular localization "protects" the peptide from immunohistochemical staining. Hökfelt (*personal communication*) found that different TRH antisera show variability in their ability to produce immunohistochemical staining. The estimate of total rat hypothalamic TRH by radioimmunoassay (RIA) has given levels 10 to 20 times those previously reported by *in vivo* bioassay (187); the discrepancy is probably based on the presence of somatostatin, which inhibits TRH-induced TSH rise (224).

Extrahypothalamic Neural Tissue

The first reports that IR-TRH was present in the brain outside the confines of the hypothalamus were provided by Jackson and Reichlin (100) (Table 2) and Oliver et al. (166). Although such concentrations are small when compared with the levels in the hypothalamus (101), quantitatively over 70% of total brain TRH is found outside this region (165,235).

Substantial quantities of TRH are found in the spinal cord (116,231), a finding we confirmed, and immunohistochemical examination has localized TRH around the motoneurons of the spinal cord (84). Networks of TRH-positive nerve terminals have also been found by these workers in many cranial nerve nuclei (84).

As in the fetal rat (52), significant concentrations of TRH are present in the extrahypothalamic brain of the human fetus (236), TRH being detected in the cerebellum as early as 9 weeks. The cerebellum of an anencephalic infant contained a relatively high concentration of TRH (236). It should be noted, however, that the area cerebrovasculosa—an area lacking in nerve cells—taken from an anencephalic fetus has been reported to synthesize a TSH-releasing substance *in vitro* (89). Extrahypothalamic brain tissue from normal human adults killed in traffic accidents contains significant concentrations of immunoassayable TRH in the thalamus and cerebral cortex (162). Guansing and Murk (77) and Kubek et al. (125) also identified IR-TRH in the extrahypothalamic brain tissue of humans.

A fundamental issue to be resolved is whether the extrahypothalamic IR-TRH present in mammalian neural tissue is indeed authentic TRH. The overall evidence from a number of laboratories strongly supports the authenticity of the tripeptide. Oliver et al. (165) showed that IR-TRH in methanolic extracts of rat brain shows an elution pattern on Sephadex G-10 column chromatography and a migratory pattern on cellulose acetate electrophoresis similar to ^{3}H-TRH and synthetic TRH. Further, these workers showed that extracts of tissue from cerebrum, thalamus, and brainstem were capable of inducing TSH release from anterior pituitaries *in vitro,* and the IR-TRH in the extracts showed susceptibility to breakdown by rat plasma, a response also manifested by synthetic TRH. In human tissue the slopes of ^{125}I-TRH antibody binding inhibition by diluted extracts of extrahy-

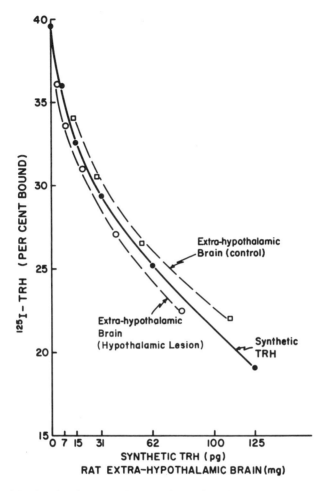

FIG. 1. Effect of dried methanol extracts of rat extrahypothalamic brain tissue from normal controls and animals with lesions of the hypothalamic "thyrotropic area" on the binding of ^{125}I to anti-TRH. Note parallelism of both these inhibition curves with that of synthetic TRH.

pothalamic brain were parallel to those of synthetic TRH, similar to our findings in the rat (Fig. 1). Elution on Sephadex G-10 column chromatography showed a pattern similar to that of synthetic TRH; and biologic activity of extrahypothalamic extracts, evaluated by pituitary TSH release *in vitro,* was qualitatively similar to that of synthetic TRH or hypothalamic extract (125). In our studies the IR-TRH present in the hypothalamus and extrahypothalamic brain tissue of the rat shows an elution pattern similar to that of synthetic TRH. However, 6 to 10% of the total IR-TRH that elutes comes off just after the void volume (Fig. 2). Whether this IR-TRH is a polymer of TRH ("big" TRH) or another molecular species is undetermined at this time. Further, it is not known if this immunoreactive moiety eluting after

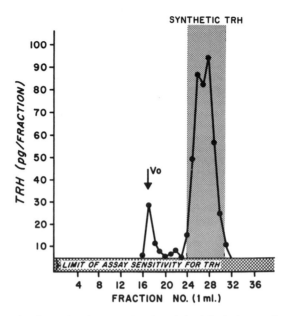

FIG. 2. Chromatography of a methanol extract of rat hypothalamic brain tissue on Sephadex G-10. Note that the bulk of the IR-TRH elutes are similar to synthetic TRH, but approximately 6 to 10% of the total TRH comes off just after the void volume ("big TRH" ?). Similar findings occur on chromatography of extra-hypothalamic brain extracts.

the void volume has biologic activity. It should be noted that at least two peaks of IR-somatostatin have been identified in fractions obtained following gel filtration of hypothalamic extracts, and that both have biologic activity (19). Kubek et al. (125) found that IR-TRH derived from human extrahypothalamic CNS tissue showed less biologic activity than IR-TRH derived from hypothalamus or synthetic TRH. These workers suggest that the reduced biologic activity of extrahypothalamic TRH might be due to interaction between TRH and neurosecretory proteins or membranes, the presence of a TRH inhibitor, or the presence of a molecular species of TRH which possesses immunologic but not biologic activity. Since somatostatin content of extrahypothalamic brain (~ 140 ng) (26) is about seven times that of TRH, it is not unlikely that brain extracts of TRH contain somatostatin and reduce the apparent biologic activity of the IR-TRH. Winokur et al. (234) reported that synthetic TRH added to rat brain homogenates *in vitro* is rapidly destroyed by incubation at 37°C, but no endogenous TRH is lost by such incubation. These workers speculate that endogenous TRH is protected by being bound to the membranes of subcellular particles or being present within synaptic vesicles in the synaptosomes. An alternative interpretation of their findings is that endogenous IR-TRH is not the authentic tripeptide.

Recently Youngblood et al. (242) reported that IR-TRH present in extrahypothalamic brain tissues does not show chromatographic identity with synthetic TRH, and they suggest that the TRH material purported to be present in such locations may be immunoassay artifact. These findings underline the importance of establishing the authenticity of IR-TRH present outside the hypothalamus; clearly the nature of the extrahypothalamic brain TRH requires further study. However, in this review, with the reservations already stated, it is considered that IR-TRH measurements in mammalian brain tissue do represent authentic TRH. Where further proof of identity other than immunoreactivity has been provided, this is mentioned.

The unexpected discovery of TRH in the CNS outside the hypothalamus raises a number of important questions.

Could the TRH in the Extrahypothalamic Brain Be Derived from the Hypothalamus?

In an attempt to determine the source of extrahypothalamic TRH, we studied the effects of classic thyrotropic area lesions which bring about a reduction in hypothalamic TRH by two-thirds. The extrahypothalamic brain TRH content was unaffected in rats so treated, providing support for the intriguing hypothesis that synthesis occurs *in situ* (104) (Table 1). Complementary studies to these experiments by Brownstein et al. (29), using hypothalamic deafferentation, demonstrated that such procedures not only leave the levels of TRH in the extrahypothalamic brain unaltered but cause a marked reduction in hypothalamic content, suggesting that much of hypothalamic TRH may be synthesized by cells outside this region. It is possible that TRH could reach extrahypothalamic brain sites by means of cerebrospinal fluid (CSF), it having been postulated that the releasing hormones are secreted into the ventricular system. However, the fact that neither "thyrotrophic area" lesions of the hypothalamus (104) nor hypothalamic deafferentation (29) alter extrahypothalamic brain TRH, yet markedly reduce hypothalamic TRH, suggests that TRH lying outside the hypothalamus is synthesized *in situ*. Whether ventricular transport of hypophysiotropic hormones from the hypothalamus still occurs as a subsidiary source under certain physiologic circumstances cannot be excluded. TRH can reach the anterior pituitary from CSF and is effective in stimulating pituitary TSH secretion (68). Kizer et al. (119) demonstrated that the circumventricular organs of the rat all contain large concentrations of LH-RH and somewhat lesser quantities of TRH. The circumventricular organs are a group of specialized ependymal midline structures which comprise the organum vasculosum of the lamina terminalis (OVLT), the ME, the subfornical organ (SFO), the subcommissural organ (SCO), and area postrema (AP). The origin of the releasing factors in these tissues is uncertain, but the possibilities include synthesis *de novo*, transport via ventricular CSF, or axoplasmic flow to nerve terminals in the circumventricular organs. The possibility that these tissues may concentrate the releasing hormones from the CSF is supported by the specialized structure and functional capacity of these ependymal cells (122).

A third route by which TRH could reach the extrahypothalamic brain is vascular. It seems unlikely that the systemic circulation is an important means by which TRH (and other hypothalamic hormones) could reach the extrahypothalamic brain since only meager levels are measurable in the peripheral blood (see later). Recent studies by Bergland and associates (15,168) provided support for the previous studies of Popa and Fielding (178) and Torok (217) that blood may flow from the pituitary in a retrograde fashion to the brain. Bergland's group demonstrated in a number of mammalian species the abundance of shunts, as well as numerous capillary connections, between neural and glandular pituitary. The pattern of arterial supply and venous flow drainage allow for the potential of flow reversal between the pituitary and the systemic circulation. The paucity of venous connections from the adenohypophysis to the surrounding systemic venous structures led Bergland to speculate that blood flow in the short portal vessels may be from adenohypophysis to neurohypophysis and not neurohypophysis to adenohypophysis as is commonly thought. The efferent routes from the neurohypophysis include: (a) the inferior hypophysial veins from the infundibular process to the cavernous sinus; (b) portal vessels extending from the median eminence to the adenohypophysis; and (c) confluent capillaries extending from the median eminence to the hypothalamus. This newer concept of retrograde flow from the pituitary to the brain raises the possibility that not only pituitary hormones (167) but also hypophysiotrophic hormones may return to the hypothalamus and to the extrahypothalamic brain. Thus both pituitary and hypothalamic brain function may be influenced through this vascular connection. It is possible that some of the peptides of hypothalamic and pituitary origin present outside the hypothalamic-pituitary area might be derived via this retrograde vascular route.

Although we showed that lesions of the hypothalamic "thyrotrophic area" do not alter the *content* of the extrahypothalamic brain, this is not categorical proof that TRH *secretion* from the extrahypothalamic brain is unaltered. As discussed in detail by Wurtman and Fernstrom (238) in relationship to precursor amino acid control of serotonin and catecholamine synthesis, any conclusion about secretion rate derived from measurement of tissue content must be qualified because certain problems cannot be resolved at the present time. These include considerations of size and distribution of different pools which may turnover at different rates: The releasable pool of TRH may represent only a small percentage of the total TRH content so that profound changes in this pool might go unrecognized if only total brain TRH is measured. Other factors influencing extrahypothalamic brain TRH may include anatomic distribution among neurons, glia, extracellular space, and the various intracellular compartments and organelles.

What Is the Function of Extrahypothalamic TRH?

It seems clear that hypothalamic TRH has an important role in regulation of TSH secretion from the anterior pituitary, but the anatomically widespread distribution of TRH throughout the CNS supports an additional role for this substance in neuronal function. The location of TRH in several cranial nerve nuclei of the brainstem and motor nuclei of the spinal cord (84) suggests a transmitter action for this peptide especially in the motor system. This suggestion is supported by pharmacologic studies. Hypophysectomized mice pretreated by paragyline, a monoamine oxidase inhibitor, show enhancement of the motor activity induced by L-DOPA when TRH is concomitantly administered (177), thus indicating that the TRH effect is independent of pituitary thyroid function. Other CNS effects of TRH include potentiation of the excitatory action of acetylcholine (Ach) on cerebral cortical neurons (240), antagonism of barbiturate-induced sleeping time (179), enhancement of cerebral norepinephrine (NE) turnover (88,117), potentiation of behavioral changes following increased 5-OH-tryptamine (5-OHT) accumulation in rats (70), and alteration of rotational activity in the rat (believed to be a dopamine-mediated action) (39). Thus TRH may directly or indirectly influence the action of the commonly accepted neurotransmitters dopamine (DA), NE, 5-OHT, and Ach (see also Horita et al., *this volume*). The psychobiologic effects in man (233) and its possible effect in human depression may reflect its action in modulating neurotransmitter function (see also Prange et al., *this volume*).

TRH has also profound effects in thermoregulation. In the cat TRH produces hypothermia in much lower doses than NE, (140) raising the possibility that the hypothermic effect of NE in this animal might be mediated through TRH. In the rabbit TRH induces hyperthermia (87) and a CNS stimulation similar to amphetamine. These authors have also shown that in this animal TRH is analeptic to pentobarbitol but *not* to morphine, although morphine-induced hypothermia is reversed. TRH may have some interaction at the opiate receptor as a blocker since shaking behavior may be induced in the rat reminiscent of morphine withdrawal or antagonism (230). Further there is *central* inhibition of morphine (as well as pentobarbital) stimulated growth hormone (GH) release in the rat (23). As in the rabbit, intraventricular TRH causes marked hyperthermia in the rat that is reversed by bombesin (see also later in section on comparative endocrinologic studies) (22). Other behavioral effects of TRH include the suppression of feeding and drinking activity in rats following intraventricular injection (226).

Other studies supporting a neurotransmitter role for TRH include an effect on the electrical activity of single neurons. TRH has been shown to have a depressant action on central neurons (48,192) but an excitatory action on spinal motoneurons (161). In homogenates of hypothalamic tissue, TRH is present in synaptosomes. TRH is released when such synaptosomes are exposed to depolarizing concentrations of K^+ in the presence of 1 to 2 mM Ca^{2+} (229). IR-TRH has also been reported in the synaptic vesicles and synaptosomes of the extrahypothalamic brain of the rat (234). High-affinity binding sites for TRH in the synaptic membrane fraction of extrahypothalamic brain tissues have been demonstrated. These receptors have properties similar to those for pituitary membranes (32). In addition, there are active synthesizing (74) and enzyme-degrading (72) systems for TRH present in extrahypothalamic brain tissue.

These anatomic, behavioral, neurophysiologic, and biologic studies support a role for TRH as a neurotransmitter or in the modulation of neurotransmitter function. This kind of function is not unique to TRH, since LH-RH and somatostatin have a number of neurological effects in addition to their regulation of the pituitary. LH-RH, for example, stimulates sexual activity in rats in whom gonadal function is held constant (153,176). Somatostatin is anatomically located in the dorsal root ganglia and posterior horns (83), a site which supports the view that somatostatin functions as a sensory depressant (83). Further, this peptide has effects distinct from, and in many cases directly opposite to, those of TRH; e.g., it enhances the depressant effect of barbiturate but reduces the mortality due to strychnine (24). As with TRH, LH-RH and somatostatin have a depressant action on the excitability of neurons in several areas of the CNS as shown by microiontophoretic studies (192). Similarly, active enzymatic degrading systems exist in brain tissue for these peptides (72). It thus appears than an extrahypothalamic neuronal function exists for all the hypophysiotrophic hormones of the hypothalamus unrelated to their effects in regulating pituitary function. TRH has many typical chemical characteristics of a neurotransmitter, having a low molecular weight and being water soluble as well as rapidly inactivated in tissue and blood. However, ^{3}H-TRH is *not* taken up by synaptosomes *in vitro* unlike the proved neurotransmitter ^{3}H-DA (169). The failure of axonal terminals to take up ^{3}H-TRH does not *exclude* a role for TRH in neurotransmission, since cholinergic neurons have been shown to release Ach and take up choline after Ach metabolism in the synaptic cleft area (90). Clearly further work is required to determine whether TRH fulfills Bloom's criteria for a central neurotransmitter (17), but the tripeptide almost certainly plays an important role in brain function.

Is Secretion of Extrahypothalamic TRH Regulated by the Same Factors That Control Hypothalamic TRH Secretion?

It has been shown that following insulin-induced hypoglycemia in the rat, TRH depletion from the hypothalamus is accompanied by a fall of TRH content in forebrain and brainstem (115). Further, nyctohemeral variation in rat hypothalamic TRH levels (hypothalamic TRH concentration at its zenith at 1,200 hr) is associated with similar changes in the amygdala, though not in the forebrain (40). These findings could indicate that factors regulating TRH secretion in the hypothalamus might also operate in the extrahypothalamic brain. Clearly, however, further studies are required to examine this important point more directly. Shambaugh et al. (205) were unable to find any circadian variation in human lumbar CSF levels. However, the TRH rise reported by Collu et al. (40) in brain TRH at 1,200 hr might have been missed in this study. Further it is not known whether TRH levels in lumbar CSF are similar to, or change with, levels in the ventricles.

As Martin et al. (131) showed, axon collaterals from the tuberoinfundibular neurons extend to extrahypothalamic brain sites. These workers speculate that release of TRH (and other hypothalamic peptides) from nerve terminals in extrahypothalamic brain regions may subserve important biologic functions affecting the electric activity of distant CNS neurons. Thus those factors affecting hypothalamic secretion might concomitantly affect TRH turnover in the extrahypothalamic brain. Extrahypothalamic TRH derived by vascular or ventricular transport or synthesized *in situ* could be regulated similar to TRH present in the hypothalamus, but this remains to be determined.

A possibility that must be considered is that the primary site of synthesis of TRH might be in the extrahypothalamic brain, and that hypothalamic and ME TRH comes from outside the hypothalamus via axonal or ventricular transport. This hypothesis is supported by the hypothalamic deafferentation studies of Brownstein et al. (29). Recently it was reported that rat cerebral cortex fragments can synthesize TRH *in vitro* (124).

Neurohypophysis

In the rat brain, the concentration of TRH in the posterior pituitary is exceeded only by that in the hypothalamus (101,102,165) (Table 2). The concentration of TRH in the posterior lobe was 20 times that of the anterior pituitary in one study (560 $\pm$ 9 versus 28 $\pm$ 2 pg/mg protein; $p < 0.001$) (104) and is much higher than that of the pars intermedia (Jackson and Reichlin, *unpublished*). There is also a high concentration of TRH in the chicken posterior pituitary as well as the pituitary complexes of lower vertebrates. The significance of the latter finding is uncertain; however, in the bony fish there is evidence [reviewed by Sawyer (202)] that the neurohypophysis may be an homolog of the median eminence of higher animals. In addition, networks of TRH-positive fibers have been observed extending into the posterior pituitary of the rat (84). The presence of hypophysiotrophic hormones in the posterior lobe or neurohypophysis is not limited to TRH, for somatostatin-positive fibers were also observed by Hökfelt et al.

(82) in the rat posterior pituitary and we demonstrated LH-RH immuno-positive fibers extending into the frog neurohypophysis (1). These findings support the concept of a third hypothalamo-hypophysial system.

When rats were given lesions to the "thyrotrophic area" of the hypothalamus, the posterior pituitary content of TRH was markedly depleted (104). These findings indicate the posterior pituitary TRH content might reflect hypothalamic TRH secretion (Fig. 3).

Bar-Sella et al. (5) showed that injected ^{125}I-T$_3$ is taken up and concentrated in neural lobe pituicytes. These workers speculated that substances in the posterior pituitary may affect the function of the anterior pituitary following transmission via the short portal vessels, which supply the posterior lobe as well as the dorsal shoulders and caudal pole of the anterior pituitary. Such concepts derive support from studies by Bergland et al. (15) on the vascular organization within the mammalian hypophysis. They showed the abundance of shunts as well as numerous capillary connections between neural and glandular pituitary (Fig. 3). The pattern of arterial supply and venous drainage allow for the potential of flow reversal within parts of the pituitary and between the pituitary and the systemic circulation. Bergland et al. (15) postulate that the neurohypophysial capillary bed may actively and selectively determine the destination of both hypothalamic and pituitary secretions, conveying some to the glandular pituitary, others to distant target organs, and yet others to the brain. Whereas blood vessels of the anterior

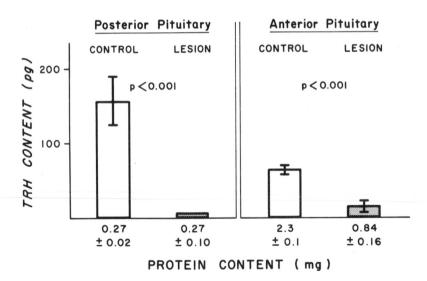

FIG. 3. Effect of lesions of the hypothalamic "thyrotropic area" on the posterior and anterior pituitary content of TRH in the rat. Lesion of the hypothalamus markedly reduces the TRH content in *both* lobes. These findings suggest the possibility of a hypothalamo-hypophysial tract containing TRH fibers directly innervating the posterior lobe, but a conduit through the adenohypophysis is an alternative hypothesis (see also text for discussion).

ME primary plexus connects with adenohypophysial secondary plexus vessels by both direct and portal routes, vessels of the posterior ME are continuous with neurohypophysial vessels within the infundibular stem. This newer concept of retrograde flow from the pituitary to the brain has important implications with regard to the brain content of hypothalamic and pituitary hormone, as well as suggesting that the posterior pituitary may play a role in the regulation of anterior pituitary secretion.

In vitro studies of the isolated neurohypophysis have been undertaken as a means of studying neurohypophysial secretion of vasopressin. Using Locke's medium, Hong and Poisner (86) provided evidence that the cold-induced *in vitro* release of vasopressin occurs by the process of exocytosis and not by generalized cell damage. A calcium-dependent potassium stimulation of somatostatin secretion from rat neurohypophysis *in vitro* has been demonstrated (171). Such calcium-dependent secretion is consistent with the "stimulus-secretion-coupling" hypothesis of Douglas (46). Since TRH, like somatostatin, is also present in high concentration in the neurohypophysis, similar methodology can be used to study the secretion of TRH from vertebrate neurohypophyses not only in relation to ions but also in response to monoamines and hormones.

In view of the presence of large quantities of TRH in the mammalian neurohypophysis (101,102), Skowsky and Swan (210) studied the perfusion of rat pituitaries with pulse doses of TRH. They found a dose-related initial rise of arginine vasopressin (AVP) within 2 min, followed by a more sustained secondary fall in AVP below base-line levels 14 to 20 min after administration of TRH. Further, Skowsky et al. (209) reported elevated basal AVP levels in hypothyroid humans and failure to normally suppress AVP levels in hypothyroid patients given an oral water load. Following full exogenous thyroid replacement, base-line AVP was normalized and was suppressed normally after the oral water load. TRH administration to normal or hypothyroid patients was reported to produce a fall in AVP 30 to 60 min after injection (212). AVP was not, however, examined during the first 10 min so that an initial brisk rise might have been missed. It is certainly possible that the large quantities of TRH in the posterior lobe may modulate the physiologic release of AVP. However, TRH may also affect water balance through a direct effect on the thirst center. Vijayan and McCann (226) gave TRH directly into the third ventricule of the rat and reported a suppressive effect on water intake at doses of 0.6 nmoles or greater.

Other CNS Sites

TRH has been reported present in mammalian pineal and retina tissue. These findings are discussed later in the section *Phylogenetic Distribution of TRH.*

Extra-CNS Distribution

TRH immunoreactivity has been reported throughout the gastrointestinal tract and pancreas of the rat in low concentrations (152). The actual anatomic location, source, and significance remain to be determined. The "pancreatic TRH" was shown by these workers to have *in vivo* bioactivity in the mouse.

FACTORS REGULATING TRH CONTENT IN THE CNS OF MAMMALS

Although TRH levels in hypothalamic and brain tissue are of interest, they provide no information with respect to secretion rate since content is the summation of synthesis and release. It is possible for both increased and decreased secretion to occur while the content remains unchanged. Either increased or decreased tissue content could indicate both increased *and* decreased secretion rate. Nonetheless, a number of studies have been undertaken to examine factors that might affect hypothalamic and brain content of TRH, and these are considered here.

Thyroid Status

Thyroid hormone has a negative feedback at the pituitary thyrotrope cell on thyroid-stimulating hormone (TSH) production, but its action at the hypothalamic level on *endogenous* TRH secretion is not well understood. Evidence against a negative feedback at that site was suggested by the report from Wilber and Porter (232), who found no reduction in TRH biological activity in hypophysial portal blood after electrical stimulation of the hypothalamus in rats pretreated with T_3, and by the acute release of IR-TRH into the systemic circulation of cold-exposed rats pretreated with T_4 (151). However, thyroxine implants in the hypothalamus of the rat and cat are reported to *inhibit* thyroid function (34,120).

Studies on hypothalamic content of TRH in animals with different thyroid states have given variable results. Sinha and Meites (207), on the basis of bioassay, found rat hypothalamic TSH-releasing activity to be increased following thyroidectomy and unaltered by T_4 administration. However, it is now known that somatostatin, which is present in the rat hypothalamus in substantial quantities (170), inhibits the effect of TRH on the release of TSH (224). Accordingly, the estimates of hypothalamic TRH content obtained by bioassay probably underestimate the levels of TRH and are of questionable significance unless steps are taken to remove somatostatin. Bassiri and Utiger (9) reported that thyroidectomized rats given daily T_4 replacement for 2 weeks had significantly higher IR-TRH levels in the hypothalamus than animals not given T_4. However, in another experiment they found that T_4 treatment to rats caused a reduction in hypothalamic TRH content, and overall these authors were unimpressed with the effect of thyroid hormone on TRH content; more recent studies from that laboratory showed no consistent effects of thyroid status on hypothalamic brain content of TRH (115). In our studies (*in preparation*) of hypothalamic TRH content, we found no evidence of any reduction in rat hypothalamic TRH content with doses of T_4 as high as 20 $\mu g/100$ g body weight/day, indicating the absence of negative feedback of thyroid hormone on hypothalamic TRH levels. Further, in only one of three experiments did we find a significant reduction of hypothalamic TRH levels in hypothyroid animals (treated by thyroidectomy). The extrahypothalamic brain content of TRH was unaltered in different thyroid states. Roti et al. (195) reported that thyroidectomy in the rat significantly decreases hypothalamic IR-TRH levels and that T_4 (but not TSH) treatment restores the TRH content to normal. However, extrahypothalamic brain content of TRH was reported by these workers to be unaltered by hypothyroidism in these experiments. Overall the content of TRH is relatively undisturbed in the rat hypothalamus by changing the thyroid status. Nevertheless, it seems clear that hypothalamic TRH secretion is important in the maintenance of normal thyroid function since rats who received ablations of the hypothalamic "thyrotrophic area" developed chemical hypothyroidism associated with a reduction of the hypothalamic content of TRH to a third of that in control rats (104).

A more recent means of studying the physiologic role of TRH in the regulation of thyroid function has been the administration of anti-TRH antibody. Passive immunization with anti-TRH has been shown to reduce the basal TSH levels in normal (79,123) and hypothyroid (79) rats. In our own studies, anti-TRH given intraperitoneally blocked the cold-induced TSH rise but did not lower the serum TSH in hypothyroid animals decapitated 2 hr after the anti-TRH administration (155). Subsequent studies using the same dose of anti-TRH administered intravenously through an indwelling cannula demonstrated a 50% reduction in the serum TSH which persisted 120 min. Failure by all workers to observe full suppression of TSH secretion could indicate insufficient anti-TRH serum, excess TRH secretion in hypothyroidism, or some autonomy of the pituitary thyrotrope. However, it should not readily be assumed that a 50% reduction in TSH secretion represents a 50% reduction in TRH secretion; the observed lowering of TSH levels could represent a near-maximal transient neutralization in TRH. In this context it should be pointed out that the TRH $T_{1/2}$ is 2.5 min whereas the TSH $T_{1/2}$ is much longer at 16 min (57).

Cold Exposure

In the rat acute and chronic cold exposure leads to an increase in thyroid function (25), but only the acute response occurs rapidly enough to imply activation by a neuroendocrine reflex (187). Abrupt lowering of the ambient temperature in unanesthetized rats results in a rise in circulating TSH levels within 5 to 10 min (187). Chronic thyroregulatory response to prolonged cold exposure in the rat may or may not involve the hypothalamus. The response to chronic cold exposure (159) may involve increased tissue metabolism as well as enhanced enterohepatic thyroxine turnover secondary to increased food intake (64). Bakke and Lawrence (4), however, found no rise in serum TSH in rats chronically cold-adapted for 4 to 6 weeks.

To determine if the enhanced TSH secretion of cold exposure reflected increased TRH secretion, blood levels of IR-TRH have been examined in animals subjected to acute cold exposure. Montoya et al. (151) reported a marked increase in blood IR-TRH, from 40 to 220 pg/ml, associated with a rise of TSH. Interestingly, he reported that pretreatment with thyroid hormone suppressed the TSH rise but did not affect the TRH response. Such findings, as mentioned earlier, are in keeping with the primary site of action for thyroid hormone being at the pituitary. However, it is by no means certain that the IR-TRH measured by Montoya came from the hypothalamus, and the possibility of TRH secretion from the extrahypothalamic brain requires consideration. Regardless of where circulating IR-TRH is derived, it seems probable that increased *hypothalamic* secretion of TRH is required to activate pituitary-thyroid function due to acute cold exposure, since lesions of the preoptic region (43) block this response (see also later discussion on deafferentation). The finding of an acute rise of blood TRH has not been generally confirmed. Eskay et al. (53) did report a very slight rise, but Emerson and Utiger (50), Harris et al. (79), and we (155) found *no* increase in blood TRH, although a TSH rise was recorded comparable to that reported by Montoya et al. Passive immunization with anti-TRH blocks the TSH rise to acute cold exposure in the rat (79,155,214) and provides support for the view that the TSH is mediated via enhanced TRH secretion, but whether this results in increased circulating levels of TRH is controversial. No significant change in hypothalamic TRH content was reported by Jobin et al. (109) following acute or chronic cold exposure to the rat. However, we found that hypothalamic content of TRH in rats exposed to 4°C for 14 days was significantly lower than that present in the hypothalami of controls kept at room temperature (130).

Following hypothalamic deafferentation, the cold-induced rise of TSH is partially (81) or completely (2) blocked. These findings suggest that hypothalamic connections with the extrahypothalamic brain are required for full activation of pituitary-thyroid function. It appears that the acute TSH rise in response to cold is dependent on central noradrenergic agonist activity (2,149,218). In the human neonate cold can activate TSH secretion (60), but in other age groups cold does not stimulate thyroidal function, although a slight but significant TSH rise has been reported in normal man (219). The explanation for the failure to stimulate TSH secretion may be the concomitant increased secretion of somatostatin.

It has been reported that prolactin (PRL) is released in response to acute cold (79,110). Since pretreatment with dexamethasone abolished the PRL rise but only delayed the TSH response, Jobin et al. (110) concluded that TRH was not involved in the PRL rise they found. This interpretation is supported by passive immunization studies with anti-TRH that reportedly prevented the cold-induced TSH increase but left the PRL elevation unaffected (79).

Nutritional Status

It has been recognized for many years that starvation in the rat leads to depressed pituitary-thyroid function (42,182). In the neonatal rat caloric restriction results in a hypothyroid state associated with a reduction in the hypothalamic content of TRH but a preservation of pituitary thyrotrope sensitivity *in vitro* to synthetic TRH (204). Adult rats fasted for 2 days showed a decreased serum TSH, T_4, free T_4, T_3 and free T_3, suggestive of central hypothyroidism (80). The hypothalamic content of TRH and the TSH response to TRH stimulation was not apparently altered in these animals. The possibility that starvation might impair thyroid function as a result of decreased hypothalamic secretion of TRH because of specific dietary deficiency of its amino acid precursor histidine (18,30), an essential amino acid in the rat (157), was suggested to us by reports that the synthesis of brain serotonin (59,129,148a), DOPA (239), and acetylcholine (38) was influenced by dietary consumption of the respective precursors tryptophan, tyrosine, and choline. It has also been reported that hypothalamic serotonin release, as inferred from changes in the anterior pituitary secretion of prolactin (113) can be augmented by the intravenous injection of tryptophan or 5-hydroxytryptophan (35). To test the hypothesis that dietary histidine regulates TRH synthesis and secretion, we studied the effects of histidine deficiency on (a) pituitary-thyroid function (as an index of hypothalamic TRH secretion) and (b) the hypothalamic content of immunoassayable TRH. The extrahypothalamic brain content of TRH was also studied because of the possible function of TRH as a neurotransmitter (94).

We found (94) that rats given a histidine-deficient diet ad libitum showed a 50% reduction in blood and brain histidine levels without significantly altering pituitary-thyroid function or the TRH content of hypothalamus or brain (Table 3). In this study it was found that a gradient of histidine from blood to brain of approximately 2:1 was demonstrated in histidine-deficient and control animals, suggesting that dietary availability regulated the brain content of this amino acid. In our experiments it was concluded that in the rat dietary availability of histidine is not rate-limiting for TRH synthesis

TABLE 3. Serum and brain levels of histidine and TRH, and pituitary-thyroid function in rats on a histidine deficient diet

Parameter	Experiment 1		Experiment 2	
	Histidine-free Ad libitum	Control Ad libitum	Histidine-free Ad libitum	Control Pair-fed
Length of study (days)	4		9	
Diet				
Access to diet				
Mean daily food consumption (g)	16 ± 4[a]	30 ± 3	12 ± 1	11 ± 1
Initial body weight (g)	304 ± 6	298 ± 6	293 ± 6	290 ± 4
Cumulative change in body weight (g)	−25 ± 3[b]	+15 ± 4	−38 ± 4	−38 ± 3
Serum histidine (µg/ml)	4.8 ± 0.9[a]	11.6 ± 0.6	5.9 ± 0.5[b]	9.9 ± 0.5
Extrahypothalamic brain histidine (µg/g)	2.4 ± 0.6[c]	4.7 ± 0.7	2.1 ± 0.3[d]	3.8 ± 0.4
Extrahypothalamic brain weight (g)	1.48 ± 0.07	1.48 ± 0.05	1.80 ± 0.04	1.68 ± 0.11
Extrahypothalamic brain TRH content (ng/whole tissue)	19.9 ± 0.6	19.8 ± 1.0	16 ± 0.5	14 ± 0.6
Hypothalamic weight (mg)	3.9 ± 0.4	4.1 ± 0.8	28.4 ± 3	30.2 ± 2.0
Hypothalamic TRH content (ng/whole tissue)[e]	2.9 ± 0.4	2.6 ± 0.3	5.1 ± 0.2	5.2 ± 0.3
Stalk-median eminence weight (mg)	0.59 ± 0.17	0.45 ± 0.09	0.59 ± 0.12	0.70 ± 0.08
Stalk-median eminence TRH content (ng/whole tissue)	1.4 ± 0.1	1.1 ± 0.1	1.5 ± 0.2	1.6 ± 0.2
Anterior pituitary weight (mg)	—	—	6.25 ± 0.53	6.45 ± 0.25
Anterior pituitary TRH content (pg)	—	—	25 ± 4	31 ± 8
Posterior pituitary weight (mg)	—	—	1.19 ± 0.15	1.08 ± 0.04
Posterior pituitary TRH content (pg)	—	—	129 ± 16	138 ± 18
Serum TSH (mU/dl)	3.1 ± 0.4	4.5 ± 1.5	4.2 ± 0.4	4.8 ± 0.3
Serum T_4 (µg/dl)	4.5 ± 0.4[c]	5.7 ± 0.4	4.6 ± 0.4	4.8 ± 0.3
Serum T_3 (ng/dl)	90 ± 8	98 ± 6	86 ± 10	91 ± 12

From ref. 94.

Results are expressed as mean ± SEM.

Compared with respective control group: [a] $p < 0.01$; [b] $p < 0.001$; [c] $p < 0.05$; [d] $p < 0.02$.

[e] For hypothalamic TRH content only the hypophysiotropic area was removed in Exp. 1. This accounts for the much smaller weight and lower overall TRH content compared with Exp. 2.

and secretion over a period of 9 days. We did not determine the effect of more prolonged histidine deprivation since histidine deficiency in the diet induced anorexia, and more prolonged histidine lack would be associated with the nonspecific effects of caloric deprivation. It is possible that rats treated by forced feedings of normal caloric content with a histidine-deficient diet for more prolonged periods (6 weeks or longer) may show effects on brain TRH synthesis and secretion.

The lack of effect of histidine deficiency on TRH synthesis contrasts with the effect of this dietary regimen in markedly lowering the brain content of histamine and carnosine, both putative neurotransmitters, and suggests that by some mechanism histidine is preferentially deviated to TRH formation.

The possible reduction of TRH secretion from the hypothalamus in starvation in the rat may reflect the reduced availability of the amino acid precursors for DA or NE synthesis. Administration of precursors of serotonin to rats has produced either no change or a reduction of serum TSH (218) and a diminution of the TSH response to cold (218). The latter report suggests an inhibition of TRH secretion from the hypothalamus since the TSH rise to exogenous TRH administration was found to be unimpaired by these workers. An inhibitory effect of 5-OHT on TRH secretion supports previous *in vitro* studies on TRH secretion from mammalian hypothalamus (14,73). Studies of DOPA administration suggest a possible inhibitory effect on TSH secretion primarily at the pituitary level (31). There are no data on a function for Ach in the regulation of TRH secretion, although the studies of Nemeroff et al. (160) raised this as a possibility. The effects of dietary availability of the amino acid precursors of 5-OHT (tryptophan), NE and DA (tyrosine), and Ach (choline) on TRH secretion await study.

MEASUREMENT OF TRH IN BIOLOGIC FLUIDS

Since TRH levels in neural tissue may not truly reflect the secretion rate, attempts have been made to assay TRH in biologic fluids as an index of hypothalamic and/or nervous system secretion of TRH. Unfortunately such investigations have been beset with severe methodologic problems. In this section we review the current status of measurement of TRH in biologic fluids.

Blood

Although TRH has been demonstrated in the portal blood of the rat by bioassay (232) and immunoassay (166), and its concentration was shown to be increased by electrical stimulation of the hypothalamus (232), there is considerable doubt as to the physiologic applicability of this preparation quite apart from the impracticality of measuring hypophysial portal blood under controlled physiologic conditions. Oliver et al. (166) demonstrated

IR-TRH in the portal blood of only 10 of 15 rats, and the levels showed a wide variation, ranging from 30 to 700 pg/ml. These authors considered the low levels of TRH in portal blood to result from either degradation in the blood during collection or surgical stress.

There are considerable difficulties in measuring TRH in the systemic circulation of rat and man due to its rapid degradation by proteolytic enzymes (180) and its low concentration in blood. Bassiri and Utiger (7) demonstrated that human serum heated at 60°C for 30 min or exposed to pH 3.0 or 10.0 did not inactivate TRH. Whereas TRH biological activity was destroyed by incubation of TRH in serum at 37°C, it was preserved after incubation in serum 60°C. These authors concluded that serum contains heat-, acid-, and alkali-labile substance(s) which inactivates the biological and immunological activity of TRH in a similar manner. The inactivation of TRH by rat blood is also prevented if the blood is frozen and then thawed prior to incubation with TRH (53). Various agents have been proposed in an effort to prevent TRH degradation in blood. 2,3-Dimercapto-propanol (BAL), a compound which reacts with disulfide groups, in quantities of 0.5 to 40 mg/ml (4 to 32 mM) prevented TRH inactivation by serum (221). However, we found that this substance interferes with the affinity of the anti-TRH for ^{125}I-TRH; similar findings were reported by Eskay et al. (53). Benzamidine, reported to prevent TRH breakdown in serum (107), likewise interferes with the TRH RIA (53). TRH inactivation was not inhibited by trasylol (100 or 1,000 units/ml) or iodoacetamide (0.002 or 0.02 M) and only slight inhibition of inactivation occurred with 0.1 M EDTA (221). Certain TRH analogs, especially L-pyroglu-L-His-o-methyl-ester (223), retard TRH activation by rat plasma and probably act as competitive inhibitors of the serum TRH inactivator(s). Since these compounds do not fully inhibit TRH breakdown, their use would have to be combined with other measures such as heating (7). 8-Hydroxyquinoline, a chelator of heavy metals, like BAL and EDTA, shows some effect in retarding the breakdown of TRH (132). The addition of Tween-20 to the 8-hydroxyquinoline may enhance its effectiveness (145). BAL, EDTA, and 8-hydroxyquinoline, used in the assay to measure plasma renin, partially act by inhibiting the activity of converting enzyme, a peptidase that hydrolyzes a bond between histidine and phenylalanine (132). It seems likely that the plasma inactivators of TRH are likewise peptidases breaking the bonds between pGlu and His and/or His and ProNH$_2$. Although Nair et al. (156) suggested that the TRH inactivator is an amidase rather than a peptidase, the studies of Visser et al. (227), using a specific RIA for pGlu-His-Pro, does not support that view. More recently it was reported that bacitracin prevents the breakdown of TRH in hypothalamic tissue culture but not in plasma (138). Direct assay of rat blood (0.1 ml) containing BAL (10 mM) or benzamidine (100 mM), or which is frozen quickly and then thawed, gave undetectable levels of TRH (53). Oliver et al. (163)

reported TRH levels in human plasma of 19.8 ± 3.1 pg/ml. These workers collected 5 ml blood in BAL (5 mg), extracted the plasma with charcoal (30 mg), and desorbed TRH from the charcoal with 75% ethanol. In our studies to examine TRH levels in rat blood, on decapitation 5 ml of trunk blood was immediately added to 15 ml ethanol and mixed thoroughly. Following centrifugation the supernatant was evaporated to dryness and then resuspended in 0.5 ml buffer; 0.2-ml aliquots (equivalent to 2 ml blood or 1 ml plasma) were assayed directly. The IR-TRH concentration found was 13 ± 3 pg/ml (102). If exogenous TRH is first added to the ethanol followed by blood, the TRH recovery is complete. However, if TRH is added to the blood and then immediately transferred to the ethanol, the recovery is 50 to 60%. Eskay et al. (53) also reported that 50% of synthetic TRH added to rat blood is degraded within seconds. These workers extracted 5 to 8 ml trunk blood with 3 volumes of methanol; the methanol extract was evaporated to dryness; and aliquots (equivalent to 0.5 to 1.5 ml blood) were assayed—a procedure similar to our own. They found IR-TRH levels of 8 to 11 pg/ml with a recovery of 77%. Saito et al. (201) reported plasma TRH levels of 4 to 19 pg/ml in the human following methanol extraction. Although with the charcoal separation procedure we adjust for nonspecific binding, we find that putting an ethanol or methanol extract from more than 0.2 ml blood in the RIA (incubation volume 0.4 ml) causes interference in the binding of antibody to label unless the blood extract has been further purified. Thus at the present time these estimates of plasma TRH require further confirmation. Similar criticisms may also be made regarding the plasma TRH estimates of Eskay et al. (53) and Saito et al. (201).

Using affinity chromatography Emerson and Utiger (50) found plasma TRH levels in male rats to range from 7 to 30 pg/ml. These workers coupled anti-TRH immunoglobulin G (IgG) to Sepharose 4B. Blood was collected in heparin and dimercaptopropanol, the plasma extracted with methanol, and the redissolved dried methanol extract applied to the anti-TRH column. Recovery of TRH was approximately 45%. Using similar methodology Montoya et al. (151) found mean blood TRH levels to be 40 pg/ml, rising to 222 pg/ml with acute cold exposure associated with a rise in circulating TSH levels. However, Emerson and Utiger (50) found no increase in plasma TRH levels in their animals, although a significant increase in TSH was recorded in all animals exposed to cold exposure. In our own studies (155) and in those of Harris et al. (79), a rise in plasma TRH was not detected following acute cold exposure, although a significant rise in plasma TSH occurred. Eskay et al. (53) reported a very slight but significant rise in plasma TRH with acute cold exposure using the methodology described earlier.

Affinity chromatography represents a significant advance in the ability to purify the IR-TRH moiety in biologic fluids. However, the discrepancy in the plasma TRH response to cold exposure found by Montoya and Emerson, who each utilized affinity chromatography, is disquieting. It must be pointed out, however, that affinity chromatography which concentrates TRH does *not* separate the authentic tripeptide from cross-reacting substances in the RIA but only from interfering materials. It should also be noted that both these groups used ^{3}H-TRH to determine recovery, and we found that commercially available labeled TRH is impure even after purification. Moreover, about one-third of such ^{3}H-TRH, although chromatographically identical with TRH in several solvent systems, is not degradable by serum possibly owing to stereochemical impurity (13). Studies of the effect of thyroid status on blood levels of TRH have also been reported. Thyroid status had no effect in the experiments of Montoya and of Emerson. In the original report by Oliver et al. (166), IR-TRH was reported to be undetectable in the plasma of hypothyroid rats, 60 to 70 pg/ml in normal rats, and elevated to 150 pg/ml in T_4-treated animals. Mitsuma et al. (145) reported IR-TRH levels to be less than 60 pg/ml in normal human subjects, undetectable in thyrotoxicosis and hypothalamic hypothyroidism, 40 to 400 pg/ml in primary hypothyroidism, and 100 to 600 pg/ml in pituitary hypothyroid patients. These high levels have not yet been confirmed by other laboratories. In our studies of human blood from patients with a wide variety of thyroid pituitary or hypothalamic disturbances, levels of IR-TRH following ethanol extraction did not exceed 20 pg/ml. Further, based on estimates of secretion rate derived from measurement of urinary excretion and metabolic clearance rate, we calculate the plasma TRH levels to be less than 5 pg/ml (99), a value below the level of sensitivity of all assays for TRH so far reported.

Urine

The first report of a TRH-like material in urine (as well as in blood) of mammals was that of Shibusawa et al. (206). However, other workers (183) failed to confirm this finding, and no further studies of urine were carried out until the TRH immunoassay era. TRH appears in urine after injection of exogenous hormone in man (8,61,96,108) in quantities ranging from 5.5 to 14.5% of the dose administered; in the rat 15% of the dose was excreted (99). When added to urine, exogenous TRH shows little or no breakdown (8,102,132).

Dilution of the IR material showed parallelism with synthetic TRH, and the addition of exogenous synthetic TRH to rat urine gave complete recovery. Montoya et al. (150) reported IR-TRH in rat urine, purified by affinity chromatography (anti-TRH IgG conjugated to Sepharose 4B), at a level of 4.3 ng/24 hr, rising to 6.8 ng/24 hr ($p < 0.05$) on exposure to 4°C. Further, we (61,96,97) and others (163) reported endogenous IR-TRH levels in human urine. We found that the excretion of IR-TRH was significantly greater in normal males than in normal females whether expressed in absolute terms or in relation to body weight or surface area. Oliver et al. (163)

also found the daily urinary excretion of IR-TRH to be greater in men than women. These workers considered that their gel filtration studies of urine extract on Sephadex G-10 and electrophoretic studies on Whatmann 3MM paper indicated identity with synthetic TRH, although close examination of their figures suggests slight discrepancy between the urine extract and synthetic TRH. However, Jeffcoate and White (108) concluded that the IR-TRH material in human urine was not authentic TRH, on the basis of chromatographic studies and impairment of degradation by serum. Further Vagenakis et al. (222) claimed "that urine TRH as measured by radioimmunoassay is probably not TRH but is a nonspecific effect of urea on the immunoassay." We reexamined the nature of the IR-TRH in urine in further detail (95). Urea shows no interference in our assay in concentrations of 4 g/100 ml or less, a quantity far in excess of that usually found in either maximally concentrated human or normal rat urine. In our studies IR-TRH was separated from urea by affinity chromatography (using anti-TRH bound to controlled pore glass) and on Sephadex G-10 chromatography. Urine IR-TRH concentration was found to be unaltered in urine treated with urease. Emerson et al. (49) also reported that urea could not account for the measured TRH immunoreactivity they found in human urine following affinity chromatography.

In our own studies, column chromatography of urine on Sephadex G-10 yielded a major peak of IR-TRH similar to that of added ^{3}H-TRH and synthetic TRH (Fig. 4, peak 2); in addition, two variable peaks of IR-TRH were obtained, one immediately following the void volume (peak 1) and the other after the major TRH area (peak 3). Chromatography of an extract of hypothalamus and extrahypothalamic brain showed that up to 10% of the IR-TRH elutes in peak 1, with the rest in peak 2, indicating some heterogeneity of hypothalamic and extrahypothalamic brain also (Fig. 2). On electrophoresis, 30% of IR-TRH in urine migrated similarly to synthetic TRH in saline. Exogenous TRH in urine, added or following intravenous injection, showed some alteration of electrophoretic mobility. Further, the urine retarded the degradation of synthetic TRH by serum.

Analogous findings were obtained by Emerson et al. (49). On Sephadex G-10 filtration, the urine IR-TRH showed heterogeneity, although there was some overlap with synthetic TRH. These authors did not apparently observe the distinct peaks we found, possibly owing to different antibody affinity and sensitivity. They found that urine IR-TRH was degraded by serum similar to synthetic TRH, whereas we found it less susceptible to breakdown. Emerson et al. (49) conclude that the urine IR-TRH is not authentic TRH and suggest it might be a metabolite such as pGlu-His-Pro, which shows some cross-reactivity with one of their anti-TRH antibodies. Visser et al. (227), who incubated synthetic TRH with serum, did not demonstrate the production of deamidated TRH using a specific assay for this substance. However, Dupont et al. (47) found that 50% of ^{3}H-TRH, following intravenous injection in the rat, was converted to the TRH-free acid, as determined by thin-layer electro-

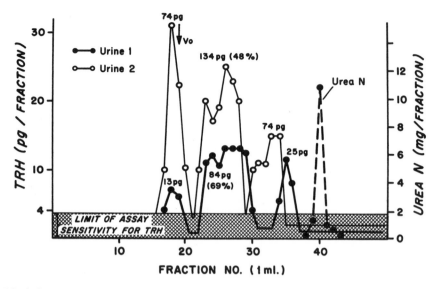

FIG. 4. Chromatography of rat urine on Sephadex G-10 reveals three peaks of IR-TRH. Peak 1 ("big TRH" ?) comes off with the void volume (see also Fig. 2); peak 2 coincides with synthetic TRH; and peak 3 comes off beyond peak 2 but before urea, which therefore is not a factor in these immunoassay measurements. The relative proportion of these peaks varies in different urine specimens (as shown for urines 1 and 2), and their nature is yet to be determined.

phoresis of methanol extracts of plasma. An alternative interpretation of the findings of Emerson et al., as well as our own, is that a fraction of IR-TRH in urine is authentic endogenous TRH with concentrations somewhat lower than our initial estimates (99), that there are other immunoreactive TRH moieties in urine, that urea is *not* a cause of IR-TRH artifact in whole urine, and that urine modifies several characteristics of native TRH. Our claim that the tripeptide is present in the urine, although it might not account for *all* the IR-TRH, is supported by the work of Leppaluoto et al. (127). These workers, using a two-step ion-exchange chromatographic method for purification of urine TRH, estimated authentic TRH in rat urine to be around 3.5 ng/day and in human urine 12 ng/day.

CSF

Beginning with the anatomical studies of Lofgren and others (see ref. 122 for review), attention has been drawn to the ependymal cell lining of the third ventricle as a possible route for the transfer of hypophysiotrophic hormones from the hypothalamus to the pituitary. Any TRH in the CSF could come from either the hypothalamus or other parts of the brain and could play a physiologic role in regulating the anterior pituitary. Although intraventricular administration of TRH can achieve release of TSH from the anterior pituitary

(68), the physiologic importance of this mode of transmission remains uncertain. Since there is no barrier to movement between the extracellular space of the brain and CSF, assay of TRH levels in the CSF may be a direct reflection of brain TRH secretion. Using a bioassay, Knigge and Joseph (121) reported values of TRH at 18.5 ng/ml in rat third ventricular fluid removed at death. Such high levels have not yet been confirmed by other workers, so the significance of these findings remains in doubt. TRH biologic activity *in vitro* has been concentrated from CSF removed from the cistern or third ventricle of human cadavers within 2 to 5 hr of death (88a). Human lumbar CSF TRH was reported by Oliver et al. (164) to range between 65 and 290 pg/ml. Shambaugh et al. (205) reported levels of around 40 pg/ml with no sex difference and no diurnal rhythm. By contrast, CSF cortisol levels obtained concurrently by these workers were twofold higher in the morning than in the afternoon.

Conclusions Regarding TRH in Biologic Fluids

The nature and authenticity of IR-TRH in blood and urine are controversial. Its origin (hypothalamus versus extrahypothalamic neural tissue), its physiologic significance, the type of secretion (tonic versus cyclic), and the physiologic factors that regulate the levels are all unknown. In the CSF, TRH levels reported from different laboratories are variable; and even if authentic, the source (hypothalamus versus brain versus spinal cord) is unclear. At this time measurement of IR-TRH in peripheral blood, urine, and CSF cannot be utilized to impute the status of hypothalamic or brain function.

PHYLOGENETIC DISTRIBUTION OF TRH

Function

The function of TRH in the regulation of pituitary-thyroid function in inframammalian species is uncertain (see refs. 92,93 for review). In aves (birds) TRH activates thyroid function, but in amphibia there is no definite evidence of a role for the tripeptide in thyroid function, although in most circumstances an intact hypothalamus is required (45).

A critical role for TRH in tadpole metamorphosis was proposed by Etkin (54). He suggested that development of the tadpole hypothalamus is under positive feedback control by thyroid hormone, and that a gradually rising level of circulating thyroid hormone during prometamorphosis induces maturation of the hypothalamic tissue concerned with the synthesis of TRH. This positive feedback system results in the stimulation of thyroid activity required for metamorphosis. However, Etkin and Gona (56) failed to induce metamorphosis in the tadpole with TRH administration. TRH has also been given to the neotenic Mexican axolotl (salamander), a species whose plasma does not degrade TRH *in vitro,* and in spite of achieving high circulating levels of the exogenous material in the blood (measured by RIA) metamorphosis was not induced (216).

These findings raise the possibility that in amphibia the mammalian TRH is not a physiologic TSH-releasing factor in these species. Alternative explanations are possible. The TRH may induce simultaneous release of prolactin, which in the tadpole, at least, blocks metamorphosis (55). Indeed antiserum to bullfrog prolactin injected into prometamorphic tadpoles of *R. catesbeiana* accelerates metamorphic climax (36). However, TRH given to the red eft, a species that undergoes water drive or second metamorphosis, which is known to be specifically controlled by prolactin (69), had no effect on metamorphosis (66). Clemons et al. (37) reported that TRH induces prolactin release in the bullfrog, and they suggested that TRH may have functioned as a prolactin-releasing factor before it became a stimulator for TSH release. Mammalian TRH has been shown to release α-MSH from the pituitary of *R. esculenta* (225), but the significance of this is uncertain.

In the lungfish TRH in high doses was not found to have any effect in stimulating thyroid function (67). However, evidence for a thyrotropin-inhibitory factor (TIF) from the hypothalamus was provided by Peter (175) for the goldfish and other teleosts, and by Rosenkilde (194) for some species of amphibia also. Bromage (20) raised the interesting possibility that TRH may function as a TIF in teleost fishes.

The evidence thus suggests that the hypothalamus is of some importance in the regulation of thyroid function in lower animals, but that the degree of autonomy of the thyroid gland is much greater than in mammalian species. In amphibia there is evidence for a thyrotropin-releasing factor, but this might be different from TRH.

Anatomic Location

Hypothalamus and Extrahypothalamic Brain

In view of the reported absence of a role for TRH in the regulation of thyroid function in inframammalian species, we examined the hypothalami of a number of vertebrates (including the snake, frog, and salmon) for TRH content and found high concentrations (101) with values up to 10 times that found in rat hypothalamus (Fig. 5). Raised TRH levels in amphibian hypothalamus were also reported by Taurog et al. (216). Further, high concentrations of TRH were also found in the extrahypothalamic brain of these vertebrates, and evidence for its authenticity was shown by the ability of a frog brain extract to release rat TSH *in vivo* (101). The neurohypophysis of vertebrates contains high levels of TRH (see also earlier section) (Fig. 5).

We also showed TRH to be present in the whole brain of the larval lam-

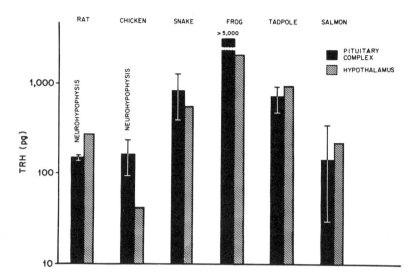

FIG. 5. Concentration of TRH (pg/mg tissue) (mean ± SEM) in the pituitary complex (or neurohypophysis of rat and chicken) and hypothalamus of a number of vertebrates. Four animals of each species were studied.

prey, in the head end of the amphioxus (101), and in the circumesophageal ganglia of the invertebrate snail (76). As the lamprey lacks TSH, and the amphioxus and snail lack a pituitary, we suggest that the TSH-regulating function of TRH may be a late evolutionary development representing an example of an organism acquiring a new function for preexisting chemical substance or hormone, analogous to the evolution of neurohypophysial hormones. In a sense, the pituitary has "co-opted" TRH as a regulatory hormone.

Pineal

We also found TRH to be present in the frog (*Rana pipiens*) pineal in high concentrations, influenced by the degree of photoillumination; changing seasons are associated with swings in pineal TRH concentrations as much as 10- to 20-fold (106). Comparable findings were reported by Kühn and Engelen (126), who, with an *in vivo* bioassay in the rat, demonstrated a seasonal variation in the PRL- and TSH-releasing activity in the hypothalamus of the frog. The function of TRH in the frog pineal is unknown, but the circannual rhythm and the effect of illumination bespeak a role in neurotransmission; this is supported by evidence that TRH has an excitatory action on frog motoneurons (161). TRH is also found in other vertebrate pineals, including that of the snake, where substantial quantities were recorded. However, in the rat pineal we have found meager quantities that apparently are not influenced by the degree of photoillumination (*unpublished observations*).

Retina

The retina is embryologically derived from an outgrowth of the diencephalon; and apart from the photoreceptor layer, it can be regarded as gray matter. IR-TRH has been reported in rat retina in levels ranging from 100 to 300 pg/mg protein, the highest levels occurring during the day at 1200 to 1800 hr, and lower levels occurring at night (203). Interestingly, TRH levels in the hypothalamus and amygdala have been reported to peak at 1200 hr (40). In the frog retina we found TRH levels at 10 times the concentration noted by Schaeffer et al. (203) in the rat. Of possible relevance to retinal TRH is the fact that amino acid neurotransmitter substances, including GABA, taurine, glycine glutamate, and aspartate, abound in the vertebrate retina (158)

Blood

Unlike the situation in mammals, TRH circulates in the blood of the *Rana pipiens* in high concentration (22 to 132 ng/ml) and shows rapid degradation *in vitro* with a $T_{\frac{1}{2}}$ of 1.8 min at 26°C and 0.95 min at 37°C. An extract of frog blood containing 100 ng IR-TRH produced a TSH rise in the rat *in vivo* comparable to that produced by synthetic TRH 100 ng, whereas a sample of the same frog blood, allowed first to incubate at 37°C, contained only 12 pg IR-TRH in the extract and caused no elevation in the rat TSH (105). Such findings support the authenticity of frog blood TRH.

Skin

Since the brain of *R. pipiens* weighs only 100 to 150 mg and contains approximately 100 ng TRH, it seemed unlikely to us that brain TRH could account for the bulk of blood TRH. Examination of organ distribution showed huge quantities of immunoreactive and bioactive TRH in the skin (mean 48 ng/mg protein), concentrations three to four times that of the hypothalamus (Fig. 6); thoracic and gastrointestinal organs, on the other hand, contained very low levels of TRH (Table 4). Since frog skin weighs approximately 10 g, we estimate the skin to contain over 50 μg TRH. In the frog, the skin is an important organ in salt and water balance and excretion, and generally in maintaining homeostasis (128). The specific function of skin TRH is unknown, but the massive quantities of TRH present in the integument of this species suggests a role for this peptide in skin function. It appears that blood TRH is derived from the skin in this species, and that the skin is an active peptide-secreting organ. Support for the authenticity of the TRH present in the frog skin is provided by our studies on extracts using high-performance liquid chromatography (HPLC) after affinity chromatographic purification (Fig. 7), and by the work of Yasuhara and Nakajima (241) who described the occurrence of a tripeptide chemically characterized as pyroglutamyl-

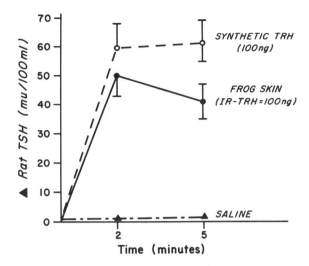

FIG. 6. Effect of an extract of skin (containing 100 ng IR-TRH) from the frog (*Rana pipiens*) on the release of TSH in the rat *in vivo*. Two other groups of five rats received either 100 ng synthetic TRH or saline alone. The material was administered intravenously under barbiturate anesthesia. Results show mean ± SEM rise in serum TSH. The skin extract exhibited biologic potency close to that achieved by synthetic TRH. The slight reduction in TSH at 5 min compared with synthetic TRH may reflect the presence of somatostatin in the skin extract. No TSH rise occurred in the saline-treated animals.

TABLE 4. *TRH concentration in various Rana pipiens tissues removed from a group of four animals[a]*

Organ	TRH (μg/g protein)
Hypothalamus	14.9 ± 1.0
Extrahypothalamic brain	7.7 ± 1.2
Spinal cord	2.3 ± 1.1
Splanchnic nerve	0.072 ± 0.03
Skin[b]	26.1 ± 15.4
Retina[c]	3.3 ± 0.4
Heart	0.057 ± 0.009
Lung	0.058 ± 0.018
Tongue	0.28 ± 0.13
Stomach	0.041 ± 0.007
Intestine	0.023 ± 0.004
Liver	0.019 ± 0.005
Spleen	0.025 ± 0.009
Kidney	0.019 ± 0.007
Gonad	0.015 ± 0.006
Muscle	0.021 ± 0.010
Blood	0.045 ± 0.007 μg/ml whole blood

From ref. 103.

[a] The blood TRH level is given for comparison. Results are shown as mean ± SEM.

[b] Protein content of skin is 15.7 ± 0.4% wet weight (N = 6). The mean skin: blood TRH concentration gradient is 91:1.

[c] Tissue obtained from a separate group of six frogs.

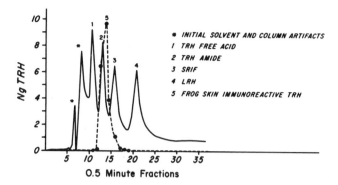

FIG. 7. HPLC of frog skin. Characterization of frog skin immunoreactive TRH on HPLC after preliminary purification by anti-TRH affinity chromatography. The elution pattern of radioimmunoassayable TRH (dotted line) isolated from *Rana pipiens* skin extract by affinity chromatography is shown. For comparison the elution patterns of pyroGlu-His-Pro (TRH-free acid), TRH, LH-RH, and somatostatin are also shown. Isocratic separation on Whatman partisil SCX column, with 10% ethanol in 0.2 M ammonium acetate pH 4.6. (From Jackson and Reichlin, *unpublished*.)

histidyl prolineamide in an extract of skin from the Korean frog, *Bombina orientalis*.

Significance of Frog Skin TRH

There are a number of other peptides present in the skin of amphibians that share amino acid sequences with peptides found in the nervous system and gastrointestinal tract of mammals (51). Caerulein (*Hyla* sp.; *Xenopus laevis*) and phyllocaerulein (*Phyllomedusa* sp.) are related to gastrin and cholecystokinin (CCK); physallaemin (*Physalaemus* sp.) and uperolein (*Uperoleia* sp.) are related to the undecapeptide substance P found in the dorsal root ganglia, brain, and gastrointestinal tract of mammals; in the spinal cord it appears to play a role in sensory excitation (85). Xenopsin is an octapeptide chemically related to the tridecapeptide neurotensin isolated from bovine hypothalamus (33), which in mammals produces hypotension, vascular permeability, and gut contraction; prolongs barbiturate sedation (similar to somatostatin; opposite effect of TRH); and following parenteral administration increases circulating levels of glucagon, glucose, GH, and prolactin in rats (193). Substance P shares similar vascular as well as GH- and PRL-releasing effects with neurotensin, but unlike the latter does not produce hypothermia when given intracisternally to the rat (21). Bombesin (*Bombina bombina*)—which is also present in mammalian gastrointestinal tract and brain, and circulates in human plasma—has potent hypothermic effects in the rat; it is 10,000 times more active than neurotensin in lowering core temperature. Bombesin prevents the hyperthermia induced by intracisternal TRH and the cold-induced TSH rise in the rat. Conversely, TRH administration prevents the hypothermia effect of bombesin (21,22).

The cells of origin of these peptides found in amphibian skin (caerulein, phyllocaerulein, physallaemin, uperolein, xenopsin, bombesin, and its related peptides litorin, ranatensin, and alytesin) have not been determined for certain, but it seems likely that they arise in anuran cutaneous glands that are derived from the specialized ectoderm of the region adjacent to the embryonic neural plate and neural crest (172). TRH also is likely to be present in these skin glands, but immunohistochemical studies for TRH as well as the other peptides are required. Thus the probable cells of origin of these amphibian skin peptides are related to the amine precursor uptake decarboxylation (APUD) system. Pearse (172) proposed that these peptide-secreting cells in the skin have evolved in parallel with the nervous system as a response to the (hostile) external environment. The cells in frog skin producing TRH and other peptides can be considered part of the diffuse neuroendocrine system (173). The cells of this system are dedicated to the production of amines and peptides, and the sole common link between them is their proved or postulated identity as modified neurons (173) so that despite their gross location the presumptive cells in the skin cutaneous glands of *R. pipiens* concerned with the production of TRH are in essence part of the nervous system.

Regulation of Frog Skin TRH

Recently we examined the neurotransmitter regulation of frog skin TRH (98). Areas of skin most densely populated with cutaneous poison glands were removed from the dorsum and incubated in buffer. NE (10^{-5} to 10^{-3} M) evoked a significant dose-related release of TRH into the medium and a re-

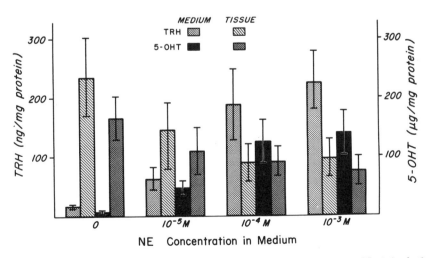

FIG. 8. Effect of NE on the release of TRH and 5-OHT from frog skin *in vitro* during a 15-min incubation. There was a marked dose-related discharge of TRH and 5-OHT into the medium paralleled by a reduction in the tissue content of these substances. (From ref. 154.)

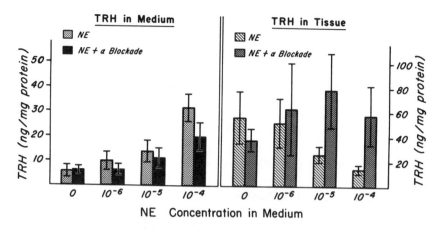

FIG. 9. Effect of phenoxybenzamine (α-blockade) *in vivo* on the stimulation of TRH release from frog skin by NE *in vitro*. In α-blocked animals the release of TRH into the medium was partly suppressed and the tissue was not depleted compared with the control frogs. Phenoxybenzamine was administered into the dorsal lymph sac of each test animal in a dose of 200 μg 15 min prior to skin removal. (From ref. 154.)

duction in tissue content of TRH (Fig. 8). These TRH responses were paralleled by changes in medium and skin serotonin (5-OHT). *In vivo* pretreatment with phenoxybenzamine (α-blockade) antagonized the ability of NE to release 5-OHT *in vitro,* and some inhibition of TRH release was also observed (Fig. 9). In contrast, *in vivo* pretreatment with propranolol (β-blockade) did not alter the NE-induced release of 5-OHT or TRH. The noradrenergic stimulation of TRH in frog skin is consistent with the neurotransmitter regulation of TRH from mammalian hypothalamic fragments previously demonstrated by Grimm and Reichlin (73). This suggests that the skin "neural cells" containing TRH are subject to the same basic regulatory mechanisms which affect the "neural cells" in mammalian hypothalamus that secrete TRH. The secretion of TRH from frog skin may provide a model for studying TRH regulation in vertebrate neural tissue.

BIOSYNTHESIS OF HYPOPHYSIOTROPIC HORMONES

Until the discovery of the chemical nature of the releasing hormones, scientific studies of their biosynthesis and of the factors controlling their synthesis were inaccessible to analysis. At the time of the discovery of TRH in 1969, it appeared reasonable to consider, as proposed by Geschwind (65), that there are two possible routes of synthesis. One, analogous to the synthesis of parathyroid hormone (118), implies synthesis of peptide as a prohormone in the classic mode of large protein biosynthesis followed by posttranslational, enzymatic cleavage of an active fragment. This mechanism of biosynthesis, first demonstrated by Sachs and collaborators (174,196–200,215,228), was further supported by more recent studies of neurophysin biosynthesis by

Gainer and colleagues (27,62,63). Other brain neuropeptides (e.g., β-endorphin) appear to be synthesized similarly from a precursor macromolecule, as shown by Crine et al. in a pituitary incubation system (41). One can readily speculate that this mechanism could well explain the biosynthesis of LH-RH, a decapaptide, and somatostatin, a cyclic peptide consisting of 14 amino acids. Moreover, in the case of each of these hormones a macromolecular form has been identified in tissue extracts: "big LH-RH" (141) and "big somatostatin" (114). On the other hand, in the case of TRH, a tripeptide amide, alternative mechanisms of biosynthesis are theoretically possible. The most attractive alternative hypothesis, as outlined by Mitnick and Reichlin (142,144,185,187,189), is that TRH is synthesized by a nonribosomal mechanism analogous to the formation of several other biologically significant small peptides of mammalian tissues, including the tripeptides glutathione (y-Glu-Cys-Gly), ophthalamic acid (y-Glu-a-amino-*n*-butyrylglycine), and the dipeptides carnosine (β-alanyl-L-histidine) and homocarnosine (y-aminobutyryl-L-histidine). Other oligopeptides more recently identified in brain are GABA-Lys and α-aminobutyryl-cystathione (174*a*). An inclusive list of brain oligopeptides is provided by Reichelt and Edminson (181), who also summarized evidence for brain synthesis of a novel series of peptides with N-terminal acetyl-asp. All of these peptides are synthesized by enzymes (208; also see ref. 185 for further references), which in some cases have been well characterized. Whether the product is of prohormone synthesis with cleavage or enzymatic synthesis, posttranslation mechanisms are likely involved in cyclization of the amino terminal acid (220) and the formation of a carboxy-terminal amide. Suchanek and Kreil recently proposed a novel mechanism by which COOH-terminal amides might be synthesized (212*a*). Mellitin, a polypeptide formed by queen bee venom sacks, has a terminal amide that cannot be demonstrated in peptides formed in a wheat germ-translated cell-free system. Rather, the peptide so formed has a terminal glutaminylglycine rather than a glutaminamide. They propose that "a COOH-terminal glycine represents the recognition site for a venom gland enzyme that exchanges glycine by ammonia." They further propose that glutamine may be the donor of the ammonia residue by a transamidation reaction. It may also be postulated that y-glutamyl-cycle enzymes are involved (71). A third possible mechanism that has to be considered in relation to TRH biosynthesis was emphasized by McKelvey (135,136)—synthesis by aminoacyl-tRNA transferases (211). By this mechanism an amino acid moiety can be adenylated with ATP, combined with transfer RNA, and then coupled with an existing peptide or protein.

TRH Biosynthesis

As initially reported by Reichlin and collaborators (142,144,185,187,189) fragments of rat hypothalamic tissue incubated in amino acid precursors were found to incorporate labeled amino acids into peptides that had the same chromatographic behavior as authentic TRH. Many other peptides were found in the same system. Grimm and Reichlin (73) also found that mouse hypothalamic fragments, incubated in labeled histidine, incorporated this amino acid into a substance with the mobility of TRH on thin-layer chromatography, and that the product, labeled with ^{14}C-histidine, chromatographed to constant specific activity with ^{3}H-TRH.

Subsequently, McKelvy (133,135,136) and McKelvy and Grimm-Jorgensen (74,75,136,137,139) criticized the earlier work from this laboratory on rat TRH biosynthesis on the basis that the proof of identity of the labeled product had not been rigorous enough and that only a small fraction of the radioactivity moving with TRH on electrophoresis or thin-layer chromatography was authentic TRH.

The problems in identification of a labeled product were emphasized in recent publications by McKelvy and collaborators. Their studies were carried out using much more sophisticated chemical separation methods than were the first studies done in our laboratory. *In vitro* incorporation of precursors into a compound that migrates with TRH, at least in some chromatographic systems, was reported by Guillemin and by Knigge and collaborators (see ref. 185 for review), but the same reservations about isolation of product undoubtedly apply to these reports as well. Using guinea pig hypothalamic cultures, McKelvy showed that ^{3}H-proline was incorporated into a compound that moved with TRH in at least nine separate chromatographic steps and formed an *n*-trifluoroacetyl *n*-butyl-ester derivative that had chromatographic properties identical with those of TRH. Using the whole newt brain, Grimm-Jorgensen and McKelvy conducted a similar study by extensive chromatographic procedures including derivatization and proved the identity of the compound. From these experiments and those of Grimm-Jorgensen and Reichlin, it seems reasonable to conclude the organ incubate and culture is capable of forming new TRH, but that the most rigorous separation methods are needed to establish the identity of the compound in view of the large number of new peptides that are formed by such systems. In rat brain fragment incubations we found (142,187) that puromycin (an inhibitor of translation) did not block the incorporation of amino acids into a peptide separable as TRH by thin-layer chromatography and electrophoresis. Since the identity of the isolated compound as TRH is now in doubt because of the more recent findings alluded to, the significance of this result can now be questioned. On the other hand, Grimm-Jorgensen and McKelvy (74,75) found that newt brain TRH formation was blocked by neither incubation with puromycin nor by diphtheria antitoxin, a potent ribosomal poison also indicating a non-ribosomal form of biosynthesis. Kubek et al. (124) reported that rat hypothalamic fragments incubated *in vitro* with ^{3}H-proline incorporated the amino acid into a product separated by affinity chromatography on anti-TRH columns. Although this may well be TRH, the occurrence of some non-TRH compounds that react with anti-TRH antisera make it essential to carry out more extensive separation methods than simple affinity chromatography. In this system, incorporation of counts into "TRH" was not blocked by cycloheximide, indicating a nonribosomal form of biosynthesis.

TRH Biosynthesis in Cell-Free Preparations

Following our observation that puromycin did not block the incorporation of amino acids into a material that had the mobility of TRH in several chromatographic systems, we considered the possibility that TRH was formed by a nonribosomal enzymatic synthetic process analogous to that responsible for the formation of glutathione.

Procedures adapted from those used to study glutathione were used to study TRH biosynthesis (143,188). These included incubation of the soluble fraction of hypothalamic tissue in the presence of Mg^{2+}, ATP, and precursor amino acids (glutamic acid, histidine, and proline). A product was isolated from the incubate by a series of chromatographic steps, including charcoal adsorption and elution; thin-layer chromatography (TLC), carboxy methyl cellulose, and Sephadex chromatography; and electrophoresis, all showing correspondence to synthetic TRH. It was proposed therefore that TRH was formed by a "synthetase" analogous to the enzyme that synthesizes glutathione. Further studies were made of the influence of a number of factors, including prior thyroid status on "TRH" formation, using electrophoresis to separate the product; it was concluded that thyroid deficiency decreased TRH synthesis, and that thyroxine feeding enhanced TRH synthesis. The observations were interpreted to indicate that thyroxine exerted a "positive" feedback effect on TRH synthesis and, by inference, on TRH secretion.

Unfortunately these results that appeared so clear-cut have not been confirmed by a number of other workers who have either published their studies (10–12,44) or who have communicated these results in personal communications (McKelvy, LaBrie, Rosenberg, Barnea). Bauer and co-workers (10–12) reported that the incubation procedure led to the enzymatic degradation of TRH. In an attempt to circumvent this problem, an inhibitor of TRH degradation was added to the reaction mixture. In the presence of the inhibitor, substantial amounts of labeled TRH were isolated from the reaction mixture, but Bauer believes that the product arose by a "substitution reaction" consequent to enzymatic degradation. In the studies of Dixon and Acres (44), initial separation of product on charcoal and electrophoresis revealed counts corresponding to TRH, but the material did not behave like TRH in other separation systems. These authors also were unable to identify synthesis of TRH by isolated rat hypothalamic fragments incubated *in vitro*. McKelvy and Grimm-Jorgensen also failed to identify labeled TRH in freeze-dried porcine or rat hypothalamic tissue, or in fresh rat hypothalamic extract supernatants separated by low-speed centrifugation (*personal communication*).

The latter workers used whole newt brain for studies of TRH synthesis by extracts. Newt brain has a high concentration of extrahypothalamic TRH, and for this reason it was presumed that it would provide a richer source of TRH-synthesizing structures. In their studies a 5,000-g supernatant was incubated in amphibian Ringer Hepes at 22°C in the presence of 0.1 mM ATP and ^{3}H-proline, 25 μCi/ml; it showed progressive incorporation of radioactivity into "TRH" over a 30-min period. The identity of the product was confirmed by electrophoresis in acid and alkaline media, and by dinitrophenylation. The DNP derivative was separated by electrophoresis and was shown to have chromatographic behavior identical to that of authentic DNP-TRH. In the newt extract preparation, formation of TRH was blocked by RNAse pretreatment of the extract. On the basis of this observation they concluded that biosynthesis was by an RNA-dependent mechanism; but since they previously showed in whole newt brain that biosynthesis was blocked by neither cycloheximide nor diphtheria toxin, they proposed that synthesis might take place by an active transfer acyl-tRNA mechanism mediating peptide bond formation.

Reports that TRH formation by soluble hypothalamic extracts could not be confirmed in a number of laboratories began at the time that our laboratory moved to Boston in 1972. In collaboration with Dr. Richard Saperstein and Miss Stella Mothon, efforts were made to set up the originally described experiments as close as possible to the original technique. In a number of trials using fresh rat hypothalamic extracts, freeze-dried rat, and porcine hypothalamic extracts, we were unable to demonstrate consistently and in a convincing way that new counts appeared in "TRH" as isolated by charcoal adsorption, electrophoresis, and TLC (185).

The three major areas of concern were the problem of degradation of product, the problem of degradation of ATP by ATPases of hypothalamic tissue, and the unambiguous demonstration of product as authentic TRH. These problems apply to all studies of hypothalamic hormone biosynthesis by soluble systems. The first issue addressed appeared to be the problem of enzymatic degradation of product. The more general problem of enzymatic breakdown of neuropeptides was recently reviewed in detail by Marks (129a). The hypothalamic incubation system we used was found to degrade TRH actively, and the rate of inactivation proved to be a function of the concentration of extract added (185). A series of compounds were studied in an attempt to find one that would protect TRH from degradation and would not interfere with biosynthesis (185). TRH degradation was blocked by a number of amidated and nonamidated peptides including TRH, deamido TRH (kindly supplied by Dr. Will White, Abbott Laboratories), LRH, deamido LRH, angiotensin amide, angiotensin I, angiotensin II, and somatostatin (kindly provided by Dr. M. Goetz, Ayerst Laboratories). The reaction was not blocked by vasopressin, oxytocin nor by so-called MIF (Pro-Leu-Gly-NH$_2$). Our conclusion with respect to the degradation system was that hypothalamic tissues degrade TRH by one or more peptidases capable of attacking the amide bond as well as the peptide bond, as has been shown for chymotrypsin.

The second problem is that of ATPase concentration. We found that ATP was rapidly destroyed by the incubation system—within 10 min virtually all of it was gone. Even with the addition of an ATP-generating system, the concentration of ATP, initially 3.2 mM, fell to 1.6 mM by 15 min and 0.1 mM at the end of 0.5 hr. If in fact ATP is a necessary cofactor for the formation of TRH by a soluble system, its rapid degradation would require either the addition of even larger amounts of ATP or the separation of ATPase from other extract components.

Taking into account a number of these factors, we carried out further studies of cell-free biosynthesis using a variety of ATP-generating systems, as well as the addition of peptides that interfere with TRH breakdown. These are summarized in an earlier paper (185), which indicated that such experiments gave inconsistent and only minimal amounts of TRH product, even by less-specific chromatographic procedures.

We therefore spent some time in developing more reliable methods for isolating synthesized product because we recognized that only minute amounts of new peptide could conceivably be detected in the usual kinds of incubation system. The approach chosen was to utilize an anti-TRH affinity column followed by further purification of eluted product by high pressure liquid chromatography using a method modified from that of McKelvy (134). We found earlier that the combination of affinity chromatography followed by electrophoresis gave good separation of newly synthesized LH-RH by whole rat hypothalamic incubates (185). Rat hypothalamic fragments incubated in ^{3}H-proline were found to incorporate less than 10^{-5} of total tissue counts into a compound retained on an anti-TRH affinity column. When this material was further separated, it was evident that less than 35 total counts were isolated as TRH; this represents 10^{-6} times the total tissue counts and is illustrative of the extremely small yields of new peptide formation in such preparations. It is also illustrative of the low turnover of new compound *in vitro*.

In addition to studies of rat hypothalamic incubates, we also utilized incubations of frog skin poison gland strips described above in relation to *in vitro* control of TRH secretion. On the basis of blood turnover studies, we anticipated that this tissue would have a high rate of TRH turnover. Working in collaboration with Dr. Gregory Mueller, incubating frog skin in frog Ringers solution in the absence of added cofactors, we attempted to isolate labeled product from incubates at 1, 2, and 24 hr. Total immunoassayable TRH remained the same in the skin preparations, and we were unable to identify any newly labeled TRH in the skin. It should be emphasized that, as mentioned earlier, endogenous TRH in frog skin shows a similar elution pattern to synthetic TRH on HPLC (Fig. 7).

McKelvey's laboratory has been active in pursuing the mechanism of TRH biosynthesis. In summary, this group developed a series of peptide inhibitors of TRH degradation, showed that bacitracin blocks hypothalamic degradation by soluble hypothalamic extracts (138), and carried out studies of *in vitro* labeling of TRH by soluble preparations separated from low-speed supernatants of guinea pig and rat hypothalamic extracts with "additions appropriate for ribosomal protein synthesis." They report that the rate of TRH production assessed by measurements of immunoreactive TRH was greater than that derived from TRH labeling with ^{3}H-proline (135) and suggest that two pathways may exist for the formation of TRH: *de novo* biosynthesis and the formation of a precursor with subsequent breakdown. In this system they further report that the antibiotics cycloheximide and puromycin abolished the labeling of TRH (135). These findings favor a pathway of biosynthesis by classic pathways.

Recently Schaeffer et al. (203) reported that there is TRH in rat retina and that its concentration varies with altered lighting conditions. They also stated that injecting rats with cycloheximide, 20 mg/kg, prevented the light-induced rise in TRH, "suggesting that protein synthesis is necessary for the daytime increase." This could be because TRH is synthesized on ribosomes or that the synthetic machinery for TRH is so synthesized.

For comparison, brief mention should be made of the status of knowledge of biosynthesis of the other hypothalamic hypophysiotrophic hormones. The *in vitro* incorporation of radioactive precursor amino acids into LH-RH has been reported by several groups (78,111,112,146–148,185,188), and data have been presented indicating that incorporation is enhanced by prior castration. Rat hypothalamic fragments have been reported to generate LH-RH activity after incubation (213), and extracts of hypothalamic tissue have been reported to generate biological LH-RH activity after incubation *in vitro* (58). All of these studies are characterized by strikingly small amounts of newly synthesized material and by the lack of critical proof of identity. The only studies testing a specific mode of biosynthesis of LH-RH are those of Johansson et al. (111,112), who suggest a enzymatic, nonribosomal mode of biosynthesis. There are too few data available to form an adequate conclusion as to the mode of biosynthesis of this hormone.

Bioassays were used to demonstrate the cell-free biosynthesis of GH-RF (190) and PRF (144) by Reichlin and collaborators. With the now-available knowledge that hypothalamic extracts degrade somatostatin very rapidly, it is possible that the claim for biosynthesis of GH-RF may be due to loss of associated somatostatin activity. No other reports of studies of this type have appeared. Finally, mention should be made of the recent report by Kantner et al. (114) that ^{3}H-phenylalanine was incorporated into both hypothalamic and pancreatic slices *in vitro,* and that in both sites there was a macromolecular precursor.

SUMMARY AND CONCLUSIONS

TRH is readily detectable by immunoassay in the hypothalamus and stalk median eminence (SME) of mammals including man. Evidence that hypothalamic TRH regulates pituitary-thyroid function is shown by the fact that ablation of the "thyrotrophic area" causes hypothyroidism associated with a 70% fall in hypothalamic content of TRH. When compared with the hypothalamus, the concentration of TRH in mammalian extrahypothalamic brain is low, but quantitatively close to 80% of brain TRH lies in this region. Hypothalamic "thyrotrophic area" lesions do not affect extrahypothalamic brain content of TRH, suggesting that TRH located there is synthesized *in situ;* since deafferentation lowers hypothalamic but not extrahypothalamic TRH, it is possible that TRH located in the hypothalamus originates from outside this brain region. IR-TRH-like material is present in mammalian blood, urine, and CSF, but its nature, source, and physiologic significance are uncertain and controversial.

Although TRH is unable to stimulate pituitary thyroid function in species lower than aves, it has been reported to cause prolactin secretion in the bullfrog; and it may be speculated that this action is the first role acquired by TRH in the regulation of pituitary function. The significance of its reported stimulation of α-MSH from the amphibian pars intermedia is unclear. In spite of the apparent absence of any effect on thyroid function, large quantities of TRH are found in the hypothalamus and brain of submammalian vertebrates including amphibia and fish. TRH is also present in whole brain of the larval lamprey, which does not produce TSH, and in neural tissue of the invertebrate snail, which lacks a pituitary.

In contradistinction to studies in mammalian species, in the leopard frog we found large quantities of circulating IR-TRH that is biologically and chromatographically identical to native TRH. The origin of this TRH appears to be skin wherein its concentration is three to four times that of hypothalamus. Skin TRH is located in cutaneous glands which are embryologically derived from neuroendocrine-programmed ectoblast (173). APUD cells, so located, which synthesize a wide variety of neural peptides such as TRH, can be considered to constitute a third division of the nervous system (172). There is evidence that the cutaneous TRH in the frog is under α-adrenergic control similar to that operative in the mammalian hypothalamus, suggesting that the basic mechanism underlying TRH control may remain intact during evolution.

The elucidation of the mechanism of biosynthesis of TRH has proved to be difficult, primarily because only minute amounts of product are formed in incubation systems concomitantly with a host of other peptides. Two possible pathways have been proposed, one by enzymatic nonribosomal biosynthesis analogous to the synthetase-mediated synthesis of glutathione (Glu-Cys-Gly) and the other by an mRNA-directed ribosomal formation of a large prohormone with subsequent splitting of the TRH peptide, analogous to the formation of vasopressin and oxytocin from neurophysin. The actual mechanism underlying TRH synthesis still remains to be determined.

The widespread distribution of TRH in neural tissue remote from the hypothalamus suggests a role for this substance in neuronal function apart from pituitary regulation, and there is considerable evidence in favor of such a hypothesis. First, TRH is located in extrahypothalamic brain sites where it has apparent independence from hypothalamic regulation. Secondly, TRH is found in tissues of vertebrate and invertebrate species in which TRH clearly has no role in the regulation of any pituitary-thyroid axis that might be present. Thirdly, *in vitro* synthesis and degrading systems, as well as high-affinity binding sites for TRH in the synaptic membrane fraction, have been located in rat extrahypothalamic brain tissues. Fourthly, neurophysiologic and behavioral effects for this tripeptide have been reported.

The evidence from phylogenetic studies suggests that the role of TRH in pituitary regulation is a late evolutionary development representing an example of an organism acquiring a new target for a preexisting chemical substance, and that the primitive function of this hormone is that of a neural peptide. It appears that TRH (like LH-RH and somatostatin) are part of a family of neural peptides, including substance P, neurotensin, endorphines, and many others with hypophysiotropic regulation being only one aspect of their overall function. The hypothalamus itself is subsidiary to the brain, which might be considered a huge peptide-secreting organ regulating both neural and endocrine function. The neuroendocrine system, in the form of APUD cells secreting neural peptides, extends into other parts of the body, including the gastrointestinal tract and skin; and it conceptually breaks down the previously held rigid confines of the nervous system. Preliminary findings suggest that study of these remote areas of the nervous system may in turn provide knowledge on the regulation of brain function.

ACKNOWLEDGMENT

This work was supported in part by a grant from the NIH (AM 16684). Deamido TRH was kindly supplied by Dr. Will White, Abbott Laboratories. The somatostatin was kindly provided by Dr. M. Goetz, Ayerst Laboratories.

REFERENCES

1. Alpert, L. C., Brawer, J. R., Jackson, I. M. D., and Reichlin, S. (1976): Localization of LH-RH in neurons in frog brain (Rana pipiens and Rana catesbeiana). *Endocrinology*, 98:910–921.
2. Annunziato, L., DiRenzo, G., Lombardi, G., et al. (1977): The role of central

noradrenergic neurons in the control of thyrotropin secretion in the rat. *Endocrinology*, 100:738–744.

3. Arimura, A., Sato, H., Dupont, A., Nishi, N., and Schally, A. V. (1975): Somatostatin: Abundance of immunoreactive hormone in rat stomach and pancreas. *Science*, 189:1007–1009.

4. Bakke, J. L., and Lawrence, N. L. (1971): Effects of cold-adaptation, rewarming and heat-exposure on thyrotropin (TSH) secretion in rats. *Endocrinology*, 89:204–212.

5. Bar-Sella, P., Stein, O., and Gross, J. (1973): Electron microscopic radioautography of ^{125}I-triiodothyronine in rat posterior pituitary and median eminence. *Endocrinology*, 93:1410–1422.

6. Bassiri, R. M., and Utiger, R. D. (1972): The preparation and specificity of antibody to thyrotropin releasing hormone. *Endocrinology*, 90:722–727.

7. Bassiri, R. M., and Utiger, R. D. (1972): Serum inactivation of the immunological and biological activity of thyrotropin-releasing hormone (TRH). *Endocrinology*, 91:657–664.

8. Bassiri, R. M., and Utiger, R. D. (1973): Metabolism and excretion of exogenous thyrotropin-releasing hormone in humans. *J. Clin. Invest.*, 52:1616–1619.

9. Bassiri, R. M., and Utiger, R. D. (1974): Thyrotropin-releasing hormone in the hypothalamus of the rat. *Endocrinology*, 94:188–197.

10. Bauer, K. (1974): Degradation of thyrotropin releasing hormone (TRH). Its inhibition by pyroglu-His-OCH₃ and the effect of the inhibitor in attempts to study the biosynthesis of TRH. In: *Lipmann Symposium: Energy, Biosynthesis and Regulation in Molecular Biology*, pp. 53–62. Gruyter, Berlin.

11. Bauer, K., and Kleinkauf, H. (1974): Degradation of thyrotropin-releasing hormone (TRH) by serum and hypothalamic tissue and its inhibition by analogues of TRH. *Z. Physiol. Chem.*, 355:1173–1176.

12. Bauer, K., Sy, J., and Lipmann, F. (1973): Degradation of thyrotropin releasing hormone (TRH) by extracts of hypothalamus. *Fed. Proc.*, 32:489 (abstract).

13. Bauer, K., and Lipmann, F. (1976): Attempts toward biosynthesis of the thyrotropin-releasing hormone and studies on its breakdown in hypothalamic tissue preparations. *Endocrinology*, 99:230–242.

14. Bennett, G. W., Edwardson, J. A., Holland, D., Jeffcoate, S. L., and White, N. (1975): Release of immunoreactive luteinising hormone-releasing hormone and thyrotropin releasing hormone from hypothalamic synaptosomes. *Nature (Lond)*, 257:323–325.

15. Bergland, R. M., Davis, S. L., and Page, R. B. (1977): Pituitary secretes to brain. *Lancet*, 2:276–277.

16. Blackwell, R. E., and Guillemin, R. (1973): Hypothalamic control of adenohypophysial secretions. *Annu. Rev. Physiol.*, 35:357–390.

17. Bloom, F. E. (1971): Possible function of monoamines as neurotransmitters. *Neurosci. Res. Prog. Bull.*, 9:209–217.

18. Bøler, J., Enzmann, F., Folkers, K., Bowers, C. Y., and Schally, A. V. (1969): The identity of chemical and hormonal properties of the thyrotropin releasing hormone and pyroglutamyl-histidyl-proline-amide. *Biochem. Biophys. Res. Commun.*, 37:705–710.

19. Brazeau, P., Vale, W., Burgus, R., Ling, N., Butcher, M., Rivier, J., and Guillemin, R. (1973): Hypothalamic polypeptide that inhibits the secretion of immunoreactive pituitary growth hormone. *Science*, 179:77–79.

20. Bromage, N. R. (1975): The effects of mammalian thyrotropin-releasing hormone on the pituitary-thyroid axis of teleost fish. *Gen. Comp. Endocrinol.*, 25:292–297.

21. Brown, M., Rivier, J., and Vale, W. (1977): Bombesin: Potent effects on thermoregulation in the rat. *Science*, 196:998–1000.

22. Brown, M., Rivier, J., and Vale, W. (1977): Actions of bombesin, thyrotropin releasing factor, prostaglandin E_2 and naloxone on thermoregulation in the rat. *Life Sci.*, 20:1681–1688.

23. Brown, M., and Vale, W. (1975): Growth hormone release in the rat: Effects of somatostatin and thyrotropin-releasing factor. *Endocrinology*, 97:1151–1156.

24. Brown, M., and Vale, W. (1975): Central nervous system effects of hypothalamic peptides. *Endocrinology,* 96:1333–1336.
25. Brown-Grant, K. (1956): Changes in thyroid activity of rats exposed to cold. *J. Physiol. (Lond),* 131:52–54.
26. Brownstein, M., Arimura, A., Sato, H., Schally, A. V., and Kizer, J. S. (1975): The regional distribution of somatostatin in the rat brain. *Endocrinology,* 96:1456–1461.
27. Brownstein, M. J., and Gainer, H. (1977): Neurophysin biosynthesis in normal rats and in rats with hereditary diabetes insipidus. *Proc. Natl. Acad. Sci. USA,* 74:4046–4049.
28. Brownstein, M. J., Palkovits, M., Saavedra, J. M., Bassiri, R. M., and Utiger, R. D. (1974): Thyrotropin-releasing hormone in specific nuclei of rat brain. *Science,* 185:267–269.
29. Brownstein, M. J., Utiger, R. D., Palkovits, M., and Kizer, J. S. (1975): Effect of hypothalamic deafferentation° on thyrotropin releasing hormone levels in rat brain. *Proc. Natl. Acad. Sci. USA,* 72:4177–4179.
30. Burgus, R., Dunn, T., Desiderio, D., and Guillemin, R. (1969): Structure moleculaire du facteur hypothalamique hypophysiotrope TRF d'orgine ovine: mise en évidence pat spectomètre de masse de la seguence Pca-His-Pro-NH₂. *C. R. Acad. Sci. (Paris),* 269:1870–1873.
31. Burrow, G. N., May, P. B., Spaulding, S. W., and Donabedian, R. K. (1976): Mutual antagonism between dopamine and TRH in pituitary hormone control. In: *Program: 5th International Congress of Endocrinology, Hamburg* p. 333, abstract 802.
32. Burt, D. R., and Synder, S. H. (1975): Thyrotropin releasing hormone (TRH): Apparent receptor binding in rat brain membranes. *Brain Res.,* 93:309–328.
33. Carraway, R. E., Demers, L. M., and Leeman, S. E. (1976): Hyperglycemic effect of neurotensin, a hypothalamic peptide. *Endocrinology,* 99:1452–1462.
34. Chambers, W. F., and Sobel, R. J. (1971): Effect of thyroxine-agar tube application to the rat hypothalamus. *Neuroendocrinology,* 7:37–45.
35. Chen, H. J., and Meites, J. (1975): Effects of biogenic amines and TRH on release of prolactin and TSH in the rat. *Endocrinology,* 96:10–14.
36. Clemons, G. K., and Nicoll, C. S. (1977): Effects of antisera to bullfrog prolactin and growth hormone on metamorphosis of Rana catesbeiana tadpoles. *Gen. Comp. Endocrinol.,* 31:495–497.
37. Clemons, G. K., Russel, S. M., and Nicoll, C. S. (1976): Effects of thyrotropin releasing hormone (TRH) and ergotamine on prolactin (PRL) secretion in vitro by bullfrog anterior pituitaries. In: *Program: 5th International Congress of Endocrinology, Hamburg,* p. 333, abstract 809.
38. Cohen, E. L., and Wurtman, R. J. (1976): Brain acetylcholine: Control by dietary choline. *Science,* 191:561–562.
39. Cohn, M. L., Cohn, M., and Taylor, F. H. (1975): Thyrotropin releasing factor (TRF) regulation of rotation in the non-lesioned rat. *Brain Res.,* 96:134–137.
40. Collu, R. DuRuisseau, P., Tache, Y., and Ducharme, J. R. (1977): Thyrotropin-releasing hormone in rat brain: Nyctohemeral variations. *Endocrinology,* 100:1391–1393.
41. Crine, P., Benjannet, S., Seidah, N. G., Lis, M., and Chrétien, M. (1977): In vitro biosynthesis of β-endorphin, γ-lipotropin, and β-lipotropin by the pars intermedia of beef pituitary glands. *Proc. Natl. Acad. Sci. USA,* 74:4276–4280.
42. D'Angelo, S. A. (1951): The effect of acute starvation on the thyrotrophic hormone level in the blood of the rat and mouse. *Endocrinology,* 48:341–343.
43. D'Angelo, S. A. (1960): Hypothalamus and endocrine function in persistent estrous rats at low environmental temperature. *Am. J. Physiol.,* 199:701–706.
44. Dixon, J. E., and Acres, S. C. (1975): The inability to demonstrate the non-ribosomal biosynthesis of thyrotropin releasing hormone in hypothalamic tissue. *Fed. Proc.,* 34:658 (abstract).
45. Dodd, J. M., Follett, B. K., and Sharp, P. J. (1971): Hypothalamic control of

pituitary function in submammalian vertebrates. *Adv. Comp. Physiol. Biochem.,* 4:113–223.

46. Douglas, W. W. (1974): In: *Handbook of Physiology. Section 7: Endocrinology,* Vol. IV, Part 1, edited by R. O. Greep and E. B. Astwood, p. 191. American Physiological Society, Washington, D.C.

47. Dupont, A., Labrie, F., Levasseur, L., Dussault, J. H., and Schally, A. V. (1976): Effect of thyroxine on the inactivation of thyrotropin-releasing hormone by rat and human plasma. *Clin. Endocrinol.,* 5:323–330.

48. Dyer, R. G., and Dyball, R. E. J. (1974): Evidence for a direct effect of LRF and TRF on single unit activity in the rostral hypothalamus. *Nature (Lond),* 252:486–488.

49. Emerson, C. H., Frohman, L. A., Szabo, M., and Thakkar, I. (1977): TRH immunoreactivity in human urine: Evidence for dissociation from TRH. *J. Clin. Endocrinol. Metab.,* 45:392–399.

50. Emerson, C. H., and Utiger, R. D. (1975): Plasma thyrotropin-releasing hormone concentrations in the rat. *J. Clin. Invest.,* 56:1564–1570.

51. Erspamer, V., and Melchiorri, P. (1973): Active polypeptides of the amphibian skin and their synthetic analogues. *Pure Appl. Chem.,* 35:463–494.

52. Eskay, R. L., Oliver, C., Grollman, A., and Porter, J. C. (1974): Immunoreactive LRH and TRH in the fetal, neonatal and adult rat brain. In: *Program: 56th Meeting of the Endocrinology Society,* p. A83 (abstract).

53. Eskay, R. L., Oliver, C., Warberg, J., and Porter, J. C. (1976): Inhibition of degradation and measurement of immunoreactive thyrotropin-releasing hormone in rat blood and plasma. *Endocrinology,* 98:269–277.

54. Etkin, W. (1963): Metamorphosis-activating system of the frog. *Science,* 139: 810–813.

55. Etkin, W., and Gona, A. G. (1967): Antagonism between prolactin and thyroid hormone in amphibian development. *J. Exp. Zool.,* 165:249–258.

56. Etkin, W., and Gona, A. G. (1968): Failure of mammalian thyrotropin-releasing factor preparation to elicit metamorphic responses in tadpoles. *Endocrinology,* 82:1067–1068.

57. Fang, V. S., Lim, V. S., and Refetoff, S. (1973): Sustained thyrotropin elevation in patients with renal failure; studies of mechanism in azotemic rats. In: *Program: 49th Meeting of the American Thyroid Association,* p. T-6 (abstract).

58. Fawcett, C. P., and Shin, S. H. (1975): Generation of hypophysiotropic activity in hypothalamic extracts in vitro. *Endocrine Res. Commun.,* 2:151–158.

59. Fernstrom, J. D., and Wurtman, R. J. (1974): Nutrition and the brain. *Sci. Am.,* 230:84–91.

60. Fisher, D. A., and Odell, W. D. (1969): Acute release of thyrotropin in the newborn. *J. Clin. Invest.,* 48:1670–1674.

61. Gagel, R. F., Jackson, I. M. D., Deprez, D. P., Papapetrou, P. D., and Reichlin, S. (1976): The significance of urinary thyrotropin releasing hormone (TRH) excretion in man. In: *Proceedings of the 7th International Thyroid Conference,* pp. 8–10. International Congress Series No. 378. Excerpta Medica, Amsterdam.

62. Gainer, H., Loh, Y. P., and Sarne, Y. (1977): Biosynthesis of neuron and peptides. In: *Peptides in Neurobiology,* edited by H. Gainer, pp. 183–219. Plenum Press, New York.

63. Gainer, H., Sarne, Y., and Brownstein, M. J. (1977): Neurophysin biosynthesis: Conversion of a putative precursor during axonal transport. *Science,* 195:1354–1356.

64. Galton, V. A. (1971): Environmental effects on the thyroid. In: *The Thyroid,* 3rd ed., edited by S. C. Werner and S. H. Ingbar, pp. 153–158. Harper & Row, New York.

65. Geschwind, I. I. (1971): Biochemical mechanisms in hormone storage and secretion. *Mem. Soc. Endocrinol.,* 19:945–950.

66. Gona, A., and Gona, O. (1974): Failure of synthetic TRF to elicit metamorphosis in frog tadpoles or red-spotted newts. *Gen. Comp. Endocrinol.,* 24:223–225.

67. Gorbman, A., and Hyder, M. (1973): Failure of mammalian TRH to stimulate thyroid function in the lungfish. *Gen. Comp. Endocrinol.,* 20:588–589.
68. Gordon, J., Bollinger, J., and Reichlin, S. (1972): Plasma thyrotropin responses to thyrotropin releasing hormone after injection into the third ventricle systemic circulation median eminence and anterior pituitary. *Endocrinology,* 91:696–701.
69. Grant, W. C., and Grant, J. A. (1958): Water drive studies on hypophysectomized efts of Diemictylus viridescens: The role of the lactogenic hormone. *Biol. Bull.,* 114:1–9.
70. Green, A. R., and Grahame-Smith, D. G. (1974): TRH potentiates behavioural changes following increased brain 5-hydroxytryptamine accumulation in rats. *Nature (Lond),* 251:524–526.
71. Griffith, O. W., and Meister, A. (1977): Selective inhibition of γ-glutamyl-cycle enzymes by substrate analogs. *Proc. Natl. Acad. Sci. USA,* 74:3330–3334.
72. Griffiths, E. C. (1976): Peptidase inactivation of hypothalamic releasing hormones. *Horm. Res.,* 7:179–191.
73. Grimm, Y., and Reichlin, S. (1973): Thyrotropin-releasing hormone (TRH): Neurotransmitter regulation of secretion by mouse hypothalamic tissue in vitro. *Endocrinology,* 93:626–631.
74. Grimm-Jorgensen, Y., and McKelvy, J. F. (1974): Biosynthesis of thyrotropin releasing factor by newt (Triturus viridescens) brain in vitro: Isolation and characterization by thyrotropin releasing factor. *J. Neurochem.,* 23:471–478.
75. Grimm-Jorgensen, Y., and McKelvy, J. F. (1976): TRF biosynthesis in vitro, effect of inhibitors of protein synthesis. *Brain Res. Bull.,* 1:171–175.
76. Grimm-Jorgensen, Y., McKelvy, J. F., and Jackson, I. M. D. (1975): Immunoreactive thyrotropin releasing factor in gastropod circumoesophageal ganglia. *Nature (Lond),* 254:620.
77. Guansing, A. R., and Murk, L. M. (1976): Distribution of thyrotropin-releasing hormone in human brain. *Horm. Metab. Res.,* 8:493–494.
78. Hall, R. W., and Steinberger, E. (1976): Synthesis of LH-RH by rat hypothalamic tissue in vitro. I. Use of a specific antibody to LH-RH for immunoprecipitation. *Neuroendocrinology,* 21:111–119.
79. Harris, A., Christianson, D., Smith, M. S., Braverman, L., and Vagenakis, A. (1977): The physiological role of TRH in the regulation of TSH and prolactin secretion in the rat. *Clin. Res.,* 25:463A.
80. Harris, A., Fang, S., Braverman, L., and Vagenakis, A. (1977): Effect of carbohydrate (CHO) protein (P) and fat (F) infusion on hepatic T3 generation in the fasted rat. In: *Program 53rd Meeting of the American Thyroid Association,* p. T-13 (abstract).
81. Hefco, E., Krulich, L., Illner, P., and Larsen, P. R. (1975): Effect of acute exposure to cold on the activity of the hypothalamic-pituitary-thyroid system. *Endocrinology,* 97:1185–1195.
82. Hökfelt, T., Efendic, S., Hellerström, C., Johansson, O., Luft, R., and Arimura, A. (1975): Cellular localization of somatostatin in endocrine-like cells and neurons of the rat with special references to the A_1 cells of the pancreatic islets and to the hypothalamus. *Acta Endocrinol. (Kbh)* [Suppl.], 5–41.
83. Hökfelt, T., Elde, R., Johansson, O., Luft, R., and Arimura, A. (1975): Immunohistochemical evidence for the presence of somatostatin, a powerful inhibitory peptide in some primary sensory neurons. *Neurosci. Lett.,* 1:231–235.
84. Hökfelt, T., Fuxe, K., Johansson, O., Jeffcoate, S., and White, N. (1975): Thyrotropin releasing hormone (TRH)-containing nerve terminals in certain brain stem nuclei and in the spinal cord. *Neurosci. Lett.,* 1:133–139.
85. Hökfelt, T., Kellerth, J. O., Nilsson, G., and Pernow, B. (1975): Substance P in spinal cord. *Science,* 190:889.
86. Hong, J. S., and Poisner, A. M. (1974): Effect of low temperature on the release of vasopressin from the isolated bovine neurohypophysis. *Endocrinology,* 94:234–240.
87. Horita, A., and Carino, M. A. (1975): Thyrotropin-releasing hormone (TRH)-

induced hyperthermia and behavioral excitation in rabbits. *Psychopharmacol. Commun.,* 1:403–414.

88. Horst, W. D., and Spirt, N. (1974): A possible mechanism for the anti-depressant activity of thyrotropin releasing hormone. *Life Sci.,* 15:1073–1082.

88a. Ishikawa, H. (1973): Study on the existence of TRH in the cerebrospinal fluid in humans. *Biochem. Biophys. Res. Commun.,* 54:1203–1209.

89. Ishikawa, H., Nagayama, T., Kato, C., and Niizuma, K. (1976). Establishment of a TSH-releasing-hormone-secreting cell live from the area cerebrovasculosa of an anencephalic foetus. *Am. J. Anat.,* 145:143–148.

90. Iverson, L. L. (1975): In: *Handbook of Psychopharmacology,* Vol. III, edited by L. L. Iverson, S. D. Iverson, and S. H. Snyder, p. 381. Plenum Press, New York.

91. Jackson, I. M. D. (1977): Extrahypothalamic distribution of TRH, LRH, and somatostatin and their function. In: *Proceedings of the 5th International Congress on Endocrinology,* Hamburg, pp. 62–66. Excerpta Medica, Amsterdam.

92. Jackson, I. M. D. (1978): Extrahypothalamic and phylogenetic distribution of hypothalamic peptides. In: *The Hypothalamus,* edited by S. Reichlin, R. J. Baldessarini, and J. B. Martin, pp. 217–231. Raven Press, New York.

93. Jackson, I. M. D. (1978): Phylogenetic distribution and function of the hypophysiotropic hormones of the hypothalamus. *Am. Zool.,* 18:385–399.

94. Jackson, I. M. D., Ampola. M. G., and Reichlin, S. (1977): Hypothalamic and brain thyrotropin-releasing hormone content and pituitary-thyroid-function in histidine-deficient rats. *Endocrinology,* 101:442–446.

95. Jackson, I. M. D., Franco, F. S., Baum, G., Soo-Hoo, F., and Reichlin, S. (1976): Is there, or is there not, thyrotropin releasing hormone (TRH) in urine? In: *Program 4th New England Endocrine Conference,* p. 19.

96. Jackson, I. M. D., Gagel, R., Papapetrou, P. D., Deprez, D., and Reichlin, S. (1975): TRH excretion and metabolism in man. *Clin. Res.,* 23:238.

97. Jackson, I. M. D., Gagel, R., Papapetrou, P., and Reichlin, S. (1974): Pituitary hypothalamic and urinary thyrotropin releasing hormone (TRH) concentration in altered thyroid states of rat and man. *Clin. Res.,* 22:342.

98. Jackson, I. M. D., Mueller, G. P., Alpert. L., and Reichlin, S. (1978): TRH secretion from frog skin is stimulated by nor-epinephrine. In: *Program: 60th Meeting of the Endocrine Society, Miami* (abstract).

99. Jackson, I. M. D., Papapetrou, P. D., and Reichlin. S. (1974): The metabolism and excretion of TRH in the rat in states of altered thyroid function. In: *Program: 50th Meeting of the American Thyroid Association,* p. T-1.

100. Jackson, I. M. D., and Reichlin, S. (1973): TRH radioimmunoassay; measurements in normal and altered states of thyroid function in the rat. In: *Program: 49th Meeting of the American Thyroid Association,* p. T4.

101. Jackson, I. M. D., and Reichlin, S. (1974): Thyrotropin-releasing hormone (TRH): Distribution in hypothalamic and extrahypothalamic brain tissues of mammalian and submammalian chordates. *Endocrinology,* 95:854–862.

102. Jackson, I. M. D., and Reichlin, S. (1974): Thyrotropin releasing hormone (TRH) distribution in the brain, blood and urine of the rat. *Life Sci.,* 14:2259–2266.

103. Jackson, I. M. D., and Reichlin, S. (1977): Thyrotropin-releasing hormone: Abundance in the skin of the frog, Rana pipiens. *Science,* 198:414–415.

104. Jackson, I. M. D., and Reichlin, S. (1977): Brain thyrotrophin-releasing hormone is independent of the hypothalamus. *Nature (Lond),* 267:853–854.

105. Jackson, I. M. D., and Reichlin, S. (1977): The skin is a massive TRH secreting organ in the frog. In: *Program: 59th Meeting of the Endocrine Society,* abstract #140, p. 126.

106. Jackson, I. M. D., Saperstein, R., and Reichlin, S. (1977): Thyrotropin releasing hormone (TRH) in pineal and hypothalamus of the frog: Effect of season and illumination. *Endocrinology,* 100:97–100.

107. Jeffcoate, S. L., and White, N. (1974): Use of benzamidine to prevent the destruction of thyrotropin-releasing hormone (TRH) by blood. *J. Clin. Endocrinol. Metab.,* 38:155–157.

108. Jeffcoate, S. L., and White, N. (1975): Clearance and identification of thyrotropin releasing hormone in human urine after intravenous injection. *Clin. Endocrinol.,* 4:421–426.

109. Jobin, M., Ferland, L., Cote, J., and Labrie, F. (1975): Effect of exposure to cold on hypothalamic TRH activity and plasma levels of TSH and prolactin in the rat. *Neuroendocrinology,* 18:204–212.

110. Jobin, M., Ferland, L., and Labrie, F. (1976): Effect of pharmacological blockade of ACTH and TSH secretion on the acute stimulation of prolactin release by exposure to cold and ether stress. *Endocrinology,* 99:146–151.

111. Johansson, N. G., Currie, B. L., Folkers, K., and Bowers, C. (1973): Biosynthesis of the luteinizing hormone releasing hormone in mitochondrial preparations and by a possible pantetheine-template mechanism. *Biochem. Biophys. Res. Commun.,* 53:502–507.

112. Johansson, N. G., Hooper, F., Sievertsson, H., Currie, B. L., Folkers, K., and Bowers, C. (1972): Biosynthesis in vitro of the luteinizing releasing hormone by hypothalamic tissue. *Biochem. Biophys. Res. Commun.,* 49:656–660.

113. Kamberi, I. A., Mical, R. S., and Porter, J. C. (1971): Effects of melatonin and serotonin on the release of FSH and prolactin. *Endocrinology,* 88:1288–1293.

114. Kantner, R., Laschansky, E., Goodner, C., and Ensinck, J. (1977): Somatostatin biosynthesis in rat hypothalamus and pancreas. *Clin. Res.,* 26:159A.

115. Kardon, F., Marcus, R. J., Winokur, A., and Utiger, R. D. (1977): Thyrotropin-releasing hormone content of rat brain and hypothalamus: Results of endocrine and pharmacologic treatments. *Endocrinology,* 100:1604–1609.

116. Kardon, F. C., Winokur, A., and Utiger, R. D. (1977): Thyrotropin-releasing hormone (TRH) in rat spinal cord. *Brain Res.,* 122:578–581.

117. Keller, H. H., Bartholini, G., and Pletscher, A. (1974): Enhancement of cerebral noradrenaline turnover by thyrotropin-releasing hormone. *Nature (Lond),* 248:528–529.

118. Kemper, B., Habener, J. F., Potts, J. T., Jr., and Rich, A. (1972): Proparathyroid hormone: Identification of a biosynthetic precursor to parathyroid hormone. *Proc. Natl. Acad. Sci. USA,* 79:643–647.

119. Kizer, J. S., Palkovits, M., and Brownstein, M. J. (1976): Releasing factors in the circumventricular organs of the rat brain. *Endocrinology,* 98:311–317.

120. Knigge, K. M., and Joseph, S. A. (1971): Neural regulation of TSH secretion: Sites of thyroxine feedback. *Neuroendocrinology,* 8:273–288.

121. Knigge, K. M., and Joseph, S. A. (1974): Thyrotrophin releasing factor (TRF) in cerebrospinal fluid of the 3rd ventricle of rat. *Acta Endocrinol. (Kbh),* 76:209–213.

122. Knigge, K. M., and Silverman, A. J. (1972): Transport capacity of the median eminence. In: *Brain-Endocrine Interaction Median Eminence: Structure and Function,* edited by K. M. Knigge, D. E. Scott, and A. Weindl, pp. 350–363. Karger, Basel.

123. Koch, Y., Goldhaber, G., Fireman, I., Zor, U., Shani, J., and Tal, E. (1977): Suppression of prolactin and thyrotropin secretion in the rat by antiserum to thyrotropin-releasing hormone. *Endocrinology,* 100:1476–1478.

124. Kubek, M., Lorincz, M., Emanuele, N., Shambaugh, G. E., and Wilber, J. (1977): Thyrotropin releasing hormone (TRH): Biosynthesis by extrahypothalamic and hypothalamic tissues in vitro. In: *Abstracts, 59th Annual Meeting of Endocrine Society, Chicago,* p. 125.

125. Kubek, M. J., Lorincz, M. A., and Wilber, J. F. (1977): The identification of thyrotropin releasing hormone (TRH) in hypothalamic and extrahypothalamic loci of the human nervous system. *Brain Res.,* 126:196–200.

126. Kühn, E. R., and Engelen, H. (1976): Seasonal variation in prolactin and TSH releasing activity in the hypothalamus of Rana temporaria. *Gen. Comp. Endocrinol.,* 28:277–282.

127. Leppaluoto, J., Ling, N., and Vale, W. (1976): Purification and measurement of urinary TRF. In: *Program: 5th International Congress of Endocrinology,* Hamburg, p. 333, abstract 807.

128. Lindemann, B., and Voute, C. (1976): Structure and function of the epidermis. In: *Frog Neurobiology,* edited by R. Llinas and W. Precht, pp. 178–185. Springer-Verlag, Berlin.

129. Little, L. D., Messing, R. B., Fisher, L., and Phebus, L. (1975): Effects of long-term corn consumption on brain serotonin and the response to electric shock. *Science,* 190:692–694.

129a. Marks, N. (1977): Conversion and inactivation of neuropeptides. In: *Peptides in Neurobiology,* edited by H. Gaines, p. 221. Plenum Press, New York.

130. Martin, J. B., and Jackson, I. M. D. (1975): Anatomical neuroendocrinology. In: *Int. Conf. Neurobiology of CNS-Hormone Interactions,* edited by W. E. Stumpf and L. D. Grant, pp. 343–353. UNC Press, Chapel Hill.

131. Martin, J. B., Renaud, L. P., and Brazeau, P. (1975): Hypothalamic peptides: New evidence for "peptidergic" pathways in the CNS. *Lancet,* 2:303–395.

132. May, P., and Donabedian, R. K. (1973): A sensitive radioimmunoassay for thyrotropin releasing hormone. *Clin. Chim. Acta,* 46:371–376.

133. McKelvy, J. F. (1974): Biochemical neuroendocrinology. I. Biosynthesis of thyrotropin releasing hormone (TRH) by organ cultures of mammalian hypothalamus. *Brain Res.,* 65:489–502.

134. McKelvy, J. F., and Epelbaum, J. (1978): Biosynthesis, packaging, transport and release of brain peptides. In: *The Hypothalamus,* edited by S. Reichlin, R. J. Baldessarini, and J. B. Martin, pp. 195–211. Raven Press, New York.

135. McKelvy, J. F. (1977): Biosynthesis of hypothalamic peptides. In: *Hypothalamic Peptide Hormones and Pituitary Regulation,* edited by J. C. Porter, pp. 77–98. Plenum Press, New York.

136. McKelvy, J. F., and Grimm-Jorgensen, Y. (1975): Studies on the biosynthesis of thyrotropin releasing hormone in vitro. In: *Hypothalamic Hormones,* edited by M. Motta, P. G. Crosignani, and L. Martini, pp. 13–26. Academic Press, New York.

137. McKelvy, J. F., and Grimm-Jorgensen, Y. (1976): Biosynthesis and degradation of hypothalamic hypophysiotropic peptides. In: *Endocrinology, Proceedings of the 5th International Congress of Endocrinology, Hamburg,* Vol. 1, edited by V. H. T. James, pp. 175–179. Excerpta Medica, Amsterdam.

138. McKelvy, J. F., Leblanc, P., Loudes, C., Perrie, S., Grimm-Jorgensen, Y., and Kordon, C. (1976): The use of bacitracin as an inhibitor of the degradation of thyrotropin releasing factor and luteinizing hormone releasing factor. *Biochem. Biophys. Res. Commun.,* 73:507–515.

139. McKelvy, J. F., Sheridan, M., Joseph, S., Phelps, C. H., and Perrie, S. (1975): Biosynthesis of thyrotropin releasing hormone in organ cultures of the guinea pig median eminence. *Endocrinology,* 97:908–918.

140. Metcalf, G. (1974): TRH: A possible mediator of thermoregulation. *Nature (Lond),* 252:310–311.

141. Millar, R. P., Aehnelt, C., and Rossier, G. (1977): Higher molecular weight immunoreactive species of luteinizing hormone releasing hormone: Possible precursors of the hormone. *Biochem. Biophys. Res. Commun.,* 74:720–731.

142. Mitnick, M., and Reichlin, S. (1971): Biosynthesis of TRH by rat hypothalamic tissue in vitro. *Science,* 172:1241–1243.

143. Mitnick, M., and Reichlin, S. (1972): Enzymatic synthesis of thyrotropin releasing hormone (TRH) by hypothalamic "TRH synthetase." *Endocrinology,* 91:1145–1153.

144. Mitnick, M., Valverde, R. C., and Reichlin, S. (1973): Enzymatic synthesis of prolactin releasing factor (PRF) by rat hypothalamic incubates and by extracts of rat hypothalamic tissue: evidence for PRF synthetase. *Proc. Soc. Exp. Biol.,* 143:418–421.

145. Mitsuma, T., Hirooka, Y., and Nihei, N. (1976): Radioimmunoassay of thyrotrophin releasing hormone in human serum and its clinical application. *Acta Endocrinol. (Kbh),* 83:225–235.

146. Moguilevsky, J. A., Enero, M. A., and Szwarcfarb, B. (1974): Luteinizing hor-

mone releasing hormone-biosynthesis by rat hypothalamus in vitro. *Proc. Soc. Exp. Biol. Med.,* 147:434–435.

147. Moguilevsky, J. A., Enero, M. A., and Szwarcfarb, B. (1974): Luteinizing hormone releasing hormone-biosynthesis by rat hypothalamus in vitro, influence of castration. *Proc. Soc. Exp. Biol.,* 147:434–437.

148. Moguilevsky, J. A., Scacchi, P., Debeljuk, L., and Faigon, M. R. (1975): Effect of castration upon hypothalamic luteinizing hormone releasing factor (LH-RF). *Neuroendocrinology,* 17:189–192.

148a. Moir, A. T. B., and Eccleston, D. (1968): The effects of precursor loading in the cerebral metabolism of 5-Hydroxyindoles. *J. Neurochem.,* 15:1093–1108.

149. Montoya, E., Lorincz, M., and Wilber, J. F. (1976): Neuropharmacological studies of thyrotropin (TSH) secretion. In: *Program of the 5th International Congress of Endocrinology, Hamburg,* p. 28.

150. Montoya, E., Seibel, M. J., and Wilber, J. (1973): Studies of thyrotropin-releasing hormone (TRH) in the rat by means of radioimmunoassay normal values and response to cold exposure. In: *Program 55th Meeting of the Endocrine Society,* p. A138.

151. Montoya, E., Seibel, M. J., and Wilber, J. F. (1975): Thyrotropin-releasing hormone secretory physiology: Studies by radioimmunoassay and affinity chromatography. *Endocrinology,* 96:1413–1418.

152. Morley, J. E., Garvin, T. J., Pekary, A. E., and Hershman, J. M. (1977): Thyrotropin-releasing hormone in the gastrointestinal tract. *Biochem. Biophys. Res. Commun.,* 79:314–318.

153. Moss, R. L., and McCann, S. M. (1973): Induction of mating behavior in rats by luteinizing hormone releasing factor. *Science,* 181:177–179.

154. Mueller, G. P., Alpert, L., Reichlin, S., and Jackson, I. M. D. (1978): Neurotransmitter regulation of TRH secretion from frog skin. (*Submitted for publication*)

155. Mueller, G. P., Franco, F. S., Reichlin, S., and Jackson, I. M. D. (1977): Elevated serum thyrotropin (TSH) of myxedema does not require continuous thyrotropin releasing hormone (TRH) secretion. *Clin. Res.,* 25:298A.

156. Nair, R., Redding, T., and Schally, A. (1971): Site of inactivation of thyrotropin-releasing hormone by plasma. *Biochemistry,* 10:3621–3624.

157. Nasset, E. S., and Gatewood, V. H. (1954): Nitrogen balance and hemoglobin of adult rats fed amino acid diets low in L- and D-histidine. *J. Nutr.,* 53:163–176.

158. Neal, M. J. (1976): Amino acid transmitter substances in the vertebrate retina. *Gen. Pharmacol.,* 7:321–332.

159. Nejad, I. F., Bollinger, J. A., Mitnick, M. A., and Reichlin, S. (1972): Importance of T3 (triiodothyronine) secretion in altered states of thyroid function in the rat: Cold exposure, subtotal thyroidectomy and hypophysectomy. *Trans. Assoc. Am. Physician,* 85:295–308.

160. Nemeroff, C. B., Konkol, R. J., Bissette, G., Youngblood, W., Martin, J. B., Brazeau, P., Rone, M. S., Prange, A. J., Jr., Breese, G. R., and Kizer, J. S. (1977): Analysis of the disruption in hypothalamic-pituitary regulation in rats treated neonatally with monosodium L-glutamate (MSG): Evidence for the involvement of tuberoinfundibular cholinergic and dopaminergic systems in neuroendocrine regulation. *Endocrinology,* 101:613–622.

161. Nicoll, R. A. (1977): Excitatory action of TRH on spinal motoneurones. *Nature (Lond),* 265:242–243.

162. Okon, E., and Koch, Y. (1976): Localisation of gonadotropin-releasing and thyrotropin-releasing hormones in human brain by radioimmunoassay. *Nature (Lond),* 263:345–347.

163. Oliver, C., Charvet, J. P., Codaccioni, J. L., and Vague, J. (1974): Radioimmunoassay of thyrotropin-releasing hormone in human plasma and urine. *J. Clin. Endocrinol. Metab.,* 39:406–409.

164. Oliver, C., Charvet, J. P., Codaccioni, J. L., Vague, J., and Porter, J. C. (1974): TRH in human CSF. *Lancet,* 1:873.

165. Oliver, C., Eskay, R. L., Ben-Jonathan, N., and Porter, J. C. (1974): Distribution and concentration of TRH in the rat brain. *Endocrinology,* 95:540–546.
166. Oliver, C., Eskay, R. L., Mical, R. S., and Porter, J. C. (1973): Radioimmunoassay for TRH and its determination in hypophysial and portal and peripheral plasma of rats. In: *Program 49th Meeting of the American Thyroid Association,* p. T4.
167. Oliver, C., Mical, R. S., and Porter, J. C. (1977): Hypothalamic-pituitary vasculature: Evidence for retrograde blood flow in the pituitary stalk. *Endocrinology,* 101: 598–604.
168. Page, R. B., and Bergland, R. M. (1977): Pituitary vasculature. In: *The Pituitary, A Current Review,* edited by M. B. Allen and V. B. Mahesh, pp. 9–17. Academic Press, New York.
169. Parker, C. R., Jr., Neaves, W. B., Barnea, A., and Porter, J. C. (1977): Studies on the uptake of ^{3}H-thyrotropin-releasing hormone and its metabolites by synaptosome preparations of the rat brain. *Endocrinology,* 101:66–75.
170. Patel, Y. C., and Reichlin, S. (1978): Somatostatin in hypothalamus, extrahypothalamic brain, and peripheral tissues of the rat. *Endocrinology,* 102:523–530.
171. Patel, Y. C., Zingg, H. H., and Dreifuss, J. J. (1977): Calcium-dependent somatostatin secretion from rat neurohypophysis in vitro. *Nature (Lond),* 267:852.
172. Pearse, A. G. E. (1976): Peptides in brain and intestine. *Nature (Lond),* 262: 92–94.
173. Pearse, A. G. E. (1977): *The Diffuse Neuroendocrine System and the "Common Peptides,"* edited by MacIntyre and Szelke, pp. 309–323. Elsevier North Holland, Amsterdam.
174. Pearson, D., Shainberg, A., Malamed, S., and Sachs, H. (1975): The hypothalamo-neurohypophysial complex in organ culture: Effects of metabolic inhibitors, biologic and pharmacologic agents. *Endocrinology,* 96:994–1003.
174a. Perry, T. L., Hansen, S., Schier, G. M., and Halpern, B. (1977): Isolation and identification of γ aminobutyryl-cystathionine from human brain and CSF. *J. Neurochem.* 29:791–795.
175. Peter, R. E. (1970): Hypothalamic control of thyroid gland activity and gonadal activity in the goldfish, *Carassius auratus. Gen. Comp. Endocrinol.,* 14:334–356.
176. Pfaff, D. W. (1973): Luteinizing hormone-releasing factor potentiates lordosis behavior in hypophysectomized ovarectomized female rats. *Science,* 182:1148–1149.
177. Plotnikoff, N. P., Prange, A. J., Jr., Breese, G. R., Anderson, M. S., and Wilson, I. C. (1972): Thyrotropin releasing hormone: Enhancement of DOPA activity by a hypothalamic hormone. *Science,* 178:417–418.
178. Popa, G., and Fielding, U. (1930): A portal circulation from the pituitary to the hypothalamic region. *J. Anat.,* 65:88–91.
179. Prange, A. J., Jr., Breese, G. R., Cott, J. M., Martin, B. R., Cooper, B. R., Wilson, I. C., and Plotnikoff, N. P. (1974): Thyrotropin releasing hormone: Antagonism of pentobarbital in rodents. *Life Sci.,* 14:447–455.
180. Redding, T. W., and Schally, A. V. (1969): Studies on thyrotropin-releasing hormone (TRH) activity in peripheral blood. *Proc. Soc. Exp. Biol. Med.,* 131:420–424.
181. Reichelt, K. L., and Edminson, P. D. (1977): Peptides containing probable transmitter candidates in the central nervous system. In: *Peptides in Neurobiology,* edited by H. Gainer. Plenum Press, New York.
182. Reichlin, S. (1957): The effect of dehydration, starvation and pitressin injections on thyroid activity in the rat. *Endocrinology,* 60:470–487.
183. Reichlin, S. (1966): Control of thyrotropic hormone secretion. In: *Neuroendocrinology,* edited by L. Martini and W. F. Ganong, pp. 445–536. Academic Press, New York.
184. Reichlin, S. (1973): Hypothalamic-pituitary function. In: *Proceedings of the 4th International Congress Endocrinology Washington* pp. 1–15. International Congress Series 273. Excerpta Medica, Amsterdam.
185. Reichlin, S. (1976): Biosynthesis and degradation of hypothalamic hypophysio-

tropic factors. In: *Subcellular Mechanisms in Reproductive Neuroendocrinology*, edited by F. Naftolin, pp. 109–127. Elsevier, Amsterdam.

186. Reichlin, S., Martin, J. B., and Jackson, I. M. D. (1978): Regulation of thyroid stimulating hormone (TSH) secretion. In: *The Endocrine Hypothalamus*, edited by S. L. Jeffcoate and J. S. M. Hutchinson. Academic Press, New York (*in press*).

187. Reichlin, S., Martin, J. B., Mitnick, M., Boshans, R., Grimm-Jorgensen, Y., Bollinger, J., Gordon, J., and Malacara, J. (1972): The hypothalamus in pituitary-thyroid regulation. *Recent Prog. Horm. Res.*, 28:229–277.

188. Reichlin, S., and Mitnick, M. A. (1973): Biosynthesis of hypothalamic hypophysiotropic hormones. In: *Frontiers in Neuroendocrinology*, edited by W. F. Ganong and L. Martini, pp. 61–88. Oxford University Press, New York.

189. Reichlin, S., and Mitnick, M. A. (1973): Biosynthesis of thyrotropin releasing hormone and its control by hormones, central monoamines and external environment. In: *Hypothalamic Hypophysiotropic Hormones*, pp. 124–135. International Congress Series 263. Excerpta Medica, Amsterdam.

190. Reichlin, S., and Mitnick, M. A. (1973): Enzymatic synthesis of growth hormone releasing factor (GH-RF) by rat incubates and by extracts of rat and porcine hypothalamic tissue. *Proc. Soc. Exp. Biol.*, 142:497–501.

191. Reichlin, S., Saperstein, R., Jackson, I. M. D., Boyd, A. E., III, and Patel, Y. (1976): Hypothalamic hormones. *Ann. Rev. Phys.*, 38:389–424.

192. Renaud, L. P., Martin, J. B., and Brazeau, P. (1975): Depressant action of TRH, LH-RH and somatostatin on activity of central neurons. *Nature (Lond)*, 255:233–235.

193. Rivier, C., Brown, M., and Vale, W.: (1977): Effect of neurotensin, substance P and morphine sulfate on the secretion of prolactin and growth hormone in the rat. *Endocrinology*, 100:751–754.

194. Rosenkilde, P. (1972): Hypothalamic control of thyroid function in amphibia. *Gen. Com. Endocrinol. (Suppl.)*, 3:32–40.

195. Roti, E., Braverman, L., Christianson, D., Bonney, M., Harris, A., and Vagenakis, A. (1977): Short-loop feedback regulation of hypothalamic TRH content in the rat and dwarf mouse. In: *Program 59th Meeting Endocrine Society, Chicago*, p. 197.

196. Sachs, H., Fawcett, C. P., Takabatake, Y., and Portanova, R. (1969): Biosynthesis and release of vasopressin and neurophysin. *Recent Prog. Hor. Res.*, 25:447–491.

197. Sachs, H., Goodman, R., Osinchak, J., and McKelvy, J. (1971): Supraoptic neurosecretory neurons of the guinea pig in organ culture. *Proc. Natl. Acad. Sci. USA*, 68:2782–2786.

198. Sachs, H., Goodman, R., Shin, S., Shainberg, A., and Pearson, D. (1973): Vasopressin and neurophysin biosynthesis in hypothalamic organ cultures. In: *Endocrinology Proceedings of the 4th International Congress of Endocrinology*, edited by R. O. Scow, pp. 573–578. Excerpta Medica, Amsterdam.

199. Sachs, H., Pearson, D., Shainberg, A., Shin, S., Bryce, G., Malamed, S., and Mowles, T. (1974): Studies on the hypothalamo-neurohypophysial complex in organ culture. In: *Recent Studies of Hypothalamic Function*, edited by K. Lederis and K. E. Cooper, pp. 50–66. Karger, Basel.

200. Sachs, H., and Takabatake, Y. (1964): Evidence for a precursor in vasopressin biosynthesis. *Endocrinology*, 75:943–948.

201. Saito, S., Musa, K., Yamamoto, S., Oshima, I., and Funato, T. (1975): Radioimmunoassay of thyrotropin releasing hormone in plasma and urine. *Endocrinol. Jpn.*, 22:303–309.

202. Sawyer, W. H. (1964): Vertebrate neurohypophysial principles. *Endocrinology*, 75:981–990.

203. Schaeffer, J. M., Brownstein, M. J., and Axelrod, J. (1977): Thyrotropin-releasing hormone-like material in the rat retina: Changes due to environmental lighting. *Proc. Natl. Acad. Sci. USA*, 74:3579–3581.

204. Shambaugh, G. E., III, and Wilber, J. F. (1974): The effect of caloric deprivation upon thyroid function in the neonatal rat. *Endocrinology*, 94:1145–1149.

205. Shambaugh, G. E., III, Wilber, J. F., Montoya, E., Ruder, H., and Blonsky, E. R.

(1975): Thyrotropin-releasing hormone (TRH): Measurements in human spinal fluid. *J. Clin. Endocrinol. Metab.*, 41:131–134.

206. Shibusawa, K., Yamamoto, T., Nishi, K., Abe, C., and Tomie, S. (1959): Urinary excretion of TRF in various functional states of the thyroid. *Endocrinol. Jpn.*, 6:131–136.

207. Sinha, D., and Meites, J. (1965): Effects of thyroidectomy and thyroxine on hypothalamic control of "Thyrotropin Releasing Factor" and pituitary content of thyrotropin in rats. *Neuroendocrinology*, 1:4–14.

208. Skaper, S. K., Das, S., and Marshall, F. D. (1973): Some properties of a homo-carnosine-carnosine synthetase isolated from rat brain. *J. Neurochem.*, 21:1429–1445.

209. Skowsky, R., Nielson, T., and Fisher, D. (1974): Arginine vasopressin (AVP) kinetics in the thyroidectomized sheep. In: *Program: 56th Annual Meeting of the Endocrine Society,* abstract 164.

210. Skowsky, R., and Swan, L. (1976): Effect of hypothalamic releasing hormone on neurohypophyseal arginine vasopressin (AVP) secretion. *Clin. Res.*, 24:101.

211. Soffer, R. L. (1973): Post-translational modification of proteins catalyzed by amino acyl-tRNA protein transerases. *Mol. Cell. Biochem.*, w:3–14.

212. Sowers, J. R., Hershman, J. M., Skowsky, W. R., and Carlson, H. E. (1976): Effect of TRH on serum arginine vasopressin in euthyroid and hypothyroid subjects. *Horm. Res.*, 7:232–237.

212a. Suchanek, G., and Kreil, G. (1977): Translation of melittin messenger RNA in vitro yields a product terminating with glutaminylglycine rather than with gluta-minamide. *Proc. Natl. Acad. Sci. USA*, 71:975–978.

213. Sundberg, D. K., and Knigge, K. M. (1977): Luteinizing hormone releasing hormone (LH-RH) production and degradation by rat medial basal hypothalami in vitro. *Brain Res.*, 139:89–99.

214. Szabo, M., and Frohman, L. A. (1976): Suppression of cold stimulated TSH secretion in the rat by anti-TRH serum. In: *Program: 58th Annual Meeting Endocrine Society,* p. 189, abstract 265.

215. Takabatake, Y., and Sachs, H. (1964): Vasopressin biosynthesis. III. In vitro studies. *Endocrinology*, 75:934–942.

216. Taurog, A., Oliver, C., Eskay, R. L., Porter, J. C., and McKenzie, J. M. (1974): The role of TRH in the neoteny of the Mexican axolotl (Ambystoma mexicanum). *Gen. Comp. Endocrinol.*, 24:267–279.

217. Torok, B. (1954): Lebend beobachtung des hypophysenkreis-laufer an hunden. *Acta Morph. Acad. Sci. Hung.*, 4:83–89.

218. Tuomisto, J., Ranta, T., Mannisto, P., Saarinen, A., and Leppaluoto, J. (1975): Neurotransmitter control of thyrotropin secretion in the rat. *Eur. J. Pharmacol.*, 30:221.

219. Tuomisto, P., Mannisto, B., Lamberg, A., and Linnoila, M. (1976): Effect of cold-exposure on serum thyrotropin levels in man. *Acta Endocrinol. (Kbh)*, 83: 522–527.

220. Twardzik, D. R., and Peterkofsky, A. (1972): Glutamic acid as a precursor to N-terminal pyroglutamic acid in mouse plasmacytoma protein. *Proc. Natl. Acad. Sci. USA*, 69:277.

221. Utiger, R. D., and Bassiri, R. M. (1973): Thyrotropin releasing hormone (TRH) radioimmunoassay. In: *Serono Foundation Conference on Hypothalamic Hypophysiotrophic Hormones,* edited by C. Gual and E. Rosemberg, p. 146. Excerpta Medica, Amsterdam.

222. Vagenakis, A. G., Roti, E., Mannix, J., and Braverman, L. E. (1975): Problems in the measurement of urinary TRH. *J. Clin. Endocrinol. Metab.*, 41:801–804.

223. Vale, W., Burgus, R., Dunn, T. F., and Guillemin, R. (1971): In vitro plasma activation of thyrotropin-releasing factor (TRF) and related peptides: Its inhibition by various means and by the synthetic peptide PCA-His-Ome. *Hormone*, 2:193–203.

224. Vale, W., Rivier, C., Brazeau, P., and Guillemin, R. (1974): Effects of somatostatin on the secretion of thyrotropin and prolactin. *Endocrinology*, 95:968–977.

225. Vaudry, H., Trochard, M. C., Leboulenger, F., and Vaillant, R. (1977): Controle de la secretion melanotrope hypophysaire chez un amphibien anoure par la thyroliberine (TRH): Etude in vitro. *C R Acad. Sci. (Paris)*, 284:961–965.
226. Vijayan, E., and McCann, S. M. (1977): Suppression of feeding and drinking activity in rats following intraventricular injection of thyrotropin releasing hormone (TRH). *Endocrinology*, 100:1727–1730.
227. Visser, T. J., Klootwijk, W., Docter, R., and Hennemann, G. (1975): A radioimmunoassay for measurement of pyroglutamyl-histidyl-proline, a proposed thyrotropin releasing hormone metabolite. *J. Clin. Endocrinol. Metab.*, 40:742–745.
228. Walter, R., Audhya, T. K., Schlesinger, D. H., Shin, S., Saito, S., and Sachs, H. (1977): Biosynthesis of neurophysin in the dog and their isolation. *Endocrinology*, 100:162–174.
229. Warberg, J., Eskay, R. L., Barnea, A., Reynolds, R. C., and Porter, J. C. (1977): Release of luteinizing hormone releasing hormone and thyrotropin releasing hormone from a synaptosome-enriched fraction of hypothalamic homogenates. *Endocrinology*, 100:814–825.
230. Wei, E., Sigel, S., Loh, H., and Way, E. L. (1975): Thyrotropin-releasing hormone and shaking behaviour in rat. *Nature (Lond)*, 253:739–740.
231. Wilber, J. F., Montoya, E., Plotnikoff, N. P., White, W. F., Gendrich, R., Renaud, L., and Martin, J. B. (1976): Gonadotropin-releasing hormone and thyrotropin-releasing hormone: Distribution and effects in the central nervous system. *Rec. Prog. Horm. Res.*, 32:117–159.
232. Wilber, J. F., and Porter, J. C. (1970): Thyrotropin and growth hormone releasing activity in hypophysial portal blood. *Endocrinology*, 87:807–811.
233. Wilson, I. C., Prange, A. J., Jr., Lara, P. P., Alltop, L. B., Stikeleather, R. A., and Lipton, M. A. (1973): TRH (Lopremone): Psychobiological responses of normal women. *Arch. Gen. Psychiatry*, 29:15–21.
234. Winokur, A., Davis, R., and Utiger, R. D. (1977): Subcellular distribution of thyrotropin releasing hormone (TRH) in rat brain and hypothalamus. *Brain Res.*, 120:423–434.
235. Winokur, A., and Utiger, R. D. (1974): Thyrotropin releasing hormone: Regional distribution in rat brain. *Science*, 185:265–267.
236. Winters, A. J., Eskay, R. L., and Porter, J. C. (1974): Concentration and distribution of TRH and LRH in the human fetal brain. *J. Clin. Endocrinol. Metab.*, 39:960–963.
237. Wurtman, R. J. (1971): Brain monoamines and endocrine function. *Neurosci. Res. Prog. Bull.*, 9:172–297.
238. Wurtman, R. J., and Fernstrom, J. D. (1972): L-Tryptophan, L-tyrosine and the control of brain monoamine biosynthesis. In: *Perspectives in Neuropharmacology*, edited by S. H. Snyder, pp. 143–193. Oxford Univ. Press, New York.
239. Wurtman, R. J., Larin, F., Mostafapour, S., and Fernstrom, J. D. (1974): Brain catechol synthesis: Control by brain tyrosine concentration. *Science*, 185:183–184.
240. Yarbrough, G. G. (1976): TRH potentiates excitatory actions of acetylcholine on cerebral cortical neurones. *Nature (Lond)*, 263:523–524.
241. Yasuhara, T., and Nakajima, T. (1975): Occurrence of Pyr-His-ProNH$_2$ in frog skin. *Chem. Pharm. Bull.*, 23:3301–3303.
242. Youngblood, W. W., Lipton, M. A., and Kizer, J. S. (1978): TRH-like immunoreactivity in urine, serum and extrahypothalamic brain: Non-identity with synthetic pyroglu-hist-proNH$_2$ (TRH). *Brain. Res.*, 151:99–116.

Central Nervous System Effects of Hypothalamic Hormones and Other Peptides, edited by Collu et al. Raven Press, New York © 1979.

Thyrotropin-Releasing Hormone in the Central Nervous System: Distribution and Degradation

Andrew Winokur and Robert D. Utiger

Departments of Psychiatry, Pharmacology, and Medicine, University of Pennsylvania School of Medicine, Philadelphia, Pennsylvania 19104

Thyrotropin-releasing hormone (TRH) was the first of the hypothalamic-releasing hormones to be isolated and to have its structure characterized (7,29). It soon became apparent, however, that TRH was capable of producing a number of effects on the central nervous system (CNS) that were independent of its hypophysiotropic actions (5,14,15,19,21,25,26). Such findings suggested that TRH was a constituent of extrahypothalamic brain tissue, and data reported from three different groups—Oliver et al. (23), Jackson and Reichlin (16), and Winokur and Utiger (30)—supported this hypothesis.

In our own studies, rat brains were dissected, according to a modification of the technique of Glowinski and Iversen, into six regions: hypothalamus, forebrain, brainstem, posterior diencephalon, posterior cortex, and cerebellum (8). Brain pieces were weighed; homogenized in 0.01 M phosphate, 0.15 M NaCl, pH 7.5; and then extracted in methanol prior to determination of TRH content by means of radioimmunoassay. The radioimmunoassay technique used was previously shown to be a sensitive and highly specific method for determining TRH content (2). Recovery of TRH added to neural tissue that was then homogenized and extracted as described above ranged from 89 to 104% in three separate experiments. The results of TRH assays of extracts from male rats are shown in Table 1. The highest content and concentration of immunoreactive TRH was found in the hypothalamus, but substantial quantities were detected in several other regions, including forebrain, brainstem, and posterior diencephalon.

Several studies were conducted to establish that extract immunoreactivity resembled TRH. The extracts from all regions of brain gave dose-response patterns indistinguishable from that produced by synthetic TRH (30). Incubation of extracts of several regions of brain with 1:5 diluted normal human serum for 60 min at 37°C resulted in loss of immunoreactivity comparable to that observed for extracts of hypothalamus and for synthetic TRH. Extract immunoreactivity and synthetic TRH appeared in the same fractions when the two materials were filtered on Sephadex G-25. Oliver et al. (23) found

TABLE 1. *Distribution of TRH in rat brain*

Region	Tissue weight (mg)	TRH		
		ng	ng/mg	% of total
Hypothalamus	32.6 ± 1.5	4.1 ± 0.2	0.129 ± 0.007	31.2
Forebrain	399.0 ± 8.9	3.5 ± 0.3	0.009 ± 0.001	25.6
Brainstem	185.0 ± 5.5	2.1 ± 0.1	0.012 ± 0.002	16.9
Posterior diencephalon	213.3 ± 8.7	1.9 ± 0.2	0.009 ± 0.005	13.8
Posterior cortex	622.8 ± 11.5	1.3 ± 0.1	0.002 ± 0.001	10.6
Cerebellum	244.0 ± 5.1	0.26 ± 0.03	0.001	2.1
Total		13.2 ± 0.4		

From ref. 12.
The brains were from 30 male rats.
Results given as mean ± SEM.

that extracts of brain regions incubated with rat pituitaries *in vitro* produced increases in TSH secretion similar to that observed with hypothalamic extracts. In addition, identical electrophoretic patterns were observed for the TRH in brain and hypothalamic extracts and synthetic TRH. Thus according to a number of physicochemical parameters, extrahypothalamic TRH is indistinguishable from hypothalamic and synthetic TRH. Despite these observations, occasional studies suggest that neural immunoreactive TRH is not in fact TRH (i.e., pyroglutamyl-histidyl-prolineamide) but rather another substance, presumably a peptide, with slightly different properties. Jeffcoate and White (17) reported that cerebral cortical immunoreactive TRH had dose-response characteristics that differed from those of synthetic TRH in their radioimmunoassay, and that the immunoreactive TRH in such extracts was chromatographically different from synthetic TRH. Kubek et al. (20) found less TRH biological activity in extracts of human brain than expected on the basis of extract TRH immunoreactivity. Resolution of these inconsistencies is not yet possible, but, as previously mentioned, in our studies no differences between extrahypothalamic TRH immunoreactivity and that of hypothalamic and synthetic TRH have been detected.

The distribution of immunoreactive TRH within discrete nuclei in the hypothalamus was examined by Brownstein et al. (6) by punching small pellets of tissue from frozen sections of brain under stereomicroscopic control. As expected, TRH was found in highest concentration in the median eminence but was also present in substantial concentrations in several hypothalamic nuclei, including the medial part of the ventromedial nucleus, the dorsomedial nucleus, the arcuate nucleus, the lateral part of the ventromedial nucleus, and the periventricular nucleus. Thus immunoreactive TRH is widely distributed within the hypothalamus and outside the hypothalamus in brain tissue.

The distribution of TRH in extrahypothalamic brain tissue of various other species was reported by Jackson and Reichlin (16). In addition, we examined the extrahypothalamic TRH content in brain regions from several species sent to us by Dr. R. E. Peter of the University of Alberta. Substantial amounts of extrahypothalamic TRH were observed in brains of all of the species examined, including the trout, chameleon, turtle, goldfish, toad, quail, and chipmunk. The pattern of distribution differed markedly from one species to another. In the goldfish and the trout, for example, the olfactory tubercle contained a higher concentration of TRH than did the hypothalamus.

Kubek et al. (20) examined TRH distribution in neural tissue obtained from human postmortem specimens. Although the hypothalamus contained the highest concentration, TRH immunoreactivity was identified throughout all areas of human brain, with the highest extrahypothalamic concentrations being found in mamillary body, amygdala, and inferior olivary nucleus. In limbic structures, amygdala and hippocampus contained relatively high concentrations as well.

With the demonstration that immunoreactive TRH was widely distributed throughout brain tissue in a number of animal species and in man, it was of interest to examine the possible localization of this peptide in spinal cord. Kardon et al. (18), in our laboratory, examined the content and distribution of immunoreactive TRH in the rat spinal cord. The mean TRH content of the entire spinal cord from 15 rats was 18.7 ± 0.7 ng (SEM), and the mean TRH concentration was 41.7 ± 1.7 pg/mg wet weight. There was little variation in TRH concentration throughout the length of the cord. The distribution of TRH within a transverse cross-section of spinal cord was studied by pooling plugs of tissue from multiple cross-sections. Figure 1 illustrates a transverse section of spinal cord containing representations of the regions from which plugs were removed. As shown in Table 2, no TRH was detected in any white matter region, a low concentration was identified in posterior horn (0.30 ± 0.02 pg/μg protein), and high concentrations in anterior horn (1.01 ± 0.15 pg/μg) and central canal (0.96 ± 0.10 pg/μg) samples. Nicoll (22) reported that application of TRH (10^{-4} M) by microiontophoresis to

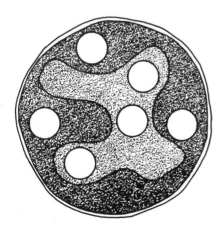

FIG. 1. Transverse section of rat spinal cord indicating regions from which tissue plugs were removed for TRH determination. Sections of thoracic spinal cord 1 to 2 cm long were removed, set in embedding medium (O.C.T. compound, Lab-Tek Products), and frozen on Dry Ice. Each piece was mounted in a cryostat at $-10°$C, and 24 or 25 transverse sections, 300 μm thick, were cut. Plugs of tissue were removed under a dissecting microscope with a needle of 240 μm inside diameter. (From ref. 18.)

TABLE 2. *Distribution of TRH in rat spinal cord*

Region	No. of samples	TRH (pg/μg protein)
Anterior horn	6	1.01 ± 0.15
Central canal	7	0.96 ± 0.10
Posterior horn	6	0.30 ± 0.02
Anterior funiculus	6	<0.30
Posterior funiculus	6	<0.33
Lateral funiculus	10	<0.25
Whole spinal cord		0.39 ± 0.06

From ref. 18.
Results given as mean $\pm$ SEM.

an *in vitro* frog spinal cord preparation produces excitatory postsynaptic potentials. Further studies are needed to determine the physiological role of TRH in spinal cord function.

Several studies demonstrated a widespread distribution of TRH throughout the CNS. These studies do not, however, provide information about the discrete localization of TRH pathways. To our knowledge, only one group, Hökfelt et al. (12,13), reported successful development of an immunohistochemical technique for TRH. Using the indirect immunofluorescence technique, they reported TRH-positive fibers in varicose enlargements which probably represented nerve terminals. Staining was most highly concentrated in the median eminence, particularly in the medial part of the external layer. High densities of TRH-positive fibers were observed in other areas of the hypothalamus, including the dorsomedial hypothalamic nucleus, the perifornical region, and the parvocellular part of the paraventricular nucleus. TRH-positive fibers were also observed in other regions of the CNS, including the organum vasculosum, the nucleus accumbens, in many brainstem nuclei, and in the spinal cord, particularly in the ventral horn and central canal regions. The localization of TRH by immunofluorescence techniques corresponds reasonably well to data derived from regional radioimmunological studies. More extensive studies utilizing immunocytochemical techniques are needed to delineate the pathways of TRH-containing neurons, to explore *in situ* localization at the ultrastructural level, and to examine interconnections with other neurotransmitter systems.

Localization of immunoreactive TRH in neural tissue has also been examined by means of subcellular distribution techniques (1,31). Differential centrifugation and density gradient separation were carried out with hypothalamic and extrahypothalamic preparations of rat brain tissue, and the TRH content determined by radioimmunoassay. As shown in Table 3, the patterns of subcellular distribution for TRH were similar for hypothalamic and extrahypothalamic brain tissue. In both cases the synaptosomal fraction contained the highest concentration of TRH. In other studies the crude mito-

TABLE 3. *Subcellular distribution of TRH in rat brain and hypothalamic tissue*

Fraction	Brain TRH[a]		Hypothalamus TRH[b]	
	ng	ng/mg protein	ng	ng/mg protein
Homogenate	89.5 ± 4.8	0.09 ± 0.02	250.2 ± 14.6	2.52 ± 0.41
Nuclear fraction	9.7 ± 0.7	0.06 ± 0.02	37.8 ± 4.5	1.41 ± 0.17
Crude mitochondrial fraction	35.6 ± 3.7	0.14 ± 0.03	86.5 ± 5.7	3.28 ± 0.87
Cytosol microsome fraction	18.8 ± 0.7	0.09 ± 0.01	48.6 ± 6.4	1.43 ± 0.21
Myelin	2.2 ± 0.3	0.05 ± 0.01	4.3 ± 1.1	2.02 ± 0.74
Synaptosomes	11.1 ± 1.5	0.31 ± 0.01	13.7 ± 0.8	7.99 ± 0.58
Mitochondria	6.4 ± 1.6	0.18 ± 0.01	15.7 ± 5.7	4.07 ± 0.95

From ref. 23.

[a] Mean ± SEM of three experiments, each of which utilized brain tissue from five rats.

[b] Mean ± SEM of four experiments, each of which utilized hypothalamic tissue from 28 rats.

chondrial fraction of brain tissue was exposed to osmotic shock, and the resultant supernatant subjected to differential centrifugation. The 96,000 × *g* precipitate (the fraction enriched in synaptic vesicles) contained the highest concentration of TRH, 2.4 times that of the initial tissue homogenate (Fig. 2). These findings indicate that TRH is highly concentrated in the nerve terminal region of neural tissue and contained in synaptic vesicles therein.

With the demonstration that TRH immunoreactivity is widely distributed throughout brain, it has been of interest to examine the inactivating activity of neural tissue. Inactivation of TRH by serum and plasma has been reported

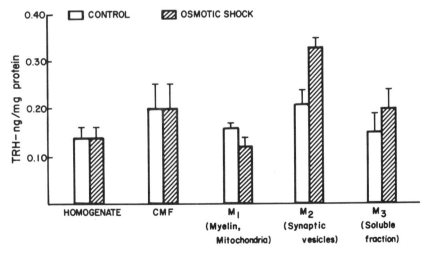

FIG. 2. TRH concentration in various subcellular fractions isolated after osmotic shock of rat brain crude mitochondrial fraction. Results are the mean ± SEM of five experiments. In the control experiments the CMF pellet was resuspended in 0.32 M sucrose rather than water. Both suspensions were then processed in an identical manner. (From ref. 23.)

by several investigators. Destruction of TRH by brain tissue was initially reported by Redding and Schally in 1969 (28). Bassiri and Utiger (3) observed that both hypothalamic and brain extracts exhibited TRH-inactivating activity. Griffiths and co-workers (9–11) demonstrated TRH-inactivating activity in hypothalamic homogenates in the rat, and in hypothalamus, thalamus, cerebral cortex, and cerebellum in the rabbit. A limited number of studies examining the mechanisms underlying TRH inactivation have been conducted. Bauer and Lipman (4) found that incubation of ^{3}H-TRH with a high-speed supernatant of freeze-dried porcine hypothalamic tissue resulted in the formation of deamido-TRH as the main degradation product. After incubation of ^{3}H-TRH proline with a high-speed supernatant fraction prepared from fresh rat hypothalamic tissue, only deamidation was found, whereas incubation with whole homogenates produced proline and prolineamide as degradation products. Prasad and Peterkofsky (27) also reported evidence of two mechanisms of TRH inactivation. The $27,000 \times g$ supernatant from hamster hypothalamic extracts were subjected to Sephadex G-100 chromatography. Two separate peaks of inactivating activity were identified, with peak 1 producing deamidation of TRH and the second peak producing pyroglutamic acid and His-Pro-NH$_2$.

These studies indicate that TRH inactivation by neural tissue is indeed a complex process which appears to involve more than one metabolic pathway. Furthermore, comparison of reports of inactivation of TRH by brain tissue and blood suggests differences in metabolism produced by the two tissues. This suggestion is further supported by the report of Oliver et al. (24) that the ontogenic development of TRH-degrading activity in rat serum and brain tissue can be clearly differentiated.

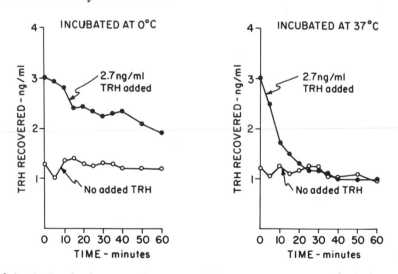

FIG. 3. Inactivation of endogenous and exogenous TRH by brain homogenates at 0°C *(left)* and 37°C *(right)*. Aliquots of a single brain homogenate without or with added TRH were incubated; aliquots were removed and immediately extracted with methanol at the times indicated. (From ref. 23.)

We studied TRH inactivation by brain tissue homogenates using a different approach. Whole brain tissue homogenates were maintained at 0°C or were incubated at 37°C for 60 min (31). At frequent intervals, aliquots were obtained and the immunoreactive TRH content determined. No disappearance of endogenous TRH immunoreactivity was observed in homogenates at 0°C or 37°C (Fig. 3). In other experiments, synthetic TRH (2.7 ng/ml) was added to the homogenate samples and incubation carried out as described above. In samples maintained at 0°C, a moderate reduction of TRH immunoreactivity was observed over 60 min. With incubation at 37°C, a marked reduction in TRH levels was observed, declining to the endogenous TRH content within 30 min. The added TRH was not labeled, so the identification of the pool of TRH being inactivated could not be determined. It seems likely, nevertheless, that the exogenous TRH pool was the one being inactivated during the incubation. In other studies, larger concentrations of synthetic TRH were added, to a 50-fold increase over endogenous levels. In all cases, a reduction to endogenous TRH levels was observed within 30 min (Fig. 4). These data suggested that endogenous TRH is stored or compartmentalized in such a manner as to be protected from degradation. Yet brain tissue contains large amounts of inactivating activity, such that an amount of exogenous TRH equivalent to a 50-fold increase over endogenous levels was rapidly and completely inactivated. This is further evidence that TRH is stored in synaptic vesicles wherein it is protected from degradation.

During the past 5 years a substantial amount of work has documented a wide distribution of immunoreactive TRH throughout the CNS and a capacity of neural tissue to inactivate this peptide. Numerous studies conducted

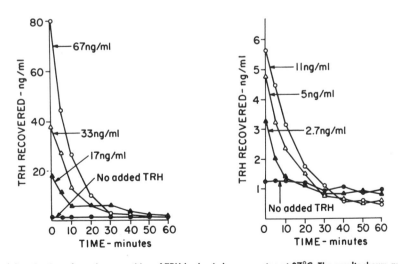

FIG. 4. Inactivation of varying quantities of TRH by brain homogenates at 37°C. The results shown are the means of three experiments in which aliquots of brain homogenates without or with added TRH were incubated and aliquots removed and immediately extracted with methanol at the times indicated. (From ref. 23.)

during the same time period have demonstrated that TRH produces a variety of physiological and behavioral effects in animals and humans. It will be a considerable challenge to integrate the data from studies of TRH localization with those demonstrating the pharmacological effects to arrive at an understanding of the physiological function(s) of TRH within the CNS.

ACKNOWLEDGMENTS

Supported by NIMH Research Scientist Development Award MH00044 (to A. W.) and by USPHS grant AM14039. The authors acknowledge the expert technical assistance of Miss Kathleen Kelley and the skilled secretarial help of Mrs. Elaine Paolini.

REFERENCES

1. Barnea, A., Ben-Jonathan, N., Colston, C., Johnston, J. M., and Porter, J. C. (1975): Differential sub-cellular compartmentalization of thyrotropin releasing hormone (TRH) and gonadotropin releasing hormone (LRH) in hypothalamic tissue. *Proc. Natl. Acad. Sci. USA,* 8:3153–3157.
2. Bassiri, R. M., and Utiger, R. D. (1972): The preparation and specificity of antibody to thyrotropin releasing hormone. *Endocrinology,* 90:722–727.
3. Bassiri, R. M., and Utiger, R. D. (1974): Thyrotropin-releasing hormone in the hypothalamus of the rat. *Endocrinology,* 94:188–197.
4. Bauer, K., and Lipmann, T. (1976): Attempts toward biosynthesis of the thyrotropin-releasing hormone and studies on its breakdown in hypothalamic tissue preparations. *Endocrinology,* 99:230–242.
5. Breese, G. R., Cott, J. M., Cooper, B. R., Prange, A. J., Jr., and Lipton, M. S. (1974): Antagonism of ethanol narcosis by thyrotropin releasing hormone. *Life Sci.,* 14:1053–1063.
6. Brownstein, M. J., Parkovits, M., Saavedra, J. M., Bassiri, R. M., and Utiger, R. D. (1974): Thyrotropin releasing hormone in specific nuclei of rat brain. *Science,* 185:269.
7. Burgus, R., Dunn, T. E., Desiderio, D., Ward, D. N., Vale, W., and Guillemin, R. (1970): Characterization of ovine hypothalamic hypophysiotropic TRH-releasing factor. *Nature (Lond),* 226:321–325.
8. Glowinski, J., and Iversen, L. L. (1966): Regional studies of catecholamines in the rat brain. *J. Neurochem.,* 13:655–669.
9. Griffiths, E. C., and Hooper, K. C. (1974): Peptidase activity in different areas of the rat hypothalamus. *Acta Endocrinol. (Kbh),* 77:10–18.
10. Griffiths, E. C., Hooper, K. C., Hutson, D., Jeffcoate, S. L., and White, N. (1976): Hypothalamic inactivation of thyrotropin-releasing hormone. *Mol. Cell Endocrinol.,* 4:215–222.
11. Griffiths, E. C., Hooper, K. C., Jeffcoate, S. L., and White, N. (1976): Inactivation of thyrotropin releasing hormone (TRH) by peptidases in different areas of the rabbit brain. *Brain Res.,* 105:376–380.
12. Hökfelt, T., Fuxe, K., Johansson, O., Jeffcoate, S., and White, N. (1975): Distribution of thyrotropin-releasing hormone (TRH) in the central nervous system as revealed with immunohistochemistry. *Eur. J. Pharmacol.,* 34:389–392.
13. Hökfelt, T., Fuxe, K., Johansson, O., Jeffcoate, S., and White, N. (1975): Thyrotropin releasing hormone (TRH)-containing nerve terminals in certain brain stem nuclei and in the spinal cord. *Neurosci. Lett.,* 1:133–139.
14. Horita, A., and Corino, M. A. (1975): Thyrotropin-releasing hormone (TRH)-induced hyperthermia and behavioral excitation in rabbits. *Psychopharmacol. Publ.,* 1:403–414.

15. Itil, T. M., Patterson, L. D., Polvan, N., Bigelow, A., and Bergen, B. (1975): Clinical and CNS effects of oral and i.v. thyrotropin releasing hormone in depressed patients. *Dis. Nerv. Syst.*, 36:529–536.
16. Jackson, I., and Reichlin, S. (1974): Thyrotropin-releasing hormone (TRH): Distribution in hypothalamic and extrahypothalamic brain tissues of mammalian and submammalian chordates. *Endocrinology*, 95:854–862.
17. Jeffcoate, S. L., and White, N. (1975): Is there any thyrotropin releasing hormone in mammalian extra-hypothalamic brain tissue? *J. Endocrinol.*, 67:42P.
18. Kardon, F. C., Winokur, A., and Utiger, R. D. (1977): Thyrotropin releasing hormone (TRH) in rat spinal cord. *Brain Res.*, 122:578–581.
19. Kruse, H. (1975): Thyrotropin releasing hormone: Interaction with chlorpromazine in mice, rats and rabbits. *J. Pharmacol.*, 6:249–268.
20. Kubek, M. J., Lorincz, M. A., and Wilber, J. F. (1977): The identification of thyrotropin releasing hormone (TRH) in hypothalamic and extrahypothalamic loci of the human nervous system. *Brain Res.*, 126:196–200.
21. Metcalf, G. (1974): TRH: A possible mediator of thermoregulation. *Nature (Lond)*, 252:310–311.
22. Nicoll, R. A. (1977): Excitatory action of TRH on spinal motor neurons. *Nature (Lond)*, 265:242–243.
23. Oliver, C., Eskay, R. L., Ben-Jonathan, N., Porter, J. C. (1974): Distribution and concentration of TRH in the rat brain. *Endocrinology*, 96:540–546.
24. Oliver, C., Parker, C. R., Jr., and Porter, J. C. (1977): Developmental changes in the degradation of thyrotropin releasing hormone by serum and brain tissues of the male rat. *J. Endocrinol.*, 74:339–340.
25. Plotnikoff, N. P., Prange, A. J., Jr., Breese, G. R., Anderson, M. S., and Wilson, I. C. (1972): Thyrotropin-releasing hormone: Enhancement of DOPA activity by a hypothalamic hormone. *Science*, 178:417–418.
26. Prange, A. J., Jr., Breese, G. R., Cott, J. M., Martin, B. R., Cooper, B. R., Wilson, I. C., and Plotnikoff, N. P. (1974): Thyrotropin-releasing hormone: Antagonism of pentobarbital in rodents. *Life Sci.*, 14:447–455.
27. Prasad, C., and Peterkofsky, A. (1976): Demonstration of pyroglutamylpeptidase and amidase activities toward thyrotropin-releasing hormone in hamster hypothalamus extracts. *J. Biol. Chem.*, 251:3229–3234.
28. Redding, T. W., and Schally, A. V. (1969): Studies on the inactivation of thyrotropin-releasing hormone (TRH). *Proc. Soc. Exp. Biol. Med.*, 131:415–420.
29. Schally, A. V., Redding, T. W., Bowers, C. Y., and Barrett, J. F. (1969): Isolation and properties of porcine thyrotropin-releasing hormone. *J. Biol. Chem.*, 244:4077–4088.
30. Winokur, A., and Utiger, R. D. (1974): Thyrotropin-releasing hormone: Regional distribution in rat brain. *Science*, 185:265–267.
31. Winokur, A., Davis, R., and Utiger, R. D. (1977): Subcellular distribution of thyrotropin-releasing hormone (TRH) in rat brain and hypothalamus. *Brain Res.*. 120:423–434.

Central Nervous System Effects of Hypothalamic Hormones and Other Peptides, edited by Collu et al. Raven Press, New York © 1979.

Behavioral and Autonomic Effects of TRH in Animals

A. Horita, M. A. Carino, H. Lai, and T. R. LaHann

Department of Pharmacology, School of Medicine, University of Washington, Seattle, Washington 98195

Two important discoveries stimulated current interest in the neuropsychopharmacology of thyrotropin-releasing hormone (TRH): (a) in man and animals TRH exerts effects independent of its hypophysiotropic function (3,4,8,20,23–25); and (b) TRH is present in brain areas other than those associated with the neuroendocrine area of the hypothalamus (6,34). Aside from its neuroendocrine function, the physiological role(s) of TRH has yet to be determined. Because of its broad distribution in brain and spinal cord and its potent neuropsychopharmacologic activity, however, its possible functions can be reasonably speculated on.

Most of the experimental pharmacology of TRH has been carried out in rats and mice (3–5,7,9,23,24,27,32). In our laboratory we found the rabbit, in spite of its larger size, to be an extremely useful and sensitive model for studying the central actions of TRH (1,8,14–16,18,19). In the course of our investigation of the behavioral effects of TRH, we discovered its centrally mediated gastrointestinal and cardiovascular effects as well. In this chapter we will report these aspects of our work in the rabbit.

BEHAVIORAL EFFECTS OF TRH

The behavioral effects of TRH intracerebroventricularly (i.c.v.) injected in conscious rabbits were described previously (14,15). Briefly, tachypnea and slight hyperthermia are produced by low doses (0.1 to 5.0 μg), and marked behavioral excitation, increased locomotor activity, a compulsive scratching behavior, severe hyperthermia, and sympathetic stimulation by high doses (50 to 100 μg). The effects resemble those produced by *d*-amphetamine (26). Unlike the behavioral effects of amphetamine, however, those of TRH in conscious rabbits exhibited unusual resistance to blockade by various catecholamine antagonists and depleting agents (19). The most consistent and potent antagonist of TRH-induced excitation that we found thus far is morphine. The increase in respiratory rate and colonic temperature produced by TRH is partially attenuated by morphine, but the behavioral excitation is totally abolished. In animals pretreated with morphine, TRH, even in high doses, was ineffective in reversing the sedative and analgesic actions of the

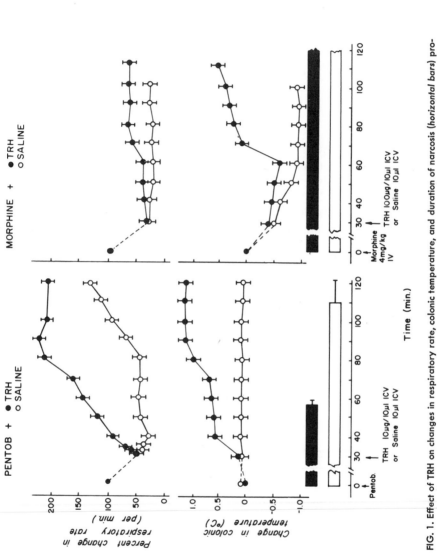

FIG. 1. Effect of TRH on changes in respiratory rate, colonic temperature, and duration of narcosis (horizontal bars) produced by pentobarbital (25 mg/kg i.v.) and morphine (4 mg/kg i.v.) in rabbits. The TRH dose was 10 μg (i.c.v.) in pentobarbital-pretreated animals and 100 μg in morphine-pretreated animals. Each line or bar represents mean responses in at least five animals. Variations are expressed as SEM.

narcotic. Figure 1 illustrates the effects of TRH on the hypothermia, respiratory depression, and narcosis produced by pentobarbital and morphine.

Perhaps the property of TRH that most dramatically affects behavior is its ability to reverse or prevent anesthesia from barbiturates or other depressants. In our studies microgram quantities of TRH administered i.c.v. to rabbits anesthetized with pentobarbital sodium markedly shortened the recovery time of the righting reflex. Doses as low as 0.1 μg i.c.v. exerted this effect, and larger doses shortened the duration of barbiturate anesthesia even more markedly (15). In other studies we compared the effects of TRH on behavior, electroencephalography (EEG) patterns, and respiratory and heart rates in conscious and barbiturate-anesthetized rabbits (1). TRH significantly altered all physiological indices except heart rate in both groups of animals, but no temporal correlations could be established among the altered responses, so that none of these changes was a consequence of a single effect of TRH. That is, a particular behavioral level was not strictly associated with specific EEG patterns, nor were respiratory changes associated with either EEG or behavioral effects of TRH.

Attempts have been made to elucidate the mechanisms of the analeptic effect of TRH. The role of cholinergic mechanisms has now been confirmed by several laboratories; atropine and scopolamine completely block the analeptic effect of TRH (4,16), and the barbiturate-induced decrease in cholinergic neuron function in several regions of the rat brain can be prevented by TRH (29). Because of the similarity between the analeptic effects of TRH and those of *d*-amphetamine in pentobarbital-anesthetized rabbits, we decided to determine whether the amphetamine-induced effect can be

TABLE 1. *Effect of atropine and methylatropine on the analeptic action of TRH and amphetamine in pentobarbital-anesthetized rabbits*

Exp.	Drug treatment			No.	Duration of anesthesia (min ± SEM)
	A	B	C		
1	—	Pentobarbital	Saline	10	110 ± 10
2	—	Pentobarbital	TRH (100 μg)	7	40 ± 3[a]
3	—	Pentobarbital	Amphetamine (0.5 mg/kg)	7	53 ± 4[a]
4	Atropine	Pentobarbital	Saline	8	111 ± 4
5	Atropine	Pentobarbital	TRH (100 μg)	5	119 ± 9[b]
6	Atropine	Pentobarbital	Amphetamine (0.5 mg/kg)	5	104 ± 11[c]
7	Methylatropine	Pentobarbital	TRH (100 μg)	4	46 ± 7[a]
8	Methylatropine	Pentobarbital	Amphetamine (0.5 mg/kg)	4	55 ± 6[a]

All animals received pentobarbital sodium 25 mg/kg i.v. The dose of atropine and methylatropine was 2.5 mg/kg i.v. Drug B was administered 30 min after A, and C 30 min after B. TRH was administered by i.c.v. injection, amphetamine by i.v. injection. Duration of anesthesia represents total time of loss of righting reflex after pentobarbital administration.

[a] $p < 0.001$ when compared with Exp. 1.

[b] $p < 0.001$ when compared with Exp. 2.

[c] $p < 0.001$ when compared with Exp. 3.

antagonized as well by anticholinergic agents. We found (Table 1) that atropine was effective in blocking the arousal of pentobarbital-anesthetized rabbits by amphetamine as well as by TRH. It is apparent that these analeptics act via cholinergic mediation. However, the excitatory effects of both drugs in conscious rabbits were not attenuated by anticholinergic agents.

The presence of a cholinergic component in the actions of amphetamine was first suggested by White and Daigneault (33) when they found that atropine blocked the EEG changes produced by amphetamine in the rabbit. More direct evidence of acetylcholine (ACh) release was provided by Deffenu et al. (11), who found increases in ACh output from the cerebral cortex after amphetamine administration. This increased output appeared to be mediated via catecholamines released from adrenergic nerve endings, since it was abolished by α-methyl-p-tyrosine (22). Schmidt (28), employing the head-focused microwave method of sacrificing rats and a pyrolysis gas-liquid chromatographic method of ACh assay, demonstrated increases in ACh turnover in rat brain cortex and hippocampus and decreases in turnover in striatum and cerebellum. Our present findings of a cholinergically mediated arousal effect of amphetamine represents behavioral evidence of ACh release produced by amphetamine. Amphetamine and TRH therefore appear to exert their analeptic effects via several transmitter systems, one of which is cholinergic.

Unlike the behavioral effects of TRH in conscious animals, the analeptic effect is sensitive to various pharmacological interventions. In addition to blockade by centrally acting anticholinergics as described above, we found attenuation or abolition of the effect by catecholamine antagonists and depletors, e.g., phenoxybenzamine, 6-hydroxydopamine (i.c.v.), and α-methyl-p-tyrosine (19). Some of these interactions may differ with species, since Cott et al. (9) found no blockade of the analeptic effect in mice. Other antagonists include GABA-mimetic agents (10) and naloxone (Horita and Carino, *unpublished results*). This opiate antagonist is especially noteworthy since it also acts as an antibarbiturate agent by itself (12,13). In rabbits we found that low doses of naloxone (1 to 2 mg/kg i.v.) blocked TRH- and amphetamine-induced arousal from barbiturate anesthesia, but higher doses (5 to 15 mg/kg) reduced the duration of anesthesia. As with atropine, the antagonism of the analeptic effect of TRH by naloxone was evident only in anesthetized animals. No blockade of the behavioral excitation or hyperthermia was demonstrable in conscious animals. The naloxone effect, however, was not produced by an atropine-like antimuscarinic action since naloxone did not affect the central effects of oxotremorine. Also, although our data are still incomplete, they suggest that the naloxone effect is not a result of opiate receptor blockade.

The various TRH-drug interaction studies have revealed several points very clearly. First, the behavioral excitation produced by TRH in conscious animals is not necessarily associated with the analeptic or arousal response seen in barbiturate-anesthetized animals. Atropine and naloxone abolish the analeptic effect of TRH in anesthetized animals, but they do not block, and may even potentiate, the excitatory actions of TRH. Secondly, the analeptic phenomenon is demonstrable with very small doses (0.1 to 1.0 μg), whereas behavioral excitation requires 25 to 50 μg TRH i.c.v. Finally, the reversal of the sedative effects (*not the anesthetic effect*) of many of the central nervous system depressants, as described earlier (14), is probably a function of the excitatory effects of the large doses of TRH employed, rather than on the specific cholinergic arousal property of TRH.

GASTROINTESTINAL EFFECT OF CENTRALLY ADMINISTERED TRH

In our experiments on the analeptic effects of TRH, the animals were placed on their backs so we could observe the recovery of the righting reflex. After administration of TRH, but not saline, i.c.v., we consistently observed that prior to the righting response the abdominal regions of the animals exhibited marked vermiform movements as if increased gastrointestinal (GI) motor activity were taking place. The later appearance of diarrhea supported this assumption. After surgically exposing the GI area of anesthetized rabbits, we confirmed visually the markedly increased activity of the intestinal tract. Various methods of measuring GI activity were then explored. Initially the "open-tip" method was tried, in which small amounts of saline are infused through a cannula inserted into the intestinal tract with the opposite end connected to a pressure transducer. Employing this method we were able to demonstrate the increased intestinal motor activity from centrally, but not intravenously, administered TRH (31). However, we felt that this method of measurement had several disadvantages, the most important being the need for surgical intervention of the enteric tract. After considerable experimentation we found it best to use the miniaturized extraluminal strain gauges sewn onto the exterior wall of the intestinal tract. The output of these strain gauges was in turn fed into a Grass model 7 polygraph. In this way it was possible to measure both longitudinal and circular muscle contractions in any part of the GI tract (21).

Although most of the GI tract exhibited increased motor activity with i.c.v. TRH administration, we selected an area of the proximal colon for our studies because of its consistency in response and sensitivity to TRH. A typical tracing of the TRH-induced increase in colonic activity is shown in Fig. 2. The exquisite sensitivity of these extraluminal strain gauges has permitted us to detect the GI effects of TRH with doses as low as 0.5 μg i.c.v. Under these conditions the TRH-induced responses displayed neither dose-response nor time-effect relationships. Doses of 0.5 to 100 μg i.c.v. produced responses of similar magnitudes and durations, the latter ranging from 60 to 90 min. Atropine (both i.c.v. and i.v.) and ganglionic blockers

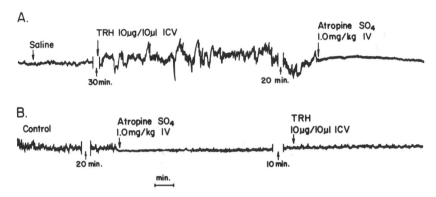

FIG. 2. Effect of i.c.v. injection of 10 μg TRH on proximal colonic contractions and its antagonism by atropine in intact rabbits anesthetized with pentobarbital.

markedly attenuated or completely blocked (whereas bilateral vagotomy always blocked) the GI responses to TRH. These findings indicate the involvement of cholinergic vagal mediation in the response.

However, even in the presence of atropine, movements of the abdominal wall were still visible in a number of animals, and diarrhea persisted. Contractility ceased (evident from the absence of transducer activity), but propulsion appeared to be present in other areas of the intestine. To determine whether such might be the case, we measured propulsive activity of the large intestine by introducing ^{51}Cr into the proximal colon and following its rate of movement in control, atropine-pretreated, and vagal-sectioned animals. The preliminary results indicate that i.c.v. administered TRH produced increased propulsive activity in the colon in both control and atropine-pretreated animals, but not in vagotomized animals. Thus it appears that TRH increases both colonic motor activity and propulsive activity; the latter may not involve a classic muscarinic cholinergic mechanism.

VASOPRESSOR EFFECT OF CENTRALLY ADMINISTERED TRH

In addition to its behavioral and GI effects, we also found a centrally mediated vasopressor response to i.c.v. (but not i.v.) administered TRH (17). Doses of 10 to 100 μg administered i.c.v. produced a response with slow onset and a long-lasting (15 to 30 min) course (Fig. 3A). In many instances Mayers wave-like fluctuations of blood pressure appeared and persisted throughout the response. Tachyphylaxis was evident after repeated administration of TRH, but most or all of the original response was restored when the second injection was made at least 3 to 4 hr after the first.

We analyzed the nature of the pressor response by employing a number of pharmacologic antagonists and depleting agents, including α- and β-adrenergic blockers, ganglionic blockers, anticholinergic agents, reserpine

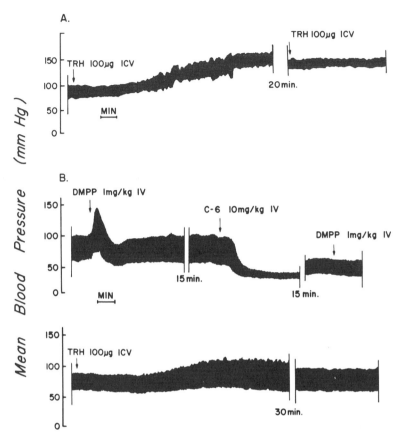

FIG. 3. Effect of i.c.v. injections of 100 μg TRH on arterial blood pressure in a (A) control and (B) hexamethonium-pretreated rabbit anesthetized with pentobarbital.

and guanethidine, and clonidine, among others. Control injections of appropriate doses of epinephrine, norepinephrine, and DMPP were employed to ensure that adequate blockade was produced by the antagonists. To our surprise none of the antagonist pretreatments prevented the TRH-induced pressor response. Doses of phenoxybenzamine sufficient to block norepinephrine totally or reverse the epinephrine pressor response reduced but did not abolish the response. Similarly, pretreatment of animals wth reserpine (5 mg/kg i.v.) 18 hr prior to TRH administration was sufficient to abolish totally the pressor responses to DMPP (1 mg/kg) but not of centrally administered TRH. Ganglionic blockade with hexamethonium, which was sufficient to block DMPP, also proved ineffective against TRH (Fig. 3B).

We also investigated the effect of spinal transections on the pressor response. It was totally blocked by transections at the C_{1-8} levels, but not at the T_{1-2} or lower segments.

The results to date indicate that centrally administered TRH exerts a centrally mediated pressor response. The response is not affected by the classic sympathetic system antagonists; therefore mechanisms other than those requiring an intact sympathetic nervous system appear to be involved. A similar pressor response to TRH was reported by Beale et al. (2) to be incapable of blockade by chlorpromazine. In its nonsympathetic nature, the pressor response to TRH resembles in some ways the response produced by electrical stimulation of the medial reticular formation in anesthetized cats (30). These authors found that this blood pressure response was also not antagonized by phenoxybenzamine, hexamethonium, or methylscopolamine. Unlike the TRH-induced pressor response, however, it was not abolished by spinal transection at C_1 but was abolished by subsequent cutting of C_{5-8}. Taking these and other experimental results into consideration, the investigators concluded that the pressor response to stimulation of the reticular formation was mediated via release of vasopressin from the neurohypophysis. However, these conclusions must still be considered speculative since neither direct measurements of plasma vasopressin nor experiments in hypophysectomized animals were conducted.

CONCLUSIONS

The i.c.v. administration of TRH in conscious and anesthetized rabbits produced interesting and provocative behavioral, gastrointestinal, and vasopressor effects. These effects represent only the tip of the iceberg, since attempts to delineate their mechanisms have revealed that they are complex and may involve not only known neural systems but also systems not usually associated with drug-induced behavioral and physiological actions. Thus although the analeptic effect of TRH, like that of amphetamine, is blocked by anticholinergics, the behavioral excitation is not antagonized by the usual antagonists of amphetamine. Similarly, although vagally mediated, only a part of the gastrointestinal effects of TRH is antagonized by anticholinergic drugs. Finally, the vasopressor response to i.c.v. administered TRH is not blocked by α-adrenergic blockers, ganglionic blockers, or catecholamine-depleting agents, so that the response is nonsympathetic in nature. All of these phenomena require that the answers be sought outside of classic autonomic and neuropharmacology; perhaps they represent the beginnings of a new and fascinating pharmacology of the neuropeptides.

ACKNOWLEDGMENTS

The work described in this chapter was supported by USPHS grants HL-15426 and MH-29503 and a grant from the Washington State Heart Association. TRH was generously supplied by Abbott Laboratories. We wish to acknowledge the valuable assistance of Tina Alma Jose and Karen Larson in these studies.

REFERENCES

1. Andry, D. K., and Horita, A. (1977): Thyrotropin-releasing hormone: Physiological concomitants of behavioral excitation. *Pharmacol. Biochem. Behav.*, 6:58–59.
2. Beale, J. S., White, R. P., and Huang, S. P. (1977): EEG and blood pressure effects of TRH in rabbits. *Neuropharmacology*, 16:499–506.
3. Breese, G. R., Cooper, B. R., Prange, A. J., Cott, J. M., and Lipton, M. A. (1974): Interactions of thyrotropin-releasing hormone with centrally acting drugs. In: *The Thyroid Axis, Drugs, and Behavior*, edited by A J. Prange, pp. 115–127. Raven Press, New York.
4. Breese, G. R., Cott, J. M., Cooper, B. R., Prange, A. J., Lipton, M. A., and Plotnikoff, N. P. (1975): Effects of thyrotropin-releasing hormone (TRH) on the actions of pentobarbital and other centrally acting drugs. *J. Pharmacol. Exp. Ther.*, 193:11–22.
5. Brown, M., and Vale, W. (1975): Central nervous system effects of hypothalamic peptides. *Endocrinology*, 96:1333–1336.
6. Brownstein, M. J., Palkovits, M., Saavedra, J. M., Bassiri, R. M., and Utiger, R. D. (1974): Thyrotropin-releasing hormone in specific nuclei of rat brain. *Science*, 185:267–269.
7. Burt, D. R., and Snyder, S. H. (1975): Thyrotropin releasing hormone (TRH): Apparent receptor binding in rat brain membranes. *Brain Res.*, 93:309–328.
8. Carino, M. A., Smith, J. R., Weick, B. G., and Horita, A. (1976): Effects of thyrotropin-releasing hormone (TRH) microinjected into various brain areas of conscious and pentobarbital pretreated rabbits. *Life Sci.*, 19:1687–1692.
9. Cott, J. M., Breese, G. R., Cooper, B. R., Barlow, T. S., and Prange, A. J. (1976): Investigations into the mechanism of reduction of ethanol sleep by thyrotropin-releasing hormone (TRH). *J. Pharmacol. Exp. Ther.*, 196:594–604.
10. Cott, J., and Engel, J. (1977): Antagonism of the analeptic activity of thyrotropin releasing hormone (TRH) by agents which enhance GABA transmission. *Psychopharmacology*, 52:145–149.
11. Deffenu, G., Bartolini, A., and Pepeu, G. (1970): Effect of amphetamine on cholinergic systems of the cerebral cortex of the cat. In: *Amphetamines and Related Compounds*, edited by E. Costa and S. Garattini, pp. 357–368. Raven Press, New York.
12. Fürst, Z., Foldes, F. F., and Knoll, J. (1977): The influence of naloxone on barbiturate anesthesia and toxicity in the rat. *Life Sci.*, 20:921–926.
13. Gilbert, P. E., and Martin, W. R. (1977): Antagonism of the effects of pentobarbital in the chronic spinal dog by naltrexone. *Life Sci.*, 20:1401–1406.
14. Horita, A., and Carino, M. A. (1975): Thyrotropin-releasing hormone (TRH)-induced hyperthermia and behavioral excitation in rabbits. *Psychopharmacol. Commun.*, 1:403–414.
15. Horita, A., Carino, M. A., and Chesnut, R. M. (1976): Influence of TRH on drug-induced narcosis and hyperthermia in the rabbit. *Psychopharmacology*, 49:57–62.
16. Horita, A., Carino, M. A., and Smith, J. R. (1976): Effects of TRH on the central nervous system of the rabbit. *Pharmacol. Biochem. Behav. (Suppl. 1)*, 5:111–116.
17. Horita, A., and Carino, M. A. (1977): Centrally administered TRH produces a vasopressor response in rabbits. *Proc. West. Pharmacol. Soc.*, 20:303–304.
18. Horita, A., and Carino, M. A. (1977): Thyrotropin-releasing hormone-induced hyperthermia and arousal in the rabbit. In: *Drugs, Biogenic Amines and Body Temperature, 3rd Symposium on the Pharmacology of Thermoregulation*, edited by K. D. Cooper, P. Lomax, and E. Schönbaum, pp. 66–74. Karger, Basel.
19. Horita, A., Carino, M. A., and Lai, H. (1977): Influence of catecholamine antagonists and depletors on the CNS effects of TRH in rabbits. *Prog. Neuropsychopharmacol.*, 1:107–113.
20. Kastin, A. J., Ehrensing, R. H., Schlach, D. S., and Anderson, M. S. (1972): Im-

provement in mental depression with decreased thyrotropin response after administration of thyrotropin-releasing hormone. *Lancet,* 2:740–742.

21. LaHann, T. R., and Horita, A. (1977): Thyrotropin-releasing hormone and the
gastrointestinal tract: The effect of central administration on colonic smooth muscle
activity. *Proc. West. Pharmacol. Soc.,* 20:305–306.

22. Nistri, A., Bartolini, A., Deffenu, G., and Pepeu, G. (1972): Investigations into the
release of acetylcholine from the cerebral cortex of the cat: Effects of amphetamine,
of scopolamine and of septal lesions. *Neuropharmacology,* 11:665–674.

23. Plotnikoff, N. P., Prange, A. J., Jr., Breese, G. R., Anderson, M. S., and Wilson,
I. C. (1972): Thyrotropin releasing hormone: Enhancement of DOPA activity by
a hypothalamic hormone. *Science,* 178:417–418.

24. Prange, A. J., Jr., Breese, G. R., Cott, J. M., Martin, B. R., Cooper, B. R., Wilson,
I. C., and Plotnikoff, N. P. (1974): Thyrotropin releasing hormone: Antagonism of
pentobarbital in rodents. *Life Sci.,* 14:447–455.

25. Prange, A. J., Jr., Wilson, I. C., Lara, P. P., Alltop, L. B., and Breese, G. R.
(1972): Effects of thyrotropin-releasing hormone in depression. *Lancet,* 2:999–
1007.

26. Quock, R. M., and Horita, A. (1976): Differentiation of neuropharmacological actions of apomorphine and d-amphetamine. *Pharmacol. Biochem. Behav.,* 5:627–631.

27. Reigle, T. G., Avni, J., Platz, P. A., Schildkraut, J. J., and Plotnikoff, N. P. (1974):
Norepinephrine metabolism in the rat brain following acute and chronic administration of thyrotropin releasing hormone. *Psychopharmacologia,* 37:1–6.

28. Schmidt, D. E. (1976): Regional levels of choline and acetylcholine in rat brain
following head focussed microwave sacrifice: Effect of (+)-amphetamine and (±)-
parachloroamphetamine. *Neuropharmacology,* 15:77–84.

29. Schmidt, D. E. (1977): Effects of thyrotropin-releasing hormone (TRH) on pentobarbital-induced decrease in cholinergic neuronal activity. *Commun. Psychopharmacol.,* 1:469–473.

30. Sharpless, S. K., and Rothballer, A. P. (1961): Humoral factors released from
intracranial sources during stimulation of reticular formation. *Am. J. Physiol.,*
200:909–915.

31. Smith, J. R., LaHann, T. R., Chesnut, R. M., Carino, M. A., and Horita, A.
(1977): Thyrotropin-releasing hormone: Stimulation of colonic activity following
intracerebroventricular administration. *Science,* 196:660–662.

32. Wei, E., Sigel, S., Loh, H., and Way, E. L. (1975): Thyrotropin-releasing hormone
and shaking behavior in rat. *Nature (Lond),* 253:739–740.

33. White, R. P., and Daigneault, E. A. (1959): The antagonism of atropine to the
EEG effects of adrenergic drugs. *J. Pharmacol. Exp. Ther.,* 125:339–346.

34. Winokur, A., and Utiger, R. D. (1974): Thyrotropin-releasing hormone: Regional
distribution in rat brain. *Science,* 185:265–267.

Central Nervous System Effects of Hypothalamic
Hormones and Other Peptides, edited by Collu et al.
Raven Press, New York © 1979.

Behavioral Effects of Thyrotropin-Releasing Hormone in Animals and Man: A Review

Arthur J. Prange, Jr., Charles B. Nemeroff, Peter T. Loosen,
Garth Bissette, Albert J. Osbahr III, *Ian C. Wilson, and Morris A. Lipton

*Department of Psychiatry, Biological Sciences Research Center, The Neurobiology Program,
University of North Carolina, School of Medicine, Chapel Hill, North Carolina 27514; and
*Division of Research, North Carolina Department of Mental Health,
Raleigh, North Carolina 27611*

The first hypothalamic-releasing hormone to be chemically characterized was TRH. This hormone is a tripeptide: pyroglutamyl-histidyl-prolineamide (8,16). Although this peptide hormone was termed TRH because of its ability to release thyroid-stimulating hormone (TSH, thyrotropin) from the anterior pituitary, it is now established that in certain species TRH releases prolactin (PRL) as well. The physiological importance of this effect is unclear (109,110).

Synthetic TRH is commercially available and radioimmunoassays (RIA) for its measurement have been developed. The development of RIAs for the tripeptide has facilitated study of the distribution of TRH in the brain, and these studies are reviewed in this volume by Winokur and Utiger (123) and Jackson (46) and elsewhere by Brownstein et al. (14,15). In brief, immunoreactive TRH has been localized by immunohistochemical and RIA procedures (13,37,52,121,122) in many brain areas, the gastrointestinal tract, plasma, cerebrospinal fluid (CSF), and urine of a variety of species.

These data concerning the localization of TRH in body tissues and fluids must be critically evaluated. Although it is clear that TRH is present in the hypothalamus, the demonstration that immunoassayable TRH in extrahypothalamic brain areas and in plasma and urine is indeed pGlu-His-Pro-NH$_2$ has not been unequivocally established. Immunoreactive TRH must be tested with bioassay procedures for potency in releasing TSH and PRL from the adenohypophysis. Youngblood et al. (126) reported that serum, brain, and urine contain substances which cross-react with TRH antiserum in their RIA. These findings are relevant to the present subject since some studies have attempted to correlate levels of TRH in biological fluids with changes in behavioral state. For example, Simonin et al. (99) reported in normal humans that plasma levels of immunoreactive TRH rise significantly after psychological stress.

Burt and Snyder (17) studied the binding of radiolabeled TRH to rat brain membranes and were able to identify both high- and low-affinity binding components for the tripeptide. The high-affinity binding component was remarkably similar to that previously reported for adenohypophyseal membranes. They demonstrated that high-affinity, saturable, TRH binding was present in several brain regions (except cerebellum) and in peripheral tissues examined (e.g., liver).

ANIMAL STUDIES

Modification of Drug-Induced Effects

Piva and Steiner (80) and Pittman (79) reviewed studies of toxicity. The tripeptide appears to be a remarkably innocuous substance (in the rat $LD_{50} = 2,500$ mg/kg i.v.).

Soon after synthetic TRH became available it was noted that the hormone potentiated the stimulant effects of L-DOPA in pargyline-treated mice and rats, a test used to screen for putative antidepressant drugs. The L-DOPA test assesses the motor response of aggregated mice pretreated with the monoamine oxidase inhibitor pargyline (40 mg/kg orally) and then given the test substance (e.g., TRH) and a fixed dose of L-DOPA (100 mg/kg), both intraperitoneally. TRH was active even after hypophysectomy (81) or thyroidectomy (82), indicating that motor stimulation by TRH is not mediated via the pituitary-thyroid axis. TRH was active in male and female mice and rats (82). This work was confirmed and extended by Huidobro-Toro et al. (42), who also showed that DOPA potentiation occurred after intracerebral injection of TRH. Moreover, TRH was found to potentiate the effects of imipramine in the DOPA test. The possibility that the action of TRH in this paradigm is mediated by actions on other organs was obviated by successive removal of the adrenals, thymus, kidney, spleen, thyroid, testes, ovaries, and pineal, as well as the demonstration that these manipulations did not prevent the activity of TRH (81,82). Nevertheless, it is interesting to note that the potency of TRH was reduced in castrated, parathyroidectomized, or pinealectomized mice.

The behavioral effects of serotonin (5-HT) accumulation have also been shown to be potentiated by TRH (33). TRH was given to rats that subsequently received tranylcypromine (an MAO inhibitor) and L-tryptophan. The TRH effect persists after hypophysectomy; TSH and thyroxine are inactive in this paradigm. Thus it appears that this action of TRH, like its action in the DOPA test, is independent of the pituitary-thyroid axis. TRH did not change brain levels of tryptophan or 5-HT, suggesting that the tripeptide may alter 5-HT receptor sensitivity. In addition, TRH augmented the hyperactivity induced by 5-methoxy-N,N-dimethyltryptamine, an agonist of central serotonergic receptors (33). TRH potentiation of the effects of increased brain 5-HT was also found by Huidobro-Toro et al. (42), who administered TRH i.p. or i.c. to mice also treated with 5-hydroxytryptophan (5-HTP) and pargyline. Pro-Leu-Gly-NH₂ (MIF-I) and angiotensin II are also active in the DOPA potentiation test (42), although only TRH is active in the 5-HTP potentiation test.

A series of reports have shown that TRH, administered peripherally or centrally, markedly antagonizes the sedation and hypothermia induced by a wide variety of centrally acting depressants (6,7,9–11,25,34,51,87–89). These include a variety of barbiturates, chloral hydrate, reserpine, chlorpromazine, diazepam, and ethanol. TRH is effective whether administered before or after the barbiturate (10,89).

The analeptic effect of TRH was demonstrated in several mammalian species: rats, mice, hamsters, gerbils, and guinea pigs (10); monkeys (25, 51); and rabbits (19,39). TRH administration to pentobarbital-treated rhesus monkeys produced increased respiratory and heart rates and arrested the progress of barbiturate-induced hypothermia. TRH-treated animals regained reflexes sooner than control animals, and sleeping time was shortened (51).

Subsequent studies showed that TRH antagonizes pentobarbital-induced sedation and hypothermia during the day, but at night only the drug-induced hypothermia was reversed by TRH. Amphetamine exhibits a similar pharmacological profile. In addition, loading doses of L-tryptophan, the amino acid precursor of serotonin, or L-DOPA, a catecholamine precursor, had no significant effect on the analeptic potency of TRH. Furthermore, TRH was shown to reverse pentobarbital-induced narcosis and hypothermia at warm (37°C) and cold (18°C) ambient temperatures (89).

Brown and Vale (11) confirmed the finding of barbiturate antagonism by TRH. They demonstrated that the i.v. administration of TRH increases the LD_{50} (decreases the lethality) of pentobarbital by 25% in intact and hypophysectomized (HPX) rats. In addition, these workers reported that mortality after a lethal dose of pentobarbital is abolished in rats treated 10 min later with TRH.

Studies with structural analogs of TRH suggest that the analeptic potency of these tripeptide congeners is unrelated to their ability to release TSH from the pituitary (25). Although the mechanism of analeptic action of TRH is not known, it is clear that the tripeptide does not exert its action by altering the metabolism of pentobarbital (10,34,51). Recently Porter et al. (83) reported that a synthetic tripeptide related to TRH [L-N-(2-oxopiperidin-6-ylcarbonyl)-L-histidyl-L-thiazolidine-α-carboxamide] is 100 times as potent as the parent compound in antagonizing methohexital-induced sedation in rats and pentobarbital- and ethanol-induced hypothermia in mice. In addition, Prasad et al. (94) showed that histidyl-proline diketopiperazine (His-Pro), a putative metabolite of TRH, is a potent antagonist of ethanol but not barbiturate-induced narcosis.

After TRH was demonstrated to antagonize the narcosis and hypothermia induced by pentobarbital, Collu and his associates (22) studied the effects of TRH on the release of pituitary hormones induced by this barbiturate. TRH antagonized pentobarbital-induced release of growth hormone (GH) in intact and thyroidectomized rats. L-Triiodothyronine (T_3) was also effective; other small peptides were not. This effect was also observed after the i.c.v. injection of TRH. The β-adrenergic receptor blocker propranolol antagonized the TRH effect but had no effect on T_3-induced inhibition of GH release. Brown and Vale (12) demonstrated that TRH, a biologically potent analog of TRH (3-methyl-His-TRH) and SRIF inhibited the *in vivo* release of GH induced by morphine sulfate and pentobarbital. These drugs presumably release GH via a central nervous system (CNS) mechanism since neither morphine nor pentobarbital stimulate GH release from *in vitro* pituitary preparations. Intact and HPX rats given morphine exhibited a rapid vibration of the tail after TRH administration. Our group (88) previously showed dissociation of analeptic and TSH releasing properties of TRH analogs. In contrast, Brown and Vale (12) reported that congeners of TRH with low TSH-releasing activity neither inhibited pentobarbital-induced GH release nor induced tail vibration in morphine-treated rats. More recently Tache et al. (104) reported that centrally or peripherally administered TRH and certain TRH analogs, many devoid of TSH releasing properties, also inhibit pentobarbital-induced release of PRL. This effect was neither blocked by propranolol nor mimicked by T_3.

Since TRH antagonizes barbiturate-induced narcosis, and since chronic phenobarbital treatment of grand mal epilepsy is sometimes limited by unwanted sedation, we studied the effects of TRH and a tetrapeptide analog of TRH (linear β-alanine TRH; pGlu-His-Pro-β-Ala-NH$_2$) on the anticonvulsant potency of the barbiturate in mice (72). The maximal electroshock seizure test, considered the model of choice for testing compounds for anti-grand mal activity (103), was employed. None of the peptides possessed significant anticonvulsant activity. However, TRH and β-ala TRH potentiated the anticonvulsant potency of phenobarbital, whereas MIF-I, TSH, and T_3 were inactive. The tetrapeptide was considerably more potent than TRH in this paradigm. Thus the peptide effects observed were probably neither nonspecific attributes of small peptides nor mediated via activation of the pituitary-thyroid axis. Since TRH and β-ala TRH are potent antagonists of the sedative properties of phenobarbital (10,88), and since they each potentiate the antiepileptic properties of this barbiturate, they may deserve testing as adjuncts to anticonvulsive therapy. It is interesting to note that this property of TRH, as well as several others, is also a pharmacological property exhibited by amphetamine (102).

Since TRH enhanced the anticonvulsant effects of phenobarbital, we examined the effects of this peptide on the anti-petit mal activity of trimethadione. TRH exerted no effect on the anticonvulsant potency of this compound against pentylenetetrazol-induced seizures (Nemeroff, Bissette, and Prange, *unpublished observations*), a laboratory model of petit mal epilepsy.

Brown and Vale (11) demonstrated that TRH reduces the strychine LD_{50} (enhances the lethality) by 28%. This effect is akin to the observations of Green and Grahame-Smith (33) after the administration of pentylenetetrazol and TRH.

Kruse (53) studied the effects of TRH on chlorpromazine (CPZ)-induced changes in behavior, muscle tone, and body temperature in the mouse and rat as well as changes in the electroencephalogram (EEG) in the rabbit. TRH antagonized CPZ-induced sedation, muscle relaxation, and hypothermia in small doses, whereas higher doses (5 to 25 mg/kg, i.p.) produced excitement, increased muscle tone, and hyperthermia. The interaction of TRH and CPZ apparently is not related to the pituitary-thyroid axis, as neither HPX nor thyroidectomy reduced but rather enhanced the neurotropic effects of TRH. In rabbits pretreated with CPZ, TRH administration resulted in behavioral and EEG arousal. This was associated with excitement, wakefulness, muscular hypertonus, and EEG desynchronization. Many of the behavioral sequelae caused by TRH alone were intensified by CPZ.

In more recent studies, Kruse (54) examined the restoration of oxotremorine tremor in mice by TRH. Oxotremorine (0.5 mg/kg s.c.) induces a primary tremor which disappears approximately 1 hr after drug administration. TRH (2.5 to 25 mg/kg) restored the tremor. This TRH effect was not altered by a variety of pharmacological blocking agents.

Green and his co-workers (34) noted the contrasting effects of TRH and cyclohexamide, a protein synthesis inhibitor, in altering the effects of centrally acting drugs. Cyclohexamide inhibits the characteristic locomotor hyperactivity induced by L-DOPA and an MAO inhibitor; as noted above, TRH enhances it. TRH also potentiated the increased locomotor activity observed in rats treated with methamphetamine and tranylcypromine but exerted no effect on apomorphine-induced hyperactivity. Cyclohexamide antagonized the methamphetamine effect and, like TRH, did not alter the effects of apomorphine. These workers also confirmed the analeptic effects of TRH, the lack of changes in plasma pentobarbital levels after TRH administration, and furthermore showed that cyclohexamide lengthens barbiturate-induced sleeping time in rats. Kulig (55) reported that TRH antagonizes the depressant effects of α-methyl-p-tyrosine on motor activity and conditioned avoidance behavior in rats.

TRH has also been reported to antagonize behavioral and endocrinological effects of certain administered peptides. Neurotensin, an endogenous tridecapeptide, produces a marked hypothermia after i.c. injection in a variety of laboratory animals (5,58,74). Although this effect of neurotensin is not antagonized by dopaminergic, cholinergic, serotonergic, or noradrenergic blocking agents, it is partially reversed by central TRH injection

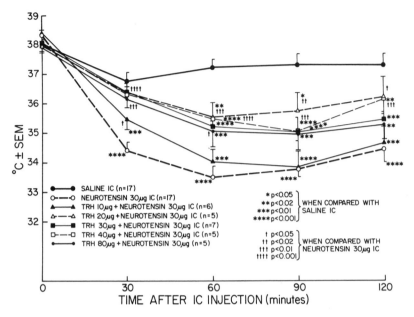

FIG. 1. Under light ether anesthesia rats were injected i.c. with saline, neurotensin (30 μg), or a fixed dose of neurotensin (30 μg) plus a variable dose of TRH (10 to 80 μg). They were then placed in individual plastic cages in a cold room (4°C) and their rectal temperatures monitored at 30-min intervals for 2 hr. As in earlier experiments, neurotensin produced a significant hypothermic response. TRH significantly but not totally abolished this effect, but the TRH-neurotensin interaction was not dose-related. Student's *t*-test (two-tailed) was utilized.

(Fig. 1). In preliminary experiments we observed that i.c. neurotensin induces a prompt, short-lived but significant decrease in the high serum TSH levels of thyroidectomized rats (Nemeroff et al., *in preparation*). Furthermore, Moss (*personal communication*) discovered that TRH antagonizes the induction of lordosis behavior by LH-RH in ovariectomized estrogen-primed female rats.

Independent Effects

TRH not only modifies the behavioral actions of certain drugs and other peptides but exerts behavioral effects in untreated animals as well. Piva and Steiner (80), in their early toxicological work, noted that rats given TRH 100 mg/kg i.v. every day for 11 days showed tremor, piloerection, tail erection, and eating-like movements of the forelegs. Schenkel-Hulliger et al. (98) later reported that even relatively small doses produced most of these symptoms. These investigators confirmed our finding (87) that lacrimation, tremor, and Straub tail phenomenon occurred in TRH-treated rats anesthetized with pentobarbital. In contrast to the numerous reports (6,7,9–11,19, 25,34,39,51,87–89) that TRH significantly shortens pentobarbital-induced sleeping time in rats, these workers reported that the duration of anesthesia was not significantly shortened. The tremorogenic effect of TRH was observed in intact, thyroidectomized, and HPX rats. Several other peptides were also examined. Given in large i.v. doses, monoiodo and diiodo analogs of TRH elicited tremor; other TRH congeners, ACTH$_{4-10}$, and LH-RH were inactive. These authors concluded that TRH administration results in a generalized state of arousal.

Wei et al. (113,114) studied the effects of injecting TRH directly into brain. Injection into certain regions (periaqueductal gray around the fourth ventricle, medial hypothalamus, and medial preoptic area) produced shaking, lacrimation, paw tremor, and intense shivering. They noted the similarity of these behavioral effects to the morphine-abstinence syndrome and hypothesized that TRH activates neural circuits which lead to heat gain. A positive correlation was demonstrated between regional TRH content and degree of response to injected TRH. Moreover, the brain areas where naloxone precipitates withdrawal shaking in morphine-dependent animals paralleled the positive sites of TRH-induced shaking. In contrast to the dissociation of pituitary and brain effects observed in the analeptic activity of TRH and TRH analogs, the potency of TRH congeners to induce shaking behavior after central injection was well correlated with potency in releasing TSH from the anterior pituitary (114). Martin et al. (67) demonstrated that TRH-induced shaking is blocked by morphine, chlorpromazine, apomorphine, and Δ^9-tetrahydrocannabinol. TRH enhances shaking behavior excited by morphine withdrawal. However, the tripeptide does not alter stereospecific binding of morphine in rat brain *in vivo* or *in vitro*. TRH appears devoid of analgesic properties.

In support of the hypothesis of Wei et al. (113), Horita and Carino (39) reported that TRH administered centrally (1 to 200 μg) or peripherally (1 to 10 mg/kg) to rabbits results in a dose-dependent hyperthermia associated with behavioral excitation and hyperactivity. The effects were reported to resemble those of *d*-amphetamine. These TRH effects were not appreciably altered by a variety of pharmacological blocking agents. One exception was phentolamine, an α-adrenergic blocking agent, which antagonized the TRH-induced behavioral arousal but did not affect the hyperthermia induced by the tripeptide. TRH reversed morphine-induced hypothermia but did not alter the behavioral effects of the opiate. In subsequent studies TRH, injected into various brain regions, produced behavioral excitation (19). After hypothalamic injection, hyperthermia was observed. In contrast to the findings of Horita and Carino (39), White and Beale (116) reported that the intracisternal (i.c.) administration of 200 μg TRH to curarized rabbits does not produce hyperthermia. Furthermore, Metcalf (70) reported that the i.c.v. injection of TRH, but not other endogenous peptides, produces a dose-related *hypothermia* in cats. As little as 3 ng TRH i.c.v. produced a 0.5°C fall in body temperature. Later studies by others demonstrated that i.c.v. TRH is a markedly more potent hypothermic agent in the cat than either norepinephrine or calcium ion (71). These workers noted in addition that i.c.v. TRH also induced profuse salivation, tachypnea, cutaneous vasodilation, and frequent defecation and vomiting. Pretreatment with α-methyltyrosine, an inhibitor of catecholamine biosynthesis, or phenotolamine did not block TRH-induced hypothermia. Thyroxine and TSH did not exhibit the pharmacological profile associated with TRH. Myers et al. (71) also stereotactically injected TRH (10 to 20 ng) into a variety of brain areas of the cat. When injected into mesencephalic sites, TRH induced polypnea, hypothermia, vocalization, salivation, defecation, and vasodilation. Hypothermia was not observed after TRH injection into the anterior hypothalamus. These workers suggested that TRH-induced hypothermia may be a consequence of the tachypnea.

Barlow and co-workers (1) reported that TRH administered i.p. caused dose-related stimulation of locomotor activity and decreases in food consumption as well as in food-reinforced, fixed-ratio, bar-press responding (F/R 30 schedule). No effects on electrical self-stimulation of the dorsal brainstem or ventral tegmentum or an active avoidance responding were noted. Further study showed that TSH, Pro-Leu-Gly-NH$_2$, and the constituent amino acids of TRH did not elicit any of the effects listed above. Destruction of CNS catecholamine systems antagonized the anorexic effects of d-amphetamine but enhanced the anorectic-like actions of TRH.

Vijayan and McCann (111) reported that TRH injection into the third ventricle of rats suppresses both food and water consumption. Smith et al. (100) found that in rats TRH administered i.c.v. stimulates muscular activity of the large intestine.

Masserano and King (68) reported that hypothalamic injections of TRH induced locomotor hyperactivity in rats, whereas no change occurred after injection into the caudate or septum. In a standard paradigm (35) designed to test substances for efficacy as discriminative stimuli in state-dependent learning, Jones et al. (47) found that rats could distinguish between TRH (20 mg/kg i.p.), amphetamine, and saline conditions on repeated testing. The peak TRH effect occurred 5 to 15 min after injection and dissipated by 1 hr after treatment. When administered into the third or lateral ventricle, relatively small doses of TRH (2.5 to 25 μg) were effective as a discriminative stimuli. Further studies revealed that TRH and d-amphetamine do not produce qualitatively similar stimulus conditions.

Crowley and Hydinger (26) administered TRH intramuscularly to juvenile male monkeys and reported that the hormone did not affect motor activity but increased behaviors of quiet rest and association and decreased environmental exploration and low-intensity dominance behaviors. Malick (66) studied the effects of TRH on the fighting behavior of mice induced by isolation. The tripeptide significantly antagonized isolation-induced fighting (ED$_{50}$ = 0.04 mg/kg i.p.). Effects were noted 30 min after administration and were still present 3 hr later. T_3, the constituent amino acids of TRH, and *d*-amphetamine were inactive in this paradigm. Amphetamine, but not TRH, increased locomotor activity in both isolated and group-housed mice.

Several investigators have attempted to elucidate the mechanism of action of TRH on the CNS by examining effects of this tripeptide on brain neurotransmitter systems. Some of these studies are reviewed in this volume by Horst (40) and Rastogi (95), and we reviewed the data in other places (91–93). Several studies have provided data supporting the hypothesis that TRH enhances brain norepinephrine turnover (23,48). Our group has not, however, been able to obtain any evidence consistent with this hypothesis (73,91–93).

Neurophysiological studies have provided further evidence for a central action of TRH. We reviewed these data elsewhere (91–93), and Renaud (97) discusses them in this volume. In brief, most workers have observed a depression of firing frequency of CNS neurons after microiontophoretically applied TRH.

King (49) reported that TRH (200 μg) injected into the lateral ventricle of cats resulted in several changes in sleep-wakefulness patterns. Sleep latency and total time awake were increased; slow wave and REM sleep were inhibited. These effects appeared not to be mediated via the pituitary-thyroid axis. White and Beale (116) recently reported that the central administration of 200 μg TRH to curarized rabbits results in an activated EEG for at least 30 min. These results are consistent with the hypothesis that TRH contributes to generalized arousal.

CLINICAL STUDIES

Behavioral Effects

Affective Disorders

In a double-blind crossover study of 10 women with unipolar depression, TRH, 0.6 mg given as an i.v. bolus, produced a rapid, partial, brief, beneficial effect. Observer and self-rating assessments showed that patients improved within a few hours after injection and reached greatest improvement the following day. Maximum improvement was about 50%, thus failing to correspond to full remission. About 1 week after injection the patients had relapsed to base-line severity (84,85).

Other investigators have attempted to discern whether TRH could be used as an efficient remedy for depression. The results have been largely disappointing (75,91–93, for review). Generalizations about the many studies performed are difficult; frequency, size of dose, route of administration, and population characteristics have varied greatly. Furlong et al. (30) suggested that differences in results might be attributed to the existence of endocrinologically distinct types of depression.

Some treatments for affective disorders are useful in depression and mania (86). Thus Huey et al. (41) examined TRH for possible antimanic effects. In a double-blind, placebo-controlled trial of five euthyroid manic men they found reliable advantages for TRH (0.5 mg i.v.) compared to saline.

Alcohol Withdrawal Syndrome

Depression is a frequent finding in alcoholism (108,115,125). We studied the effects of TRH in men in alcohol withdrawal syndrome (AWS) who showed secondary depression. In a double-blind study of 33 patients we compared the effects of TRH (0.5 mg i.v.) to the effects of two placebos, nicotinic acid and saline (60). Although all trends favored TRH, significant beneficial effects of the hormone were found only on factor I of the Hamilton Rating Scale for Depression, a measure concerned mainly with motor retardation and depressed mood. However, mean scores for the three groups were significantly different at only one time period, 3 hr after injection. At later times during a week of observation, differences between treatment groups were slight, all groups showing a tendency to improve rapidly.

Huey et al. (41) injected TRH 0.5 mg i.v. in three subjects in a state of predelirium tremens and observed no reliable beneficial effects. However, two subjects in milder stages of withdrawal showed a trend toward hormone effect revealed by improvement in a sense of well-being and increased relaxation.

Schizophrenia

In a preliminary report we described beneficial effects of TRH in four schizophrenic patients (118). We have studied 16 additional patients, 10 in a double-blind trial in which i.v. nicotinic acid was used as an active placebo (120). The tripeptide, 0.5 mg i.v., produced beneficial effects in patients in whom social withdrawal, anhedonia, and abulia were prominent. The duration of improvement was quite variable; on the average it lasted about 10 days. TRH appeared to aggravate the condition of a small subgroup of paranoid schizophrenics.

Most reports suggest that TRH exerts a behavioral effect in schizophrenia, although the effect is not always beneficial. In only three studies involving 25 patients has TRH been reported to be without effect. Drayson (29) gave repeated injections of TRH, 0.2 mg, to three patients with "cyclical psychosis." None showed significant change. Clark and his colleagues (21) performed a double-blind, placebo-controlled, crossover study of oral TRH, 300 mg per day, over 3 weeks. In the 12 schizophrenics studied they found no systematic behavioral changes. Lindstrom et al. (57) studied 10 chronic schizophrenic patients in a double-blind crossover design using TRH, 0.6 mg i.v., on 4 consecutive days. The results were substantially negative.

Three studies involving 212 schizophrenic patients have reported beneficial effects. Inanaga et al. (43) gave oral TRH, 4 mg per day, in an open study of 62 chronic schizophrenic patients who were also taking standard neuroleptics. At base line, symptoms of reduced spontaneity, abulia, apathy, and social withdrawal were prominent. In about 75% of the patients a favorable response was observed after 2 weeks. The same workers then treated 143 similar patients with oral TRH, 4 mg per day for 14 days, or with placebo in a double-blind trial (44). TRH was significantly more effective than placebo in producing overall improvement, especially in terms of enhanced motivation and social contact. In a preliminary trial Campbell (18) reported that TRH, 0.4 mg i.v., reduced hyperactivity in five of seven autistic schizophrenic children.

Two studies involving 12 patients have revealed unfavorable behavioral effects after TRH injection. In an informal trial Bigelow et al. (4) found slight worsening of depression in two of three treatment-resistant schizophrenics. Davis et al. (28) gave nine schizophrenic men TRH, 300 mg p.o. per day for 14 days, in an uncontrolled trial. Seven patients worsened, an event especially marked in paranoid patients. One withdrawn schizophrenic showed clear improvement.

Clearly the results cited do not allow definitive conclusions. Nevertheless, one can posit the suggestion that chronic schizophrenic patients, whether taking standard neuroleptics or not, tend to benefit from TRH if they are not paranoid and especially if they prominently display symptoms of social withdrawal, abulia, and anhedonia. Paranoid patients tend to be aggravated by administration of the hormone. Conclusive data, if it followed this hypothesis, would become another distinction between paranoid schizophrenics and nonparanoid schizophrenics (107). To the extent that TRH may have prodopaminergic activity (32), such findings would traduce the relevance of the dopamine hypothesis (101) for nonparanoid schizophrenics.

Other Conditions

In a double-blind crossover study of 12 patients Benkert (2) found oral TRH no more effective than placebo in male sexual impotency. Since TRH may enhance brain DA activity, several investigators have assessed the action of the hormone in Parkinson's disease. Chase and his colleagues (20) found that the tripeptide failed to produce reliable changes in neurological status. The patients, however, noted an increased sense of well-being and optimism. Lakke et al. (56) also found that the symptoms of Parkinson's disease were unaffected by TRH. The hormone reduced depression scores on a self-administered test. McCaul et al. (69) reported that two of three Parkinsonian patients taking L-DOPA, when given TRH, experienced a "dramatic improvement in well-being, including enhanced clarity of thought." Neurologic symptoms were essentially unchanged.

Tiwary and his colleagues (106) reported the results of a double-blind, crossover study of two children with hyperactivity syndrome. Both patients had shown poor responsiveness to prior methylphenidate treatment. For about 2 days after injection of TRH, 0.2 mg, all aspects of their behavior were improved.

Normal Subjects

We performed a double-blind, crossover trial of TRH, 0.5 mg i.v., and saline in 10 normal women (119). Mental changes were slight after saline, but after TRH subjects showed relaxation, mild euphoria, and a sense of increased energy. These statistically significant changes were not related to the frequency of side effects. We repeated the study in 20 additional women and obtained very similar results (Prange et al., *unpublished data*). Betts et al. (3) confirmed these findings.

Endocrine Responses

Administration of TRH offers the investigator the opportunity to observe simultaneously behavioral changes and endocrine responses, an unusual chance to study psychosomatic relationships. In this brief review only TSH responses are considered. We defined the criterion for a blunted TSH response as a maximum rise over base line (ΔTSH) of less than 5 μU/ml. The lowest ΔTSH observed in a large group of normal controls was 5.8 μU/ml. We then inspected TSH data for each patient and classified them accordingly. The results are shown in Table 1.

Blunted TSH responses were found in depressed (63) and alcoholic

TABLE 1. *TSH responses after TRH injection*

| Response[a] | Depression (N = 35) | Schizophrenia (N = 17) | Alcoholism | |
			Withdrawal (N = 12)	Postwithdrawal (N = 14)
TSH ↑	0	0	0	0
TSH ↓	10	0	6	5
TSH normal	25	17	6	9

[a] A blunted response (TSH ↓) was defined as a rise over base line, after injection of 0.5 mg TRH, of less than 5 μU/ml. This was seen in many depressed patients (10/35) and alcoholic patients (6/12, 5/14). No schizophrenic patients showed this fault. Data from each diagnostic group were compared to data from approximately equal numbers of normal subjects matched for age and sex. All normals showed a TSH rise greater than 5 μU/ml. No patient in any diagnostic group showed a rise greater than the rises shown by corresponding controls.

(60,64) patients but not in schizophrenic patients (63). In the alcoholic patients TSH blunting was observed in the withdrawal and the postwithdrawal state, more often in the former (64). In the withdrawal state TSH blunting was highly correlated with a favorable behavioral response to TRH (64).

Considering our own findings and the findings of other investigators, we sought to establish the content of TSH blunting in depressed patients (see 59,90 for review). The fault appears not to be related to previous drug intake, diagnosis, sex, age, or severity of illness. There is also no clear relationship between TSH blunting and behavioral change. Several workers have reported that some patients who demonstrate this fault during depression do not correct it upon recovery (24,50,63,65). These data indicate that the TSH response in some patients remains blunted over time in spite of marked changes in psychopathology.

Several systemic disorders can cause a blunted TSH response to TRH. Hyperthyroidism is the most common (38). In addition, TSH blunting may occur in Klinefelter's syndrome (78), 36-hr starvation (112), and chronic renal failure (27). These disorders were not present in our patients. A degree of thyroid activation is sometimes seen in depression (117); and heightened thyroid state, even within the normal range, could damp TSH response through increased negative feedback. However, no consistent correlation between thyroid indices and TSH response to TRH has been found in depressed patients. Takahashi et al. (105) provided important evidence relevant to this point by showing that patients with *low* free thyroxine indices showed the most diminished TSH responses. In our alcoholic patients we found some degree of thyroid activation in acute withdrawal, which normalized in the postwithdrawal state (64). Thus thyroid activation might play a role in TSH blunting in the former state, but it does not appear likely to account for TSH blunting seen later. Even in the acute state, however, there was no demonstrable relationship between thyroid indices and TSH blunting.

Another potential explanation for TSH blunting also needs consideration. Glucocorticoids interfere with the pituitary TSH response to TRH (77,96). To evaluate this possibility we measured serum cortisol concentrations in our patients. Base-line cortisol and TSH peak response showed a significant inverse relationship in normal subjects and in depressed patients. An inverse but statistically insignificant relationship between these variables was found in alcoholic patients. Unlike other groups, schizophrenic patients tended to show a *positive* correlation between the two parameters (61,62) (Table 2).

The findings outlined above suggest that cortisol elevation, which is known to occur in some depressed patients, may account for TSH blunting in this condition. However, the fault sometimes persists after remission from depression. In such instances the abnormality probably cannot be attributed to elevated cortisol or to any other aspect of the state of depression. In some

TABLE 2. *Correlations between cortisol at base line and TSH*

Group	Cortisol vs.	
	TSH base	TSH peak
Normal controls (N = 23)	−0.59[a]	−0.54[b]
Depression (N = 12)	−0.30	−0.68[c]
Schizophrenia (N = 13)	0.34	0.49
Alcoholism		
Withdrawal (N = 12)	0.23	−0.34
Postwithdrawal (N = 14)	0.14	−0.13

With Spearman's technique, for each group of patients and for normal controls, cortisol values at base line were tested for correlation with TSH values at base line and with TSH peak responses after TRH injection. Although depressed patients often show blunted TSH responses, the inverse relationships between TSH and cortisol tend to occur as in normals. Some of these relationships are lost in alcoholic patients. The relationships are lost in schizophrenic patients and tend in the opposite direction even though TSH responses themselves are normal in this group (Table 1).

[a] $p < 0.005$; [b] $p < 0.01$; [c] $p < 0.05$.

patients the blunted TSH response may be related to the trait of being at risk for depression rather than to the state of being depressed. This possibility parallels an observation we made concerning alcoholic patients (64). In this population, blunted TSH responses were found in the acute withdrawal and the postwithdrawal state, although less frequently in the latter (Table 1). In the latter condition behavioral symptoms had subsided and thyroid measurements had normalized. Thus it remains possible that in alcoholism, as in depression, some instance of TSH blunting are trait-related rather than state-related. A blunted TSH response may represent a common biological feature of both conditions. This in turn may parallel the genetic relationship between alcoholism in men and early-onset unipolar depression in women described by Winokur et al. (124). Clearly a blunted TSH response to TRH is not merely a nonspecific aspect of mental disorder, for the responses of schizophrenic patients were found to be normal, even though not related in normal fashion to cortisol levels.

DISCUSSION

The scope of this chapter is quite circumscribed. It is limited to TRH and focuses on behavioral effects. TRH is, of course, a member of a larger class of peptides, the hypothalamic hypophysiotropic hormones. Several members of this class have been chemically identified, and all are peptides (109). Still others, as yet unidentified, are known to exist on the basis of hypophysiotropic action of extracts of hypothalamus (91,109,110). Although these substances are by definition hormones, all identified members of the class have been shown to exert behavioral effects, at least some of which are independent of their endocrine effects. Indeed the brain contains many peptides only some of which appear to exert endocrine effects in the nervous system but many of which appear to exert behavioral effects (91). It has been suggested that the endocrine role of the hypophysiotropic peptides may have been acquired relatively late in phylogeny (45,76,91).

If one must choose a single hypothalamic hypophysiotropic hormone for discussion, TRH is probably a fortunate choice. As we said, it was the first of its class to be identified; it has been extensively studied in behavioral systems; and its endocrine effects are clearly described (109,110). Thus statements about TRH may, within limits, be taken as generic statements about hypothalamic hypophysiotropic hormones. Problems in TRH research may also be representative of problems in research pertaining to other brain peptides.

What generalizations can be made regarding the behavioral effects of TRH? First, they exist. Second, at least some clearly are not dependent on endocrine effects. Third, species differences intrude themselves in a consideration of the data. For example, centrally administered TRH appears to exert a hyperthermic effect in rabbits and a hypothermic effect in cats. TRH modifies not only the behavioral action of drugs but the behavioral actions of other peptides as well. Although TRH appears to interact with acknowledged neurotransmitter systems, not all its action can be accounted for on this basis. For example, we found that a variety of pharmacological blocking agents exert no significant effect on the analeptic activity of the tripeptide (10). It is quite possible that TRH, and other peptides, act as transmitters themselves. In another report (91) we marshalled the evidence that supports this possibility.

What theme can be stated about the behavioral actions of TRH? Here one can go no further than the suggestion that the tripeptide facilitates arousal (55). Humans given TRH often report an increased sense of well-being and an enhanced ability to cope. Not all data are in line with this generalization, at least not in an obvious way. For example, TRH inhibits fighting in mice provoked in a certain way and potentiates the anticonvulsant activity of phenobarbital. These observations are not necessarily inconsistent with the notion of enhanced arousal, for we are ignorant of how these functions relate to arousal, but they offer no clear support for it. We have suggested, and criticized, the concept that a principle of harmony may exist between the endocrine and behavioral effects of a hypothalamic hypophysiotropic hormone (91). Thus the action of TRH may be seen as ergotropic [versus trophotropic in the dichotomy of Hess (36)]; it facilitates arousal and prompts secretion of TSH and thyroid hormones, with their well-known though delayed effects of preparing the organism for activity. If a coin could have three sides, it would be interesting to think of TRH, thyroid hormones, and the sympathetic nervous system as occupying these sides.

Although in this brief review we have not emphasized the endocrine effects of TRH, we have not set them aside altogether. Indeed we sought to illustrate how the TSH response (e.g., to injected TRH) can be used as an investigative tool in psychiatry. Clearly some members of certain diagnostic groups (depression, alcohol withdrawal state) but not others (schizophrenia) show a blunted TSH response. Sometimes the blunted response appears related to another endocrine disturbance (elevated cortisol), sometimes not. Even when it is so related, both may proceed from a disturbance of central neural regulation, as Gold et al. (31) suggested, rather than one endocrine event causing the other. There is in behavioral sciences an impulse to interpret endocrine data as revealing the state of acknowledged central transmitter systems. Although this is a potentially useful exercise, its fruition is limited by the complexity of the mechanisms by which the brain influences the levels and responses of hormones measurable in the periphery. If after an endocrine challenge (e.g., TRH administration) one attends to both endocrine and behavioral responses, it is sometimes possible to find associations between the two, as we have done in men in alcohol withdrawal syndrome. The systematic search for such relationships is in the best tradition of psychosomatic medicine.

ACKNOWLEDGMENT

This research was supported in part by USPHS Career Scientist Award MH-22536 (A.J.P.), NIMH grant MH-15631, and NICHHD HD-03110.

REFERENCES

1. Barlow, T. S., Cooper, B. R., Breese, G. R., Prange, A. J., Jr., and Lipton, M. A. (1975): Effects of thyrotropin-releasing hormone (TRH) on behavior: Evidence for an anorexic-like action. *Neurosci. Abst.*, 1:334.
2. Benkert, O. (1975): Studies on pituitary hormones and releasing hormones in depression and sexual impotence. *Brain Res.*, 42:25–36.
3. Betts, T. A., Smith, J., Pidd, S., Macintosh, J., Harvey, P., and Funicane, J. (1976): The effects of thyrotropin-releasing hormone on measures of mood in normal women. *Br. J. Clin. Pharmacol.*, 3:469–473.
4. Bigelow, L. G., Gillin, J. C., Semal, C., and Wyatt, R. J. (1975): Thyrotropin releasing hormone in chronic schizophrenia. *Lancet*, 2:869–970.
5. Bissette, G., Nemeroff, C. B., Loosen, P. T., Prange, A. J., Jr., and Lipton, M. A. (1976): Hypothermia and intolerance to cold induced by intracisternal administration of the hypothalamic peptide neurotensin. *Nature (Lond)*, 262:607–609.
6. Bissette, B., Nemeroff, C. B., Loosen, P. T., Prange, A. J., Jr., and Lipton, M. A. (1976): Comparison of the analeptic activity of TRH, LHRH, ACTH$_{4-10}$ and related peptides. *Pharmacol. Biochem. Behav. (Suppl. 1)*, 5:135–138.
7. Bissette, G., Nemeroff, C. B., Prange, A. J., Jr., Loosen, P. T., Breese, G. R., Burnett, G. B., and Lipton, M. A. (1978): Modification of pentobarbital-induced sedation by natural and synthetic peptides. *Neuropharmacology*, 17:229–237.
8. Boler, J., Enzmann, F., Folkers, K., Bowers, C. Y., and Schally, A. V. (1969): The identity of chemical and hormonal properties of the thyrotropin releasing hormone and pyroglutamyl-histidyl-proline-amide. *Biochem. Biophys. Res. Commun.*, 37:705.
9. Breese, G. R., Cott, J. M., Cooper, B. R., Prange, A. J., Jr., and Lipton, M. A. (1974): Antagonism of ethanol narcosis by thyrotropin releasing hormone. *Life Sci.*, 14:1053–1063.

10. Breese, G. R., Cott, J. M., Cooper, B. R., Prange, A. J., Jr., Lipton, M. A., and Plotnikoff, N. P. (1975): Effects of thyrotropin-releasing hormone (TRH) on the actions of pentobarbital and other centrally acting drugs. *J. Pharmacol. Exp. Ther.,* 193:11–22.

11. Brown, M., and Vale, W. (1975): Central nervous system effects of hypothalamic peptides. *Endocrinology,* 96:1333–1336.

12. Brown, M., and Vale, W. (1975): Growth hormone release in the rat: Effects of somatostatin and thyrotropin releasing factor. *Endocrinology,* 97:1151–1156.

13. Brownstein, M. J., Palkovits, M., Saavedra, J. M., Basiri, R. M., and Utiger, R. D. (1974): Thyrotropin-releasing hormone in specific nuclei of rat brain. *Science,* 185:267–269.

14. Brownstein, M. J., Palkovits, M., Saavedra, J. M., and Kizer, J. S. (1976): Distribution of hypothalamic hormones and neurotransmitters within the diencephalon. In: *Frontiers in Neuroendocrinology,* edited by L. Martini and W. F. Ganong, pp. 1–23. Raven Press, New York.

15. Brownstein, M. J. (1978): Peptides in mamalian neural tissue. In: *Psychopharmacology: A Generation of Progress,* edited by M. A. Lipton, A. D. DiMascio, and K. F. Killam, pp. 397–402. Raven Press, New York.

16. Burgus, R., Dunn, T. F., Desiderio, D., and Guillemin, R. (1969): Structure moleculaire de facteur hypothalamique hypophysiotrope TRF d'origine ovine: Mise en evidence par spectrometric de masse de la sequence PCA-HIS-Pro-NH$_2$. *C R Acad. Sci. (Paris),* 269:1870–1873.

17. Burt, D. R., and Snyder, S. H. (1975): Thyrotropin-releasing hormone (TRH): Apparent receptor binding in rat brain membranes. *Brain Res.,* 93:309–328.

18. Campbell, M. (1975): Clinical trials of TRH. *Psychopharmacol. Bull.,* 11:19–20.

19. Carino, M. A., Smith, J. R., Weick, B. C., and Horita, H. (1976): Effects of thyrotropin-releasing hormone (TRH) microinjected into various brain areas of conscious and pentobarbital-pretreated rabbits. *Life Sci.,* 19:1687–1692.

20. Chase, T. N., Woods, A. C., Lipton, M. A., and Morris, C. E. (1974): Hypothalamic releasing factors and Parkinson's disease. *Arch. Neurol.,* 31:55–56.

21. Clark, M. S., Parades, A., Costiloe, J. P., and Wood, F. (1975): Synthetic thyroid releasing hormone (TRH) administered orally to chronic schizophrenic patients. *Psychopharmacol. Commun.,* 1:191–200.

22. Collu, R., Clermont, M. J., Letarte, J., Leboeuf, G., and Ducharme, J. R. (1975): Inhibition of pentobarbital-induced release of growth hormone by thyrotropin releasing hormone *Endocrine Res. Commun.,* 2:123–135.

23. Constantinidis, J., Geissbuhler, F., Gaillard, J. M., Hovaguimian, Th., and Tissot, R. (1974): Enhancement of cerebral noradrenaline turnover by thyrotropin-releasing hormone: Evidence by fluorescence-histochemistry. *Experientia,* 30:1182.

24. Coppen, A., Montgomery, S., Peet, M., and Bailey, J. (1974): Thyrotropin releasing hormone in the treatment of depression. *Lancet,* 2:433–434.

25. Cott, J. M., Breese, G. R., Cooper, B. R., Barlow, T. S., and Prange, A. J., Jr. (1976): Investigations into the mechanism of reduction of ethanol sleep by thyrotropin-releasing hormone (TRH). *J. Pharmacol. Exp. Ther.,* 196:594–604.

26. Crowley, T. J., and Hydinger, M. (1976): MIF, TRH, and simian social and motor behavior. *Pharmacol. Biochem. Behav. (Suppl. 5),* 1:79–88.

27. Czernichow, P., Dayzet, M. C., Broyer, M., and Rappoport, R. (1976): Abnormal TSH, PRL, and GH response to TSH releasing factor in chronic renal failure. *J. Clin. Endocrinol. Metab.,* 43:630.

28. Davis, K. L., Hollister, L. E., and Berger, P. A. (1975): Thyrotropin-releasing hormones in schizophrenia. *Am. J. Psychiatry,* 132:951–953.

29. Drayson, A. M. (1974): TRH in cyclical psychoses. *Lancet,* 2:312.

30. Furlong, F. W., Brown, G. M., and Beeching, M. F. (1976): Thyrotropin-releasing hormone: Differential antidepressant and endocrinological effects. *Am. J. Psychiatry,* 133:1187–1190.

31. Gold, P. W., Goodwin, F. K., Wehr, T., and Rebar, R. (1977): Pituitary thyrotropin response to thyrotropin-releasing hormone in affective illness: Relationship to spinal fluid amine metabolites. *Am. J. Psychiatry,* 134:1028–1031.

32. Goujet, M. A., Simon, P., Chermat, R., and Boissier, J. R. (1975): Profil de la TRH en psychopharmacologie experimentale. *Psychopharmacologia,* 45:87–92.
33. Green, A. R., and Grahame-Smith, D. G. (1974): TRH potentiates behavioral changes following increased brain 5-hydroxytryptamine accumulation in rats. *Nature (Lond),* 251:524–526.
34. Green, A. R., Heal, D. J., Grahame-Smith, D. G., and Kelley, P. H. (1976): The contrasting actions of TRH and cyclohexamide in altering the effects of centrally acting drugs: Evidence for the noninvolvement of dopamine sensitive adenylate cyclase. *Neuropharmacology,* 15:591–599.
35. Harris, R. T., and Balster, R. L. (1971): An analysis of the function of drugs in the stimulus control of operant behavior. In: *Stimulus Properties of Drugs,* edited by R. Pickens, pp. 111–132. Appleton-Century-Crofts, New York.
36. Hess, W. R., editor (1954): *Diencephalon, Autonomic and Extrapyramidal Functions.* Grune Publishers, New York.
37. Hökfelt, T., Elde, R., Johansson, O., Ljungdahl, A., Schultzberg, M., Fuxe, K., Goldstein, M., Nilsson, G., Pernow, B., Terenius, L., Ganten, D., Jeffcoate, S. L., Rehfield, J., and Said, S. (1978): Distribution of peptide-containing neurons. In: *Psychopharmacology: A Generation of Progress,* edited by M. A. Lipton, A. DiMascio, and K. F. Killam, pp. 39–66. Raven Press, New York.
38. Hollander, C. S., Mitsumi, T., and Nilhei, N. (1972): Clinical and laboratory observations in case of triiodothyronine narcosis confirmed by radioimmunoassay. *Lancet,* 1:609.
39. Horita, A., and Carino, M. A. (1975): Thyrotropin-releasing hormone (TRH)-induced hyperthermia and behavioral excitation in rabbits. *Psychopharmacol. Commun.,* 1:403–414.
40. Horst, W. D. (1978): The influence of TRH on the synaptic availability of biogenic amines in brain. *(This volume).*
41. Huey, L. Y., Janowsky, D. S., Mandell, A. J., Judd, L. L., and Pendery, M. (1975): Preliminary studies on the use of thyrotropin-releasing hormone in manic states, depression, and the dysphoria of alcohol withdrawal. *Psychopharmacol. Bull.,* 11:24–27.
42. Huidobro-Toro, J. P., Scotti de Carolis, A., and Longo, V. G. (1974): Action of two hypothalamic factors (TRH, MIF) and of angiotensin II on the behavioral effects of L-DOPA and 5-hydroxytryptophan in mice. *Pharmacol. Biochem. Behav.,* 2:105–109.
43. Inanaga, K., Nakano, T., and Nagato, T. (1975): Effects of thyrotropin releasing hormone in schizophrenia. *Kurume Med. J.,* 22:159–168.
44. Inanaga, K., Nakano, T., Tanaka, M., and Ogawa, N. (1978): Behavioral effects of protirelin in schizophrenia. *Arch. Gen. Psychiatry,* 35:1011–1014.
45. Jackson, I. M. D., and Reichlin, S. (1974): Distribution of pGlu-His-Pro-NH$_2$ (TRH) in hypothalamic and extrahypothalamic tissues of mammalian and submammalian chordates. *Endocrinology,* 95:816–824.
46. Jackson, I. M. D. (1978): Distribution and biosynthesis of TRH in the central nervous system. *(This volume).*
47. Jones, C. N., Grant, L. D., and Prange, A. J., Jr. (1978): Stimulus properties of thyrotropin-releasing hormone (TRH). *Psychopharmacology (in press).*
48. Keller, H. H., Bartholini, C., and Pletscher, A. (1974): Enhancement of cerebral noradrenaline turnover by thyrotropin-releasing hormone. *Nature (Lond),* 248: 528–529.
49. King, C. D. (1975): Inhibition of slow wave sleep and rapid eye movement sleep by thyrotropin releasing hormone in cats. *Pharmacologist,* 17:211.
50. Kirkegaard, C., Norlem, N., Lauridsen, U. B., Bjorum, N., and Christiansen, C. (1975): Protirelin stimulation test and thyroid function during treatment of depression. *Arch. Gen. Psychiatry,* 32:1115–1118.
51. Kraemer, G. W., Mueller, R., Breese, G. R., Prange, A. J., Jr., Lewis, J. K., Morrison, H., and McKinney, W. T., Jr. (1976): Thyrotropin-releasing hormone: Antagonism of pentobarbital narcosis in the monkey. *Pharmacol. Biochem. Behav.,* 4:709–712.

52. Krulich, L., Quiada, M., Hefco, E., and Sundberg, D. K. (1974): Localization of thyrotropin-releasing factor (TRF) in the hypothalamus of the rat. *Endocrinology*, 95:9–17.
53. Kruse, H. (1975): Thyrotropin-releasing hormone: Interaction with chlorpromazine in mice, rats, and rabbits. *J. Pharmacol. (Paris)*, 6:249:268.
54. Kruse, H. (1976): Thyrotropin releasing hormone (TRH): Restoration of oxotremorine tremor in mice. *Naunyn Schoniedebergs Arch. Pharmacol.*, 294: 39–45.
55. Kulig, B. M. (1975): The effects of thyrotropin-releasing hormone on the behavior of rats pretreated with α-methyltyrosine. *Neuropharmacology*, 14:489–492.
56. Lakke, J. P. W. F., van Praag, H. M., van Twisk, R., Doorenbos, H., and Witt, F. G. J. (1974): Effects of administration of thyrotropin releasing hormone in Parkinsonism. *Clin. Neurol. Neurosurg.*, 3/4:1–5.
57. Lindstrom, L. H., Gunne, L. M., Oest, L. G., and Person, E. (1977): Thyrotropin-releasing hormone (TRH) in chronic schizophrenia. *Acta Psychiatr. Scand.*, 55:74–80.
58. Lipton, M. A., Bissette, G., Nemeroff, C. B., Loosen, P. T., and Prange, A. J., Jr. (1976): Neurotensin: a possible mediator of thermoregulation in the mouse. In: *Drugs, Biogenic Amines and Thermoregulation*, edited by P. Lomax and E. Schonbawm, pp. 54–57. Karger, Basel.
59. Loosen, P. T., Prange, A. J., Jr., Wilson, I. C., and Lara, P. P. (1976): Pituitary responses to thyrotropin releasing hormone in depressed patients: A review. *Pharmacol. Biochem. Behav. (Suppl. 1)*, 5:95–101.
60. Loosen, P. T., Wilson, I. C., Lara, P. P., Prange, A. J., Jr., and Pettus, C. (1976): Treatment of depressive state in alcohol withdrawal syndromes by thyrotropin releasing hormone. *Arsneim. Forsch.*, 26:1164–1166.
61. Loosen, P. T., Wilson, I. C., Prange, A. J., Jr., and Lara, P. P. (1977): Thyroid stimulating hormone response after TRH and its relationship to plasma cortisol. *Psychosom. Med.*, 39:55 (abstract)
62. Loosen, P. T., Wilson, I. C., Prange, A. J., Jr., and Lara, P. P. (1977): TSH response after TRH in psychiatric patients. In: *VI World Congress of Psychiatry, Honolulu, Hawaii* (abstract)
63. Loosen, P. T., Prange, A. J., Jr., Wilson, I. C., Lara, P. P., and Pettus, C. (1977): Thyroid stimulating hormone response after thyrotropin releasing hormone in depressed, schizophrenic and normal women. *Psychoneuroendocrinology*, 2:137–148.
64. Loosen, P. T., Wilson, I. C., and Prange, A. J., Jr. Thyrotropin releasing hormone (TRH) in alcohol withdrawal syndrome. *Arch. Gen. Psychiatry (in press)*.
65. Maeda, K., Kato, Y., Ohgo, S., Chihara, K., Yoshimoto, Y., Yamaguchi, N., Kuromaru, S., and Imura, H. (1975): Growth hormone and prolactin release after injection of thyrotropin releasing hormone in patients with depression. *J. Clin. Endocrinol. Metab.*, 40:501–505.
66. Malick, J. B. (1976): Antagonism of isolation-induced aggression in mice by thyrotropin-releasing hormone (TRH). *Pharmacol. Biochem. Behav.*, 5:665–669.
67. Martin, B. R., Dewey, W. L., Chau-Pham, T., and Prange, A. J., Jr. (1977): Interactions of thyrotropin releasing hormone and morphine sulfate in rodents. *Life Sci.*, 20:715–722.
68. Masserano, J. M., and King, C. D. (1976): Comparison of thyroid releasing hormone (TRH) and amphetamine (AMP) on charges in activity levels of rats following injections into the caudate nucleus, septum and hypothalamus. *Fed. Proc.*, 35:423.
69. McCaul, J. A., Cassell, K. J., and Stern, G. M. (1974): Intravenous thyrotropin releasing hormone in Parkinson's disease. *Lancet*, 2:735.
70. Metcalf, G. (1974): TRH: A possible mediator of thermoregulation. *Nature (Lond)*, 252:310–311.
71. Myers, R. D., Metcalf, G., and Rice, J. C. (1977): Identification by microinjec-

tion on TRH-sensitive sites in the cat's brain stem that mediate respiratory, temperature and other autonomic changes. *Brain Res.,* 126:105–115.

72. Nemeroff, C. B., Prange, A. J., Jr., Bissette, G., Breese, G. R., and Lipton,
M. A. (1975): Thyrotropin-releasing hormone and its β-alanine analogue: Po-
tentiation of the anticonvulsant properties of phenobarbital. *Psychopharmacol.
Commun.,* 1:305–317.

73. Nemeroff, C. B., Diez, J. A., Bissette, G., Prange, A. J., Jr., Harrell, L. E., and
Lipton, M. A. (1977): Lack of effect of chronically administered thyrotropin-
releasing hormone (TRH) on regional rat brain tyrosine hydroxylase activity.
Pharmacol. Biochem. Behav., 6:467–469.

74. Nemeroff, C. B., Bissette, G., Prange, A. J., Jr., Loosen, P. T., Barlow, T. S.,
and Lipton, M. A. (1977): Neurotensin: Central nervous system effects of a
hypothalamic peptide. *Brain Res.,* 128:485–496.

75. Nemeroff, C. B., Loosen, P. T., Bissette, G., Manberg, P. A., Lipton, M. A.,
and Prange, A. J., Jr. (1978): Pharmaco-behavioral effects of hypothalamic
peptides in animals and man: Focus on thyrotropin-releasing hormone (TRH)
and neurotensin. *Psychoneuroendocrinology (in press).*

76. Nemeroff, C. B., and Prange, A. J., Jr. (1978): Peptides in psychoneuroendocrinology: A perspective. *Arch. Gen. Psychiatry,* 35:999–1010.

77. Otsuki, M., Dakoda, M., and Baba, S. (1973): Influence of glucocorticoids on
TRH mediated TSH response in man. *J. Clin. Endocrinol.,* 36:95–102.

78. Ozawa, Y., and Shishiba, Y. (1975): Lack of TRH-induced TSH secretion in a
patient with Klinefelter's syndrome: A case report. *Endocrinol. Jpn.,* 22:269–273.

79. Pittman, J. A. (1974): Thyrotropin-releasing hormone. *Adv. Intern. Med.,* 19:
303–325.

80. Piva, F., and Steiner, H. (1972): Bioassay and toxicology of TRH: *Front.
Horm. Res.,* 1:11–21.

81. Plotnikoff, N. P., Prange, A. J., Jr., Breese, G. R., Anderson, M. A., and Wilson,
I. C. (1972): Thyrotropin releasing hormone: Enhancement of DOPA activity
by a hypothalamic hormone. *Science,* 178:417–418.

82. Plotnikoff, N. P., Breese, G. R., and Prange, A. J., Jr. (1975): Thyrotropin
releasing hormone (TRH): DOPA potentiation and biogenic amine studies.
Pharmacol. Biochem. Behav., 3:665–670.

83. Porter, C. C., Lotti, V. J., and De Felice, M. J. (1977): The effect of TRH and
a related tripeptide, L-N-(2-oxopiperidin-6-YL-carbonyl)-L-histidyl-L-thiazolidine-
4-carboxamide (MK-771, OHT), on the depressant action of barbiturates and
alcohol in mice and rats. *Life Sci.,* 21:811–820.

84. Prange, A. J., Jr., and Wilson, I. C. (1972): Thyrotropin-releasing hormone
(TRH) for the immediate relief of depression: A preliminary report. *Psychopharmacologia,* 26:82.

85. Prange, A. J., Jr., Wilson, I. C., Lara, P. P., Alltop, L. B., and Breese, G. R.
(1972): Effects of thyrotropin-releasing hormone in depression. *Lancet,* 2:999–
1002.

86. Prange, A. J., Jr., Wilson, I. C., Lynn, C. W., Alltop, L. B., and Stikeleather,
R. A. (1974): L-Tryptophan in mania: Contribution to a permissive hypothesis of
affective disorders. *Arch. Gen. Psychiatry,* 5:56–62.

87. Prange, A. J., Jr., Breese, G. R., Cott, J. M., Martin, B. R., Cooper, B. R.,
Wilson, I. C., and Plotnikoff, N. P. (1974): Thyrotropin-releasing hormone:
Antagonism of pentobarbital in rodents. *Life Sci.,* 14:447–455.

88. Prange, A. J., Jr., Breese, G. R., Jahnke, G. D., Martin, B. R., Cooper, B. R.,
Cott, J. M., Wilson, I. C., Alltop, L. B., Lipton, M. A., Bissette, G., Nemeroff,
C. B., and Loosen, P. T. (1975): Modification of pentobarbital effects by natural
and synthetic polypeptides: Dissociation of brain and pituitary effects. *Life Sci.,*
16:1907–1914.

89. Prange, A. J., Jr., Breese, G. R., Jahnke, G. D., Cooper, B. R., Cott, J. M.,
Wilson, I. C., Lipton, M. A., and Plotnikoff, N. P. (1975): Parameters of alteration of pentobarbital response by hypothalamic polypeptides. *Neuropsychobiology,*
1:121–131.

90. Prange, A. J., Jr. (1976): Patterns of pituitary responses to thyrotropin releasing hormone in depressed patients: a review. In: *Phenomenology and Treatment of Depression,* edited by W. E. Fann, I. Karacan, A. Pikorny, and R. L. Williams, pp. 1–15. Spectrum, New York.
91. Prange, A. J., Jr., Nemeroff, C. B., Lipton, M. A., Breese, G. R., and Wilson, I. C. (1978): Peptides and the central nervous system. In: *Handbook of Pharmacology,* edited by L. L. Iversen, S. D. Iversen, and S. H. Snyder, pp. 1–107. Plenum Press, New York.
92. Prange, A. J., Jr., Nemeroff, C. B., and Lipton, M. A. (1978): Behavioral effects of peptides: basic and clinical studies. In: *Psychopharmacology: A Generation of Progress,* edited by M. A. Lipton, A. DiMascio, and K. F. Killam, pp. 441–448. Raven Press, New York.
93. Prange, A. J., Jr., Nemeroff, C. B., and Loosen, P. T. Behavioral effects of hypothalamic peptides. In: *Centrally Acting Peptides,* edited by J. Hughes, pp. 99–118. The MacMillan Press, Basingstoke, England.
94. Prasad, C., Matsui, T., and Peterkofsy, A. (1977): Antagonism of ethanol narcosis by histidyl-proline diketopiperazine. *Nature (Lond),* 268:142–144.
95. Rastogi, R. B. (1978): Involvement of brain aminergic systems in the pharmacology of TRH. (*This volume*).
96. Re, R. N., Kourides, I. A., Ridgeway, E. C., Weintraub, B. D., and Maloof, F. (1976): The effect of glucocorticoid administration on human pituitary secretion of thyrotropin and prolactin. *J. Clin. Endocrinol. Metab.,* 43:338.
97. Renaud, L. P. (1978): Effects of hypothalamic hormones on central neuronal excitability. (*This volume*).
98. Schenkel-Hulliger, L., Koella, E. P., Hartmann, A., and Maitre, L. (1974): Tremorogenic effects of thyrotropin releasing hormone in rats. *Experientia,* 30:1168–1170.
99. Simonin, R., Heim, M., Vagneur, J. P., Seban, P., and Sanmarco, J. L. (1976): Influence d'une aggression psychique aegire sur le taox sanguin du TRH chez le sujet normal. *Ann. Endocrinol. (Paris),* 37:311–312.
100. Smith, J. R., La Hann, T. R., Chesnut, R. M., Carino, M. A., and Horita, A. (1977): Thyrotropin-releasing hormone: Stimulation of colonic activity following intracerebroventricular administration. *Science,* 196:660–662.
101. Snyder, S. H. (1973): Amphetamine psychosis: A "model" schizophrenia mediated by catecholamines. *Am. J. Psychiatry,* 130:61–67.
102. Stille, G. (1953): Die bedeutung zentralerregender wurkunen fur die hemming des electrokrampfes. *Naunyn Schmiedebergs Arch. Pharmacol.,* 217:57.
103. Swinyard, E. A. (1972): Electrically induced convulsions. In: *Experimental Models of Epilepsy,* edited by D. M. Purpura, J. K. Penry, D. B. Tower, D. M. Woodburg, and R. D. Walter, pp. 434–458. Raven Press, New York.
104. Tache, Y., Du Ruisseau, P., Ducharme, J. R., and Collu, R. (1977): Antagonism of pentobarbital-induced hormonal changes by TRH in rats. *Eur. J. Pharmacol.,* 45:369–376.
105. Takahashi, S., Kondo, H., Yoshimura, M., and Ochi, Y. (1974): Thyrotropin responses to TRH in depressive illness: Relation to clinical subtypes and prolonged duration of depressive episode. *Folia Psychiatr. Neurol. Jpn.,* 28:335–365.
106. Tiwary, G. M., Rosenbloom, A. L., Robertson, M. F., and Parker, J. C. (1975): Effects of thyrotropin releasing hormone in minimal brain dysfunction. *Pediatrics,* 56:119–121.
107. Tsuang, M. T., and Winokur, G. (1974): Criteria for subtyping schizophrenia. *Arch. Gen. Psychiatry,* 31:43–47.
108. Tyndel, M. (1974): Psychiatric study of 1,000 alcoholic patients. *Can. Psychiatr. Assoc. J.,* 19:21–24.
109. Vale, W., and Rivier, C. (1975): Hypothalamic hypophysiotropic hormones. In: *Handbook of Psychopharmacology,* edited by L. L. Iversen, S. D. Iversen, and S. H. Snyder, pp. 195–238. Plenum Press, New York.
110. Vale, W., Rivier, C., Rivier, J., and Brown, M. (1978): Adenohypophysial and other extra-central nervous system roles of hypothalamic regulatory peptides. In:

Psychopharmacology: A Generation of Progress, edited by M. A. Lipton, A. DiMascio, and K. F. Killam, pp. 403–421. Raven Press, New York.

111. Vijayan, E., and McCann, S. M. (1977): Suppression of feeding and drinking activity in rats following intraventricular injection of thyrotropin releasing hormone (TRH). *Endocrinology,* 100:1727–1730.

112. Vinik, A. I., Kalt, W. J., McLaren, H., Hendricks, S., and Pimstone, B. L. (1975): Fasting blunts the TSH response to synthetic thyrotropin releasing hormone (TRH). *J. Clin. Endocrinol. Metab.,* 40:509.

113. Wei, E., Sigel, S., Loh, H., and Way, E. L. (1975): Thyrotropin-releasing hormone and shaking behavior in rat. *Nature (Lond),* 253:739–740.

114. Wei, E., Loh, H., and Way, E. L. (1976): Potency of the N^{31m}-methyl analog of TRH in the reduction of shaking movements in the rat. *Eur. J. Pharmacol.,* 36:227–229.

115. Weingold, H. P., Lachin, I. M., and Bell, A. H. (1968): Depression as a symptom of alcoholism. *J. Abnorm. Psychol.,* 72:195–197.

116. White, R. P., and Beale, J. S. (1975): Electroencephalographic (EEG) effects of thyrotropin releasing hormone on rabbits. *Neurosci. Abst.,* 1:727.

117. Whybrow, P. C., Coppen, A., Prange, A. J., Jr., Noguera, R., and Bailey, J. E. (1972): Thyroid function and the response to liothyronine in depression. *Arch. Gen. Psychiatry,* 26:242–245.

118. Wilson, I. C., Lara, P. P., and Prange, A. J., Jr. (1973): Thyrotropin releasing hormone in schizophrenia. *Lancet,* 2:43–44.

119. Wilson, I. C., Prange, A. J., Jr., Lara, P. P., Alltop, L. B., Stikeleather, R. A., and Lipton, M. A. (1973): TRH (lopremone): psychobiological responses of normal women. I. Subjective experience. *Arch. Gen. Psychiatry,* 29:15–32.

120. Wilson, I. C., Loosen, P. T., Ghate, V. R., Stikeleather, R. A., and Prange, A. J., Jr. (1978): Thyrotropin releasing hormone (TRH) in schizophrenia. *Arch. Gen. Psychiatry (in press).*

121. Winokur, A., and Utiger, R. D. (1974): Thyrotropin-releasing hormone: Regional distribution in rat brain. *Science,* 185:265–266.

122. Winokur, A., Davis, R., and Utiger, R. D. (1977): Subcellular distribution of thyrotropin-releasing hormone (TRH) in rat brain and hypothalamus. *Brain Res.,* 120:423–434.

123. Winokur, A., and Utiger, R. D. (1978): Distribution and degradation of TRH in central nervous system. (*This volume*).

124. Winokur, G., Cadoret, R., Dorzab, I., and Baker, M. (1971): Depressive disease: A genetic study. *Arch. Gen. Psychiatry,* 24:135–144.

125. Woodruff, R. A., Guze, S. B., and Clayton, P. J. (1973): Alcoholism and depression. *Arch. Gen. Psychiatry,* 28:97–100.

126. Youngblood, W. W., Lipton, M. A., and Kizer, J. S. (1978): TRH-like immunoreactivity in urine, serum and extrahypothalamic brain: Nonidentity with synthetic pGlu-His-Pro-NH₂. *Brain Res.,* 151:99–116.

Central Nervous System Effects of Hypothalamic Hormones and Other Peptides, edited by Collu et al. Raven Press, New York © 1979.

Hormonal Effects Exerted by TRH Through the Central Nervous System

R. Collu and Y. Taché

Centre de Recherche Pédiatrique, Hôpital Sainte-Justine and Université de Montréal, Montréal, Québec H3T 1C5 Canada

Until very recently hypothalamic hormones such as luteinizing hormone-releasing hormone (LH-RH), thyrotropin-releasing hormone (TRH), and growth hormone-release inhibiting factor (GIF or somatostatin) were thought to be present only in a small area of the brain and their roles limited to direct control of the anterior pituitary function. However, during the last few years more and more evidence has been accumulating to support the fact that these peptides are widely distributed not only in the brain but in the whole body (for review see ref. 33) and that they exert effects unrelated to their direct action on the anterior pituitary gland (for review see ref. 28).

In particular, TRH has been shown to modify, in intact as well as in thyroidectomized animals, the behavioral effects of centrally acting drugs and to have antidepressant properties in patients with unipolar mental depression (for review see Prange et al., *this volume*). Since several drugs such as pentobarbital (PB), morphine (M), and endorphins are capable of stimulating the secretion of growth hormone (GH) and prolactin (PRL) through a central nervous system (CNS) mechanism, it became of interest to verify whether TRH could also antagonize these hormonal changes. This was indeed the case, and results obtained in animals allowed us to elaborate a theory concerning the mechanism of abnormal hormonal responses observed in certain human pathologies following the administration of TRH.

ANTAGONISM OF PB-INDUCED GH AND PRL RELEASE

Results

Several experiments were performed with adult male rats in order to study the effects of TRH on PB-induced hormonal changes. In the first experiment, represented in Fig. 1, TRH 10 μg administered into a lateral ventricle of the brain (i.v.t.) through a chronic cannula 5 min prior to PB anesthesia (50 mg/kg i.p.) was able to block the stimulatory effect of PB on GH secre-

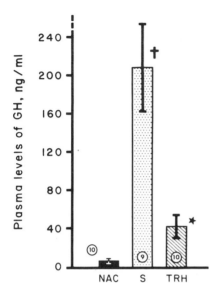

FIG. 1. Plasma GH levels in rats injected i.v.t. with either saline (S) or TRH (10 μg/rat) and anesthetized with PB. A group of animals injected with saline was not anesthetized (NAC). Columns are means ± SE. Number of rats per group are indicated at the bottom of each column. (* = p < 0.01 versus saline; † = p < 0.01 versus NAC.) (From ref. 15.)

tion. This was verified by measuring GH in plasma obtained by decapitation 15 min after PB injection. As shown in Fig. 2, PB-induced PRL secretion was also blocked by TRH. When a dose-response curve was established for these effects (Fig. 3; Table 1) it was readily apparent that PB-induced PRL secretion was much more sensitive to the antagonizing action of TRH, since doses as low as 5 ng were still effective, whereas only the highest doses (5 and 10 μg) could block PB-induced GH release.

Several analogs of TRH bearing modifications of the molecule at position 1, 2, or 3 and completely devoid of TSH-releasing action were tested in the system (Tables 1 through 3). Several were found to be effective PB antagonists. Once again PRL secretion appeared to be more sensitive to the antagonizing action since several analogs were effective in antagonizing PB-induced PRL secretion only, and when both secretions were antagonized the effect on PRL was about twice as potent as on GH release.

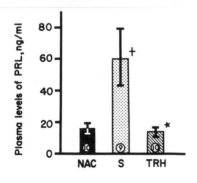

FIG. 2. Effect of TRH injected i.v.t. (10 μg/rat in 20 μl saline) on PB-induced secretion of PRL in male rats. See legend to Fig. 1 for experimental protocol and definition of symbols and abbreviations. (* = p < 0.01 versus saline; † = p < 0.01 versus NAC.) (From ref. 14.)

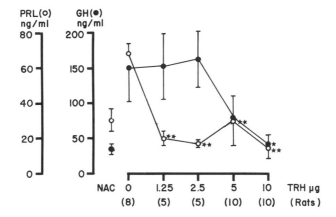

FIG. 3. Effect of decreasing amounts of TRH (μg/rat in 20 μl saline, i.v.t.) on plasma levels of PRL and GH in PB-anesthetized male rats. Animals were decapitated 15 min after PB and 20 min after TRH or saline. Hormone levels of animals injected with saline and not anesthetized (NAC) are also represented. Significant differences from control animals (TRH 0 μg) are represented as $^*p < 0.05$, $^{**}p < 0.01$ (one-way analysis of variance). Number of animals is shown in parentheses. (From ref. 14.)

In order to verify the specificity of TRH antagonizing action, two other hypothalamic factors, MIF-1 (pro-leu-gly-NH$_2$) and LH-RH, were tested in the same system. As shown in Table 4, only the release of PRL was antagonized by LH-RH.

In a final experiment designed to try to identify the mechanism of TRH-antagonizing action, groups of rats were treated either with α-methyl-*p*-

TABLE 1. *Effects of decreasing amounts of TRH and (1,3'-DCM²)TRH on plasma PRL levels in PB-anesthetized rats*

Treatment[a]	No. of rats	PRL[b] (ng/ml)
Saline	10	101 ± 12
TRH (ng/rat)		
500	5	15 ± 5[c]
250	5	23 ± 11[c]
10	5	53 ± 10[d]
5	4	57 ± 13[d]
1	4	75 ± 23
(1,3'-DCM²)TRH (ng/rat)		
50	8	37 ± 15[c]
25	5	75 ± 14
10	5	79 ± 27

From ref. 60.

[a] The rats were anesthetized with PB (50 mg/kg i.p.) 5 min after intraventricular injection of the test materials, and decapitated 15 min later.

[b] Mean ± SE.

[c] $p < 0.01$, [d] $p < 0.05$, compared with saline-treated controls.

TABLE 2. *Effects of TRH analogs on PB-induced GH and PRL release in rats*

Treatment[a]	No. of rats	GH (ng/ml)[b]	PRL (ng/ml)
Saline	15	109 ± 20	107 ± 10
TRH (p-Glu-His-Pro-NH$_2$)	10	42 ± 11^c	14 ± 3^c
TRH analogs			
Position 1 modification			
β-Ala-His-Pro-NH$_2$	5	79 ± 14	63 ± 22^d
Glu (OMe)-His-Pro-NH$_2$	5	98 ± 31	44 ± 22^c
0 = < Thr-His-Pro-NH$_2$	5	48 ± 13^d	17 ± 2^d
	5	50 ± 7^d	18 ± 2^c

Position 2 modification			
p-Glu-His (1,3'-DCM)-Pro-NH$_2$	5	24 ± 7^c	13 ± 4^c
Position 3 modification			
p-Glu-His-NHEt	4	103 ± 28	72 ± 20
p-Glu-His-N(Et)$_2$	5	80 ± 20	31 ± 15^c

p-Glu-His-N—C—NH$_2$	5	117 ± 23	93 ± 25

From ref. 60.

[a] The rats were anesthetized with PB (50 mg/kg i.p.) 5 min after intraventricular injection of the test materials (10 μg/rat) or saline (10 μl/rat), and decapitated 15 min later.

[b] Mean $\pm$ SE.

[c] $p < 0.01$, [d] $p < 0.05$, compared with saline-treated controls.

TABLE 3. *Effects of TRH analog on PB-induced PRL and GH release*

Treatment[a]	Dose (μg/rat)	GH (ng/ml)	PRL (ng/ml)
Saline		146 ± 69^b	107 ± 23
O=⟨pyridone⟩—C—His-Pro-NH$_2$	1	65 ± 26	12 ± 3^c
	0.5	65 ± 21	10 ± 2^c
	0.1	62 ± 18	16 ± 5^c

[a] Adult male rats were injected with PB (50 mg/kg i.p.) 5 min after intraventricular injection of various doses of TRH analog and decapitated 15 min later.

[b] Mean $\pm$ SE (six rats per group).

[c] $p < 0.001$ compared with saline-treated controls.

TABLE 4. *Effects of MIF and LH-RH on plasma levels of GH and PRL in PB-anesthetized rats*

Group	Treatment[a]	No. of rats	GH (ng/ml)	PRL (ng/ml)
1	Saline	7	13 ± 2[b]	49 ± 14
2	Saline + PB	8	340 ± 98[c]	167 ± 20[c]
3	MIF + PB	8	179 ± 33	157 ± 15
4	LHRH + PB	8	342 ± 102	60 ± 21[c]

[a] Rats were anesthetized with PB (50 mg/kg i.p.) 5 min after intraventricular injection of releasing factors (10 µg/rat) or saline (10 µl/rat) and decapitated 15 min later.
[b] Mean ± SE.
[c] $p < 0.001$ compared with group 2 or (in parentheses) group 1.

tyrosine (α-MT) (25 mg/100 g body weight, i.p.), an inhibitor of CNS catecholamine synthesis, or with *p*-chlorophenylalanine (PCPA) (31.6 mg/100 g i.p.), an inhibitor of CNS serotonin synthesis, respectively 4 hr, and 72 hr plus 48 hr prior to treatment with TRH (1 mg/100 g i.p.) and PB. As shown in Fig. 4, in rats pretreated with PCPA, TRH was unable to antagonize the PB-induced release of GH and PRL. Treatment with α-MT also partially reversed the antagonizing effect of TRH on PRL, but this could be due to the well-known stimulatory effect of α-MT on PRL secretion through suppression of the inhibitory dopaminergic tonus (66).

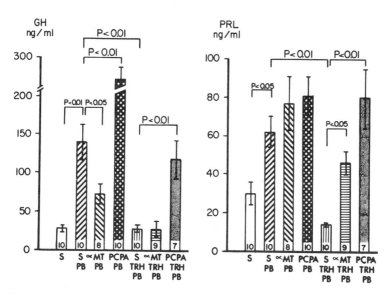

FIG. 4. Effects of α-MT and PCPA on inhibition by TRH of PB-induced GH and PRL release. The columns represent the mean ± SE. The significance of differences between the groups is expressed over the brackets (one-way analysis of variance). The number of animals in each group is shown at the base of each column. (S) Saline. (PB) Pentobarbital. (α-MT) Methyl-*p*-tyrosine. (PCPA) *p*-Chlorophenylalanine. (TRH) Thyrotropin-releasing hormone. (GH) Growth hormone. (PRL) Prolactin. (From ref. 60.)

Discussion

It is now well established that TRH is capable of inducing the release of PRL as well as GH through a direct action on the anterior pituitary gland (9,62,63). However, increasing evidence indicates that TRH antagonism of PB-induced hormonal changes represents a central mechanism, as indicated by its ineffectiveness in rats bearing lesions of the ventromedian hypothalamic nucleus or a surgically isolated mediobasal hypothalamus (44), or when it is added to anterior pituitary incubates *in vitro* (8). Secondly, TRH is incapable of antagonizing *in vivo* and *in vitro* prostaglandin E_2-induced GH release, an effect exerted directly on the pituitary gland (8). Finally, although TRH appears to be the most potent antagonist, several TRH analogs devoid of TSH-releasing action, and therefore presumably incapable of a direct pituitary influence, were also effective antagonists.

Some authors have reported that TRH induced a GH release when injected intravenously in rats anesthetized with urethane (10) and in cows (20). However, it is now clear that this effect again represents a direct action of TRH on the pituitary gland since the release of GH is enhanced in rats bearing a disconnection between the CNS and the anterior pituitary gland by either transplantation of the pituitary (50) or hypothalamic lesions (47), and is absent in calves injected intraventricularly with TRH (30).

These data indicate (Fig. 5) that TRH may influence the secretion of GH and PRL via two routes. A direct action on the pituitary gland—probably

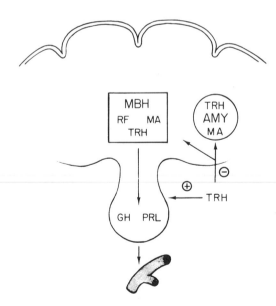

FIG. 5. Hypothetical pathways that peripherally administered TRH may follow to modify pituitary hormone secretion. (+) Stimulation. (−) Inhibition. (AMY) Amygdala. (MA) Monoamines. (MBH) Mediobasal hypothalamus. (RF) Hypothalamic releasing and release-inhibiting factors.

exerted on specific lactotroph receptors for PRL and on nonspecific somato-troph receptors for GH—results in the release of GH and PRL. The in-direct, CNS-mediated pathway exerts an inhibitory influence on the secretion of both hormones. Which effect prevails depends on the route of TRH ad-ministration and on the amount of TRH reaching central inhibitory mech-anisms. The nature of the latter is still unknown, although data obtained by us and others indicate that CNS monoaminergic pathways may be impli-cated. As extensively reviewed by Rastogi and by Horst et al. in this volume, brain aminergic systems are involved in the pharmacological effects of TRH.

The β-adrenergic receptor blocker propranolol was shown by us to be able to reverse the inhibitory effect of TRH on PB-induced GH (15) but not PRL release (14). Indeed central β-adrenergic receptors are known to exert an inhibitory influence on GH secretion in rats (17) and humans (13,18), and a stimulatory one on PRL release (39). The catecholamine de-pletor α-MT (57) did not modify the antagonistic action of TRH on GH secretion induced by PB but significantly reversed the inhibitory effect of the tripeptide on PRL release, as shown by the present data. Depletion of brain serotonin levels by PCPA, a blocker of serotonin synthesis at the tryptophan hydroxylase step (36), antagonized the inhibitory effect of TRH on PB-induced GH and PRL release. In agreement with these findings, it was recently reported that the analeptic effect of TRH is markedly attenu-ated in PCPA-pretreated, PB-anesthetized rabbits (31). Interestingly, the release of GH, but not PRL, was enhanced by pretreatment with PCPA.

These data indicate that both catecholaminergic and serotonergic central inhibitory pathways are implicated in the antagonistic effect of TRH on GH and PRL release induced by PB. However, further studies are needed to verify whether monoamines in turn activate hypothalamic inhibitory factors such as GIF and PIF. Data obtained by Brown and Vale (8) seem to exclude the participation of GIF, since prostaglandin E_2-induced release of GH—an effect exerted directly on the pituitary gland—was not suppressed by the administration of TRH *in vivo,* whereas the injection of GIF was highly effective in this respect. This was confirmed by very recent data obtained in our laboratory which show that the inhibitory action of TRH is not abolished by the prior injection of anti-GIF antiserum. Ferland et al. (25) recently published results indicating that PB may exert its GH-releasing activity through activation of a hypothalamic GH-releasing factor (GH-RF). It is possible therefore that the antagonizing property of TRH is finally exerted through inhibition of a GH-RF.

TRH is present in high and fluctuating concentrations in the brain of mammals, not only in the hypothalamus where it presumably plays the physiological role of directly stimulating the release of TSH and PRL but also in other areas such as the limbic system (16; Jackson et al., *this vol-ume;* Winokur et al., *this volume*)—which has been implicated in the control of diverse biological phenomena such as emotionality, hormone regulation, learning, sleep, and awakening (24). Because of this, it may be hypothesized that extrahypothalamic TRH may indirectly intervene in such plasma GH and PRL changes as those observed during nyctohemeral cycles in rats and humans (6,64) and during stress (22,59).

ANTAGONISM OF MORPHINE AND β-ENDORPHIN-INDUCED HORMONE RELEASE

Results

Morphine (M), a CNS depressant, is a powerful releaser of GH and PRL (8,14,55). As for PB the mechanism of M-induced hormone release is still unknown, but (again as for PB) its site of action is probably located in the CNS. In effect, M does not release GH *in vitro* (8), and its releasing effect *in vivo* is impaired in rats bearing hypothalamic ventromedial lesions (45). In view of these considerations, it was deemed of interest to verify whether TRH was capable of also antagonizing M-induced GH and PRL release. Several experiments were performed for this purpose in adult male rats. In the first experiment we used rats bearing (a) a chronic jugular catheter that allowed withdrawal of blood samples without disturbing the animal and (b) a chronic intraventricular cannula. As shown in Fig. 6, the intraventricular injection of TRH 10 μg alone induced a decrease of plasma GH levels, which remained very low (around 20 ng/ml) for 30 min and returned to

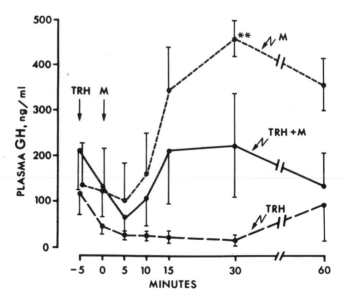

FIG. 6. Plasma GH response to TRH, M, or TRH + M in male rats bearing a chronic jugular catheter. Five rats were utilized in each group. Values are means ± SEM. ** p < 0.01 compared with values at time −5 min (one-way analysis of variance).

base line after 60 min. However, by one-way analysis of variance, no statistically significant variation could be identified. The injection of M (10 mg/kg i.v.) induced a large increase in GH levels, which reached a significant peak at 30 min. When the injection of M was preceded by the intraventricular injection of TRH (10 μg), no statistically significant GH increment could be found by analysis of variance.

Plasma PRL levels increased readily after the administration of TRH, reaching a peak at 5 min (Fig. 7). M was a more potent stimulus since PRL values climbed higher and remained elevated longer than with TRH. Pretreatment with TRH only partially prevented the M-stimulating effect.

In a subsequent experiment (Table 5), the effects of decreasing amounts of TRH were studied in rats sacrificed by decapitation 15 min after the administration of M and 20 min after the intraventricular injection of the peptide. In this model, TRH was highly effective in antagonizing M-induced GH release, whereas PRL release was unmodified. Three TRH analogs devoid of TSH-releasing action were tested in the same model and were found to be able to antagonize GH but not PRL release, although in this particular experiment PRL values did not reach high levels after M administration. Two of the analogs were found to be about 10 times more active M antagonists than TRH (Table 6).

As with PB, an experiment was performed to try to verify whether central monoaminergic pathways were involved in the antagonizing property of TRH.

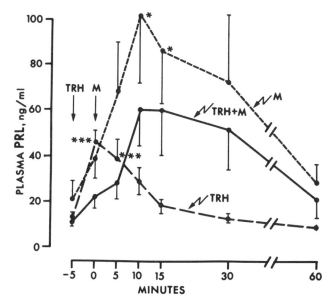

FIG. 7. Plasma PRL response to TRH, M, or TRH + M in male rats bearing a chronic jugular catheter. Five rats were utilized in each group. Values are means ± SEM. * $p < 0.05$, *** $p < 0.001$ compared with values at time −5 min (one-way analysis of variance).

TABLE 5. *Effects of decreasing amounts of TRH on plasma GH and PRL levels in morphine-treated rats*

Treatment[a]	No. of rats	GH (ng/ml)	PRL (ng/ml)
Saline	14	793 ± 90[b]	134 ± 30
TRH 10 μg	8	199 ± 75[c]	101 ± 16
TRH 1 μg	8	295 ± 136[c]	80 ± 27
TRH 500 ng	8	536 ± 201	111 ± 22

[a] The rats were injected with morphine (10 mg/kg i.p.) 5 min after the intraventricular injection of various doses of TRH, and decapitated 15 min later.
[b] Mean ± SE.
[c] $p < 0.01$ compared with saline (analysis of variance).

As shown in Table 7, TRH was unable to antagonize M-induced GH release in rats pretreated with the serotonin depletor PCPA. Once again, the release of PRL was not antagonized by TRH even in rats not pretreated with PCPA. As with PB, M-induced GH release but not PRL release was significantly enhanced by pretreatment with PCPA.

The endogenous opioid peptide β-endorphin (β-LPH61–91) was also recently shown to be a potent releaser of GH and PRL through a CNS mechanism (53,61; Dupont et al., *this volume*). As shown in Table 8, the intraventricular injection of TRH 10 μg 5 min prior to the administration of β-endorphin (50 μg, i.v.t.) completely blocked the release of GH, as measured in a blood sample obtained by decapitation 15 min after β-endorphin.

TABLE 6. *Effects of decreasing amounts of TRH analog on morphine-induced hormonal changes in rats*

Treatment[a] (μg/rat)		No. of rats	GH (ng/ml)	PRL (ng/ml)
Saline		18	363 ± 33[b]	47 ± 7
O=⟨ Thr-His-Pro-NH₂	10	7	67 ± 32[c]	62 ± 13
	10	7	7 ± 1[c]	48 ± 19
	1	6	19 ± 4[c]	39 ± 14
	0.5	7	23 ± 5[c]	27 ± 9
C-His-Pro-NH₂	0.1	6	199 ± 70[d]	26 ± 13
[1,3'-DCM²⁻]TRH	10	7	12 ± 3[c]	44 ± 10
	1	7	35 ± 7[c]	35 ± 11
	0.5	7	125 ± 66[d]	49 ± 7
	0.1	7	364 ± 58	54 ± 15

[a] The rats were injected with morphine (10 mg/kg i.p.) 5 min after the intraventricular injection of test materials, and decapitated 15 min later.
[b] Mean ± SE.
[c] $p < 0.001$, [d] $p < 0.01$, compared with saline-treated controls (one-way analysis of variance).

TABLE 7. *Effects of PCPA on inhibition by TRH of morphine-induced hormonal changes*

Group	Treatment[a]	GH (ng/ml)	PRL (ng/ml)
1	Saline-saline-M	563 ± 101[b]	155 ± 31
2	Saline + TRH + M	48 ± 12[c]	121 ± 26
3	PCPA + saline + M	1,483 ± 206[d]	95 ± 20
4	PCPA + TRH + M	507 ± 174[c]	103 ± 29

[a] Adult male rats were pretreated with saline or PCPA (31.6 mg/100 g i.p.) 72 and 48 hr prior to saline or TRH (10 μg in 10 μl saline intraventricularly). All groups were injected with morphine (M) (10 mg/kg i.p.) 5 min after TRH or saline administration and decapitated 15 min later.

[b] Means ± SE (eight rats per group).

[c] $p < 0.05$, [d] $p < 0.001$, compared with group 1 or (in parentheses) group 2.

In contrast, β-endorphin-induced PRL release was enhanced by TRH. Pretreatment of the animals with PCPA prevented the antagonizing action of TRH on GH release but not the enhancing effect on PRL release.

In vitro experiments performed in collaboration with Lis (61) and shown in Fig. 8 allowed us, however, to exclude the existence of an interaction TRH-β-endorphin at the opiate receptor level, since TRH did not displace the binding of ³H-naloxone to rat brain homogenates or affect the displacement by β-endorphin of such binding.

Discussion

As previously discussed for TRH antagonism of PB-induced GH and PRL release, the mechanism of TRH antagonism of M- and β-endorphin-induced GH release is probably localized in the CNS and is another example of the analeptic properties of the tripeptide. As recently shown by us (61), some behavioral effects of β-endorphin are also antagonized by TRH. No explanation can be offered at the present time for the lack of antagonizing effect and the enhancing action of TRH on M- and β-endorphin-induced

TABLE 8. *Effects of PCPA and TRH on opioid peptide-induced modifications of GH and PRL secretion*

Treatment	No. of rats	PRL (ng/ml)	GH (ng/ml)
Saline	8	11 ± 3	40 ± 15
PCPA	8	23 ± 11	47 ± 26
TRH	8	11 ± 3	20 ± 2
PCPA + TRH	8	13 ± 3	36 ± 15
β-Endorphin	7	145 ± 23[a]	262 ± 85[a]
PCPA + β-endorphin	8	188 ± 26[a]	347 ± 62[a]
TRH + β-endorphin	6	322 ± 48[a(a)]	54 ± 30[b]
PCPA + TRH + β-endorphin	6	303 ± 49[a(a)]	185 ± 73

[a] $p < 0.001$, [b] $p < 0.01$, compared with saline or (in parentheses) β-endorphin.

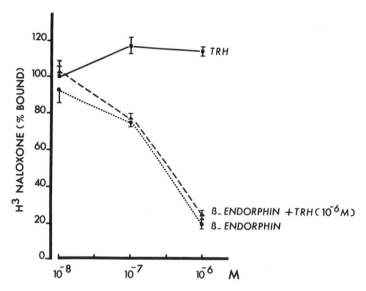

FIG. 8. Influence of various doses of TRH and β-endorphin on specific binding of ³ H-naloxone in rat brain homogenates. (From ref. 61.)

PRL release, respectively. This is the opposite of the effect observed under PB anesthesia, where PRL release is considerably more sensitive than GH release to the inhibitory action of TRH, and may indicate the existence of a basic difference between PB and opiate releasing mechanisms of the two pituitary hormones. As with PB, depletion of brain serotonin levels by PCPA antagonized the inhibitory effect of TRH on M- and β-endorphin-induced GH release, whereas *in vitro* studies eliminated the participation of brain opiate receptors in the antagonism TRH-β-endorphin. These data suggest that brain serotonergic inhibitory pathways are involved in the antagonizing action of TRH on GH release. The existence of an inhibitory serotonergic mechanism of control of GH secretion, evidenced also by the enhancing effect of PCPA pretreatment on GH release induced by PB or M, is contrary to what is currently known about the effects of serotonin on GH release (11). These conflicting results can, however, be reconciled on the basis of a hypothesis accepting the existence in the CNS of both stimulatory and inhibitory serotonin pathways exerting their effects at different brain sites, as already suggested for the control of LH-RH (37) and ACTH (65).

ANTAGONISM OF SUCKLING-INDUCED HORMONE RELEASE

Results

Suckling is a powerful stimulus for the release of PRL and GH (64): we therefore recently verified whether TRH was capable of antagonizing this

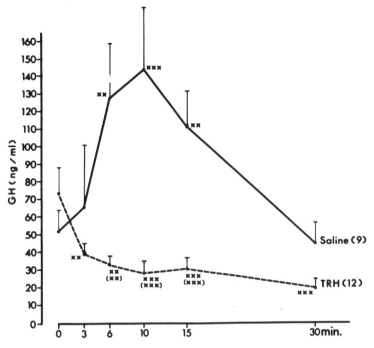

FIG. 9. Plasma GH response to suckling in saline or TRH-pretreated mothers. Saline or TRH was injected i.p. at time 0 min, and the pups were immediately allowed to resume suckling. Values are means ± SEM. Numbers of animals are in parentheses. * $p < 0.05$, ** $p < 0.01$, *** $p < 0.001$ compared with values at time 0 min or (in parentheses) with respective values of saline-pretreated mothers.

effect. For this purpose, primiparous female rats were cannulated in the jugular vein with a chronic catheter allowing the collection of blood samples without disturbing the animal 2 to 7 days following delivery. The experimental procedure was started a few days later when the animals had recovered the initial weight. In the meantime the number of pups was reduced to eight for each mother. On the experimental day the mothers were separated from the pups for 6 hr, saline or TRH (1 mg/100 g body weight, i.p.) was injected at time 0, and the pups were immediately allowed to resume suckling. As shown in Fig. 9, in saline-injected animals suckling induced a rapid and important release of GH, which peaked at 10 min. Pretreatment with TRH not only blocked the stimulatory effect of suckling but induced a significant fall of plasma GH values, which were still lower than base line 30 min later. Plasma PRL values also increased significantly following suckling in saline-pretreated rats and were still rising at the end of the experimental procedure (Fig. 10). Although PRL levels were almost always lower in TRH-pretreated rats, the stimulatory effect of suckling was not clearly antagonized. To verify the effect of TRH in nonsuckled mothers, saline or TRH 10 μg was injected intraventricularly at 0 min but the pups

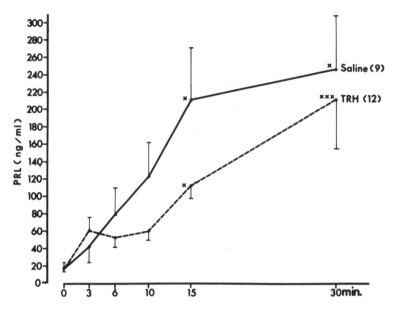

FIG. 10. Plasma PRL response to suckling in saline or TRH-pretreated mothers. Refer to Fig. 9 for experimental protocol and significance of symbols.

were not returned to their mothers. As shown in Fig. 11, injection of saline induced a small but temporary and not significant fall of plasma GH values. In contrast, following the administration of TRH a significant and prolonged reduction of GH levels was observed. The injection of saline was without significant effect on PRL, whereas TRH induced a rapid, important, and prolonged rise of the hormone values (Fig. 12).

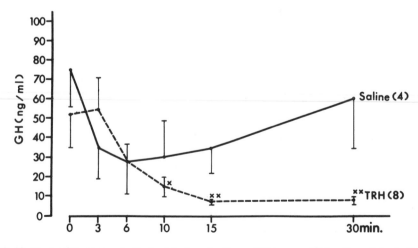

FIG. 11. Plasma GH response to the i.p. injection of saline or TRH in nonsuckled mothers. Refer to Fig. 9 for significance of symbols.

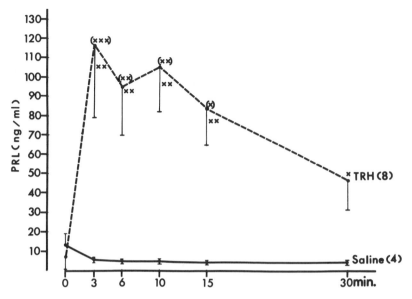

FIG. 12. Plasma PRL response to the i.p. injection of saline or TRH in nonsuckled mothers. Refer to Fig. 9 for significance of symbols.

Discussion

Although the mechanism of suckling-induced PRL (and also GH) rise is far from being completely elucidated, CNS serotonergic pathways seem to be implicated (46), whereas hypothalamic TRH apparently has no physiological role in this respect (4). Therefore TRH antagonism of suckling-induced GH release is another example of the inhibitory effect exerted by the tripeptide probably through central monoaminergic mechanisms. In this preparation the inhibitory property of peripherally administered TRH on GH secretion was clearly apparent also in nonsuckled mothers. In these, however, PRL secretion was stimulated. This indicates that on this animal model—probably secondary to hormonal sensitization of lactotroph receptors (38)—the direct stimulatory effect exerted by small amounts of TRH reaching the pituitary largely prevails over the centrally exerted inhibitory action. Incidentally, this may explain why in male rats a small PRL rise may or may not follow the peripheral administration of the peptide depending on the amount injected (*unpublished observations*). This may also explain why no antagonism of suckling-induced PRL rise was clearly evidenced. However, if one considers the fact that these two stimuli are exerted through different mechanisms, an enhancing effect should have resulted from the combined action of suckling and TRH. In contrast, in TRH-administered and suckled mothers PRL values were at best equivalent to those of TRH-administered, nonsuckled mothers for the first 15 min, and only after 30 min were they significantly higher. This may indicate that during suckling

TRH exerts an inhibitory influence also on PRL release through an extrapituitary site of action.

ABNORMAL PITUITARY HORMONE RESPONSE TO TRH: AN INDEX OF CNS DYSFUNCTION

TRH is capable of inducing the release of TSH and PRL in normal men (5,34). Although base-line plasma GH levels are not modified (1,49), the release induced by L-DOPA, arginine, and insulin is inhibited (40,41).

A paradoxical rise of plasma GH levels has been reported to occur following the administration of TRH in patients suffering from various disorders, such as acromegaly or gigantism (32,54), renal failure (27), mental depression (42), anorexia nervosa (43), and chronic liver disease (51,67). No clear-cut explanation for the inhibitory effect in normal subjects and the paradoxical stimulation of GH secretion in various pathological states has yet been provided.

We recently had the opportunity to study the pituitary response to TRH in children with primary hypothyroidism and in normal volunteers treated with a blocker of serotonergic receptors. Based on results obtained in these two conditions, as well as on previously reported clinical and experimental data, we propose that an abnormal pituitary response to TRH may be considered as an index of CNS dysfunction.

Results

Pituitary Response to TRH in Children with Primary Hypothyroidism

TRH (7 μg/kg i.v.) was given as a bolus to 11 children with clinical and laboratory evidence of untreated primary hypothyroidism (8 females and 3 males, age 5 to 16 years) and to 7 euthyroid children (4 females and 3 males, age 5 to 16 years) who underwent investigation for dwarfism later found to be of nonendocrine origin. Four hypothyroid children were also tested with LH-RH (100 μg i.v.) for delayed puberty.

GH response to TRH in euthyroid children is shown in Fig. 13. None had a significant increment of plasma GH levels as defined by an increase to at least twice the base-line levels and greater than 5 ng/ml. Actually, GH values decreased in all subjects, although statistical significance was not reached. In 7 of the 11 hypothyroid children, a significant GH increment was observed between 10 and 60 min. Figure 14 shows the mean GH values of the 7 responders, with a significant mean peak being reached at 30 min. None of the 4 hypothyroid children tested with LH-RH had a significant GH increment, although all of them had a paradoxical response to TRH (Fig. 14). PRL response to TRH is shown in Fig. 15. Base-line values were significantly higher

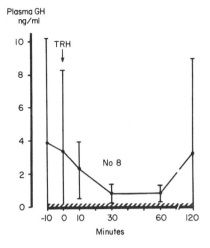

FIG. 13. Plasma GH response to TRH in seven euthyroid children. Each point represents the mean ± SD. (From ref. 19.)

in hypothyroid children, and the response to TRH was greatly enhanced, PRL levels remaining at a plateau between 10 and 60 min.

As expected, hypothyroid children had higher TSH base line (mean ± SE: 443 ± 68 versus 4 ± 1 μU/ml, $p < 0.001$) and higher peak values than euthyroid subjects (mean ± SE: 942 ± 221 versus 16 ± 2 μU/ml; $p < 0.001$).

Hypothyroid subjects generally have a poor response to the usual GH

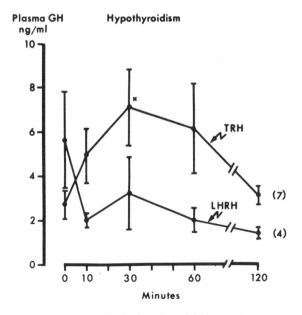

FIG. 14. Plasma GH response to TRH and LH-RH in hypothyroid children. Each point represents the mean ± SEM. * $p < 0.05$ versus 0 min values. (From ref. 19.)

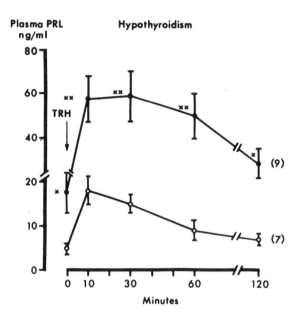

FIG. 15. Plasma PRL response to TRH in euthyroid (○) and hypothyroid children (●). Each point represents the mean ± SEM. * $p < 0.05$, ** $p < 0.01$ versus corresponding values of euthyroid children. (From ref. 19.)

stimuli (7,35); it was surprising therefore to find that 7 of 11 hypothyroid children had a significant increment of plasma GH values following the administration of TRH, particularly since no significant increment but rather a decrease was observed in euthyroid subjects. The paradoxical response to TRH appears to be specific since LH-RH administration was ineffective in 4 children in whom a significant GH increment followed the TRH injection. In accord with these data, Hamada et al. (29) reported an increase in serum GH levels in 6 of 13 adult hypothyroid subjects tested with TRH.

Our results indicate that hypothyroid children have higher base-line PRL levels and a greatly enhanced response to TRH. A higher peak PRL response to TRH but normal base-line levels have been observed in adult subjects with primary hypothyroidism (56). Elevated circulating levels of PRL were documented by Costin et al. (21) in two 8-year-old girls presenting with myxedema and precocious puberty. After treatment of the hypothyroidism, PRL response to TRH and circulating levels returned to normal (21,56).

Pituitary Response to TRH in Normal Volunteers Under Basal Conditions and Following Methysergide

Six healthy male volunteers, age 19 to 28 years, were included in this study. They were tested twice at a 48-hr interval with TRH (100 μg i.v.). After the first TRH test they were given methysergide, a blocker of sero-

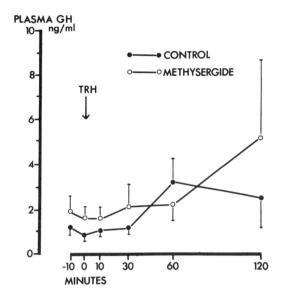

FIG. 16. Plasma GH response to TRH in normal volunteers during either a control period or methysergide administration. Each point represents the mean ± SEM. (From ref. 12.)

tonergic receptors, 2 mg p.o. every 6 hr for 48 hr. Four hours after the last dose of methysergide the second TRH test was performed.

GH response is shown in Fig. 16. Although no statistically significant changes in plasma GH levels occurred after TRH injection either during

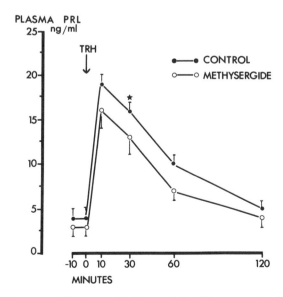

FIG. 17. Plasma PRL response to TRH in normal volunteers during either a control period or methysergide administration. Each point represents the mean ± SEM. * $p < 0.05$ versus the corresponding value of the methysergide period. (From ref. 12.)

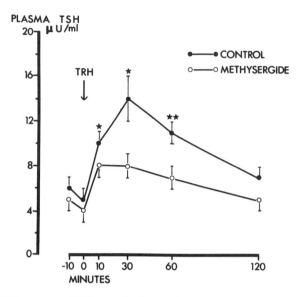

FIG. 18. Plasma TSH response to TRH in normal volunteers during either a control period or methysergide administration. Each point represents the mean ± SEM. * p < 0.05, ** p < 0.01 versus the corresponding value of the methysergide period. (From ref. 12.)

the control or the methysergide period, one volunteer had a peak GH value of 7 ng/ml at 30 min and a second volunteer a peak of 23 ng/ml at 120 min of the second TRH test (under methysergide).

Plasma PRL levels increased after TRH injections; however, the increment was somewhat smaller after methysergide (Fig. 17). TSH response to TRH is shown in Fig. 18. An increment in plasma TSH levels was observed after TRH during the control as well as during the methysergide period. However, a statistically significant reduction in TSH release occurred following the administration of the serotonergic blocker.

The administration of another blocker of serotonergic receptors, cyproheptadine, was also recently reported to antagonize the TRH-induced release of TSH while enhancing the PRL response (23). The discrepancy between data obtained with methysergide and those with cyproheptadine can be explained in terms of differences in pharmacological activities. In effect, cyproheptadine is a less specific drug since it possesses antiserotonergic, antihistaminergic, anticholinergic, and antidopaminergic properties (26,58).

Discussion

As previously mentioned, abnormal pituitary responses to TRH consisting primarily in a paradoxical rise in plasma GH levels have been reported in several unrelated diseases. Primary hypothyroidism may now be added to a lengthening list. Although some authors have suggested that TRH may have a nonspecific GH-releasing effect on a tumoral pituitary gland (32), this mechanism of an abnormal response may hold true only for acromegaly. Indeed, previously discussed experiments showing that TRH may induce changes in plasma pituitary hormone levels acting either directly on the pituitary gland or through a CNS monoaminergic pathway indicate that another mechanism may be responsible for the abnormal pituitary responses in humans. In normal rats, and presumably in normal humans, peripherally administered TRH acts preferentially through the CNS to inhibit the release of GH induced, respectively, by pentobarbital or morphine, and L-DOPA, arginine, or insulin. PRL release is, in contrast, directly activated through pituitary receptors, although the indirect route may exert a limiting influence. In lesioned rats and presumably in subjects suffering from previously mentioned disorders, the TRH indirect route being inoperable, an enhanced release of PRL and/or a paradoxical rise of plasma GH values is observed following intravenous administration of TRH. Several data obtained in humans favor such a hypothesis. Firstly, results obtained in normal volunteers treated with methysergide or cyproheptadine clearly show that alterations of monoaminergic (mainly serotonergic) functions may modify the pituitary response to TRH. This indicates that even in humans an indirect pathway may be implicated in the pituitary response to TRH. In this respect, the enhancement of TRH-induced PRL release following cyproheptadine is particularly interesting since it reproduces the pattern observed in patients with primary hypothyroidism and, more recently, in subjects with severe liver disease (51). Secondly, the existence of a dysfunction of CNS monoaminergic pathways, presumably implicated in the indirect TRH route of pituitary regulation, has been suggested to occur in acromegaly, anorexia nervosa, mental depression, hypothyroidism, and renal failure (2,3,19,52). Interestingly, in hepatic failure, a disturbance of brain serotonin turnover (due to an increased passage of tryptophan, a serotonin precursor) from plasma into the CNS has been postulated (48).

From all these data it can be concluded that an abnormal response to TRH consisting essentially in a paradoxical rise of plasma GH values sometimes associated with an enhanced PRL response may be interpreted as an indication of the existence of a dysfunction of CNS monoaminergic pathways implicated in the regulation of anterior pituitary hormone secretion.

CONCLUSIONS

From the wealth of data accumulated, it can be concluded that TRH is capable of modifying the secretion of GH and PRL acting through an indirect pathway that implicates CNS monoamines. This effect is related to the analeptic properties of the peptide, which are clearly demonstrated by the antagonism of behavioral effects of PB. We have shown that behavioral effects of β-endorphin are also antagonized by TRH; and although no data have been published, to the best of our knowledge, on TRH antagonism of opiate-induced hypothermia, analgesia, and addiction, such an antagonism may indeed exist, and clinical utilization (particularly of some more potent and more specific analog) could be indicated, e.g., in cases of opiate intoxication or addiction.

The interpretation of a paradoxical hormone response to TRH as an indication of a dysfunction of CNS monoamines, as previously discussed, may open up the way for the utilization of TRH as a test not only of pituitary reserve but also of CNS integrity. The return of a "normal" hormone response—in disorders not affecting the pituitary gland (e.g., mental depression)—could then mean the restoration of a central monoaminergic tonus.

ACKNOWLEDGMENTS

This work has been supported by Medical Research Council of Canada, grant MA-4691. The authors wish to express their gratitude for the skillful technical help of Ms. H. Guillet, F. Dionne, and O. Rebouco.

REFERENCES

1. Anderson, M. S., Bowers, C. Y., Kastin, A. J., Schalch, D. S., Schally, A. V., Snyder, P. I., Utiger, R. D., Wilber, J. F., and Wise, A. J. (1971): Synthetic thyrotropin-releasing hormone, a potent stimulator of thyrotropin secretion in man. *N. Engl. J. Med.,* 285:1279–1283.
2. Aschroft, G. W., Crawford, T. B. B., Eccleston, D., Sharman, D. F., MacDougall, E. J., Stanton, J. B., and Binns, J. K. (1966): 5-Hydroxyindole compounds in the cerebrospinal fluid of patients with psychiatric or neurological disease. *Lancet,* 2:1049–1051.
3. Barry, V. C., and Klawans, H. L. (1976): On the role of dopamine in the pathophysiology of anorexia nervosa. *J. Neurol. Transm.,* 38:107–112.
4. Blake, C. A. (1974): Stimulation of pituitary prolactin and TSH release in lactating and proestrus rats. *Endocrinology,* 94:503–508.
5. Bowers, C. Y., Friesen, H. G., Hwang, P., Guyda, H. G., and Folkers, K. (1971): Prolactin and thyrotropin release in man by synthetic pyroglutamyl-histidyl-prolinamide. *Biochem. Biophys. Res. Commun.,* 45:1033–1038.
6. Boyar, R. M. (1978): Sleep-related endocrine rhythms. In: *The Hypothalamus,* edited by S. Reichlin, R. J. Baldessarini, and J. B. Martin, pp. 373–385. Raven Press, New York.
7. Brauman, H., and Corvilain, J. (1968): Growth hormone response to hypoglycemia in myxedema. *J. Clin. Endocrinol. Metab.,* 28:301–304.
8. Brown, M., and Vale, W. (1975): Growth hormone release in the rat: Effects of somatostatin and thyrotropin-releasing factor. *Endocrinology,* 97:1151–1156.
9. Carlson, H. E., Maritz, I. K., and Daughaday, W. H. (1974): Thyrotropin-releasing hormone stimulation and somatostatin inhibition of growth hormone secretion from perfused rat adenohypophyses. *Endocrinology,* 94:1709–1713.
10. Chihara, K., Kato, Y., Ohgo, S., Iwasaki, Y., Abe, H., Maeda, K., and Imura, H. (1976): Stimulating and inhibiting effects of thyrotropin-releasing hormone on growth hormone release in rats. *Endocrinology,* 98:1047–1053.
11. Collu, R. (1977): Role of central cholinergic and aminergic neurotransmitters in the control of anterior pituitary hormone secretion. In: *Clinical Neuroendocrinol-*

ogy, edited by L. Martini and G. M. Besser, pp. 43–65. Academic Press, New York.

12. Collu, R. (1978): The effect of TRH on the release of TSH, PRL and GH in man under basal conditions and following methysergide. *J. Endocrinol. Invest.* 2:121–124.

13. Collu, R., Brun, G., Milsant, F., Leboeuf, G., Letarte, J., and Ducharme, J. R. (1978): Reevaluation of levodopa-propranolol as a test of growth hormone reserve in children. *Pediatrics,* 61:242–245.

14. Collu, R., Clermont, M. J., and Ducharme, J. R. (1976): Effects of thyrotropin-releasing hormone on prolactin, growth hormone and corticosterone secretions in adult male rats treated with pentobarbital or morphine. *Eur. J. Pharmacol.,* 37:133–140.

15. Collu, R., Clermont, M. J., Letarte, J., Leboeuf, G., and Ducharme, J. R. (1975): Inhibition of pentobarbital-induced release of growth hormone by thyrotropin-releasing hormone. *Endocrinol. Res. Commun.,* 2:123–135.

16. Collu, R., Du Ruisseau, P., Taché, Y., and Ducharme, J. R. (1977): Thyrotropin-releasing hormone in rat brain: Nyctohemeral variations. *Endocrinology,* 100:1391–1393.

17. Collu, R., Fraschini, F., Visconti, P., and Martini, K. (1972): Adrenergic and serotoninergic control of growth hormone secretion in adult male rat. *Endocrinology,* 90:1231–1237.

18. Collu, R., Leboeuf, G., Letarte, J., and Ducharme, J. R. (1975): Stimulation of growth hormone secretion by levodopa-propranolol in children and adolescents. *Pediatrics,* 56:262–266.

19. Collu, R., Leboeuf, G., Letarte, J., and Ducharme, J. R. (1977): Increase in plasma growth hormone levels following thyrotropin-releasing hormone injection in children with primary hypothyroidism. *J. Clin. Endocrinol. Metab.,* 44:743–747.

20. Convey, E. M., Tucker, H. A., Smith, V. G., and Zolman, J. (1973): Bovine prolactin, growth hormone, thyroxine and corticoid response to thyrotropin-releasing hormone. *Endocrinology,* 92:471–476.

21. Costin, G., Kershnar, A. K., Kogut, M. D., and Turkington, R. W. (1972): Prolactin activity in juvenile hypothyroidism and precocious puberty. *Pediatrics,* 50:881–889.

22. Du Ruisseau, P., Taché, Y., Brazeau, P., and Collu, R. (1978): Pattern of adenohypophyseal hormone changes induced by various stressors in male and female rats. *Neuroendocrinology (in press).*

23. Egge, A. C., Rogol, A. O., Varina, M. M., and Blizzard, R. M. (1977): Effect of cyproheptadine on the TRH-stimulated prolactin and TSH release in man. *J. Clin. Endocrinol. Metab.,* 44:210–213.

24. Elephteriou, B. E. (1972): *The Neurobiology of the Amygdala.* Plenum Press, New York.

25. Ferland, L., Labrie, F., Arimura, A., and Schally, A. V. (1977): Stimulated release of hypothalamic growth hormone-releasing activity by morphine and pentobarbital. *Mol. Cell. Endocrinol.,* 6:247–252.

26. Gilbert, J. C., and Goldberg, J. I. (1975): Characterization by cyproheptadine of the dopamine-induced contraction in canine isolated arteries. *J. Pharmacol. Exp. Ther.,* 193:435–439.

27. Gonzalez-Barcena, D., Kastin, A. J., Schalch, S., Torres-Zamora, M., Perez-Pasten, E., Kato, A., and Schally, A. V. (1973): Responses to thyrotropin-releasing hormone in patients with renal failure and after infusion in normal men. *J. Clin. Endocrinol. Metab.,* 36:117–120.

28. Guillemin, R. (1978): Biochemical and physiological correlates of hypothalamic peptides: the new endocrinology of the neuron. In: *The Hypothalamus,* edited by S. Reichlin, R. J. Baldessarini, and J. B. Martin, pp. 155–194. Raven Press, New York.

29. Hamada, N., Uoi, K., Nishizawa, Y., Okamoto, T., Hasegawa, K., Morii, H., and Wada, M. (1976): Increase of serum GH concentration following TRH injection in patients with primary hypothyroidism. *Endocrinol. Jpn.,* 23:5–9.

30. Hedlund, L., Doelger, S. G., Tollerton, A. J., Lischko, M. M., and Johnson, H. D.

(1977): Plasma growth hormone concentrations after cerebroventricular and jugular injection of thyrotropin-releasing hormone. *Proc. Soc. Exp. Biol. Med.,* 156:422–425.

31. Horita, A., and Carino, M. A. (1976): Effect of PCPA and methergoline on the pentobarbital-TRH interaction in rabbits. *Fed. Proc.,* 35:268 (abstract).
32. Irie, M., and Tsushima, T. (1972): Increase of serum growth hormone concentration following thyrotropin-releasing hormone injection in patients with acromegaly or gigantism. *J. Clin. Endocrinol. Metab.,* 35:97–100.
33. Jackson, I. M. D. (1978): Extrahypothalamic and phylogenetic distribution of hypothalamic peptides. In: *The Hypothalamus,* edited by S. Reichlin, R. J. Baldessarini, and J. B. Martin, pp. 217–231. Raven Press, New York.
34. Jacobs, L. S., Snyder, P. J., Wilber, J. F., Utiger, R. D., and Daughaday, W. H. (1971): Increased serum prolactin after administration of synthetic thyrotropin releasing hormone (TRH) in man. *J. Clin. Endocrinol. Metab.,* 33:996–998.
35. Katz, H. P., Youlton, R., Kaplan, S. L., and Grumbach, M. M. (1969): Growth and growth hormone. III. Growth hormone release in children with primary hypothyroidism and thyrotoxicosis. *J. Clin. Endocrinol. Metab.,* 29:346–351.
36. Koe, B. K., and Weissman, A. (1966): p-Chlorophenylalanine: A specific depletor of brain serotonin. *J. Pharmacol. Exp. Ther.,* 154:499–503.
37. Kordon, C., and Glowinski (1972): Role of hypothalamic monoaminergic neurons in the gonadotrophin release-regulating mechanisms. *Neuropharmacology,* 11:153–162.
38. Kordon, C., Blake, C. A., Terkel, J., and Sawyer, C. A. (1973/74): Participation of serotonin-containing neurons in the suckling-induced rise in plasma prolactin levels in lactating rats. *Neuroendocrinology,* 13:213–223.
39. Krulich, L., and Marchlewska-Koj, A. (1976): On the role of central noradrenergic and cholinergic systems in the regulation of prolactin secretion in the male rat. *Fed. Proc.,* 35:555 (abstract).
40. Maeda, K., Kato, Y., Chihara, K., Ohgo, S., Iwasaki, Y., and Imura, H. (1975): Suppression by thyrotropin-releasing hormone (TRH) of human growth hormone release induced by L-DOPA. *J. Clin. Endocrinol. Metab.,* 41:408–411.
41. Maeda, K., Kato, Y., Chihara, K., Ohgo, S., Iwazaki, Y., Abe, H., and Imura, H. (1976): Suppression by thyrotropin-releasing hormone (TRH) of growth hormone release induced by arginine and insulin-induced hypoglycemia in men. *J. Clin. Endocrinol. Metab.,* 43:453–456.
42. Maeda, K., Kato, Y., Ohgo, S., Chihara, K., Yoshimoto, Y., Yamaguchi, N., Kuromaru, S., and Imura, H. (1975): Growth hormone and prolactin release after injection of thyrotropin-releasing hormone in patients with depression. *J. Clin. Endocrinol. Metab.,* 40:501–505.
43. Maeda, K., Kato, Y., Yamaguchi, N., Chihara, K., Ohgo, S., Iwasaki, Y., Yoshimoto, Y., Moridera, K., Kuromaru, S., and Imura, H. (1976): Growth hormone release following thyrotropin-releasing hormone injection into patients with anorexia nervosa. *Acta Endocrinol. (Kbh),* 81:1–8.
44. Martin, J. B. (1973–74): Studies on the mechanism of pentobarbital-induced GH release in the rat. *Neuroendocrinology,* 13:339–350.
45. Martin, J. B., Audet, J., and Saunders, A. (1975): Effect of somatostatin and hypothalamic ventromedial lesions on growth hormone release induced by morphine. *Endocrinology,* 96:839–847.
46. Mena, F., Enjalbert, A., Carbonell, L., Priam, M., and Kordon, C. (1976): Effect of suckling on plasma prolactin and hypothalamic monoamine levels in the rat. *Endocrinology,* 99:445–451.
47. Müller, E. E., Panerai, A. E., Cocchi, D., Gil-Ad, I., Rossi, G. L., and Olgiati, V. R. (1977): Growth hormone releasing activity of thyrotropin-releasing hormone in rats with hypothalamic lesions. *Endocrinology,* 100:1663–1671.
48. Munro, H. N., Fernstrom, J. D., and Wurtman, R. J. (1975): Insulin plasma amino-acid imbalance and hepatic coma. *Lancet,* 1:722–723.
49. Ormston, B. J., Kilborn, S. R., Garry, R., Amos, J., and Hall, R. (1971): Further

observations on the effect of synthetic thyrotropin-releasing hormone in man. *Br. Med. J.,* 2:199–204.

50. Panerai, A. E., Rossi, G. L., Cocchi, D., Gil-Ad, I., Locatelli, V., and Müller, E. E. (1977): Release of growth hormone by TRH in intact rats or in intact or hypophysectomized rats bearing a heterotopic pituitary. *Proc. Soc. Exp. Biol. Med.,* 154:573–577.

51. Panerai, A. E., Salerno, F., Manneschi, M., Cocchi, D., and Müller, E. E. (1977): Growth hormone and prolactin responses to thyrotropin-releasing hormone in patients with severe liver disease. *J. Clin. Endocrinol. Metab.,* 45:134–140.

52. Reichlin, S. (1974): Regulation of somatotrophic hormone secretion. In: *The Pituitary Gland and Its Neuroendocrine Control,* edited by E. Knobil and C. H. Sawyer, pp. 405–421. American Physiological Society, Washington, D.C.

53. Rivier, C., Vale, W., Ling, N., Brown, M., and Guillemin, R. (1977): Stimulation "in vivo" of the secretion of prolactin and growth hormone by β-endorphin. *Endocrinology,* 100:238–241.

54. Schalch, D. S., Gonzalez-Barcena, D., Kastin, A. J., Schally, A. V., and Lee, L. A. (1972): Abnormalities in the release of TSH in response to thyrotropin-releasing hormone (TRH) in patients with disorders of the pituitary, hypothalamus and basal ganglia. *J. Clin. Endocrinol. Metab.,* 35:609–615.

55. Simon, M., Garcia, J. F., and George, R. (1973): Effects of morphine on regional levels of brain 5-HT, NE, and DA as correlated with anterior pituitary hormone levels in plasma. *Proc. West. Pharmacol. Soc.,* 16:19–24.

56. Snyder, P. J., Jacobs, L. S., Utiger, R. D., and Daughaday, W. H. (1973): Thyroid hormone inhibition of the prolactin response to thyrotropin-releasing hormone. *J. Clin. Invest.,* 52:2324–2329.

57. Spector, S., Sjoerdsma, A., and Udenfriend, S. (1965): Blockade of endogenous norepinephrine synthesis by α-methyl-tyrosine, an inhibitor of tyrosine hydroxylase. *J. Pharmacol. Exp. Ther.,* 147:86–95.

58. Stone, C. A., Wenger, H. C., Ludden, C. T., Stavorski, J. M., and Ross, C. A. (1961): Antiserotonin-antihistaminic properties of cyproheptadine. *J. Pharmacol. Exp. Ther.,* 131:73–78.

59. Taché, Y., Du Ruisseau, P., Ducharme, J. R., and Collu, R. (1978): Pattern of adenohypophyseal hormone changes induced by chronic stress in male rats. *Neuroendocrinology* 26:208–219.

60. Taché, Y., Du Ruisseau, P., Ducharme, J. R., and Collu, R. (1977): Antagonism of pentobarbital-induced hormonal changes by TRH in rats. *Eur. J. Pharmacol.,* 45:369–376.

61. Taché, Y., Lis, M., and Collu, R. (1977): Effects of thyrotrophin-releasing hormone on behavioral and hormonal changes induced by β-endorphin. *Life Sci.,* 21:841–846.

62. Takahara, J., Arimura, A., and Schally, A. V. (1974): Stimulation of prolactin and growth hormone release by TRH infused into a hypophyseal portal vessel. *Proc. Soc. Exp. Biol. Med.,* 146:831–835.

63. Tashjian, A. H., Barowsky, N. J., and Jensen, D. K. (1971): Thyrotropin releasing hormone: Direct evidence for stimulation of prolactin production by pituitary cells in culture. *Biochem. Biophys. Res. Commun.,* 43:516–520.

64. Terry, L. C., Saunders, A., Audet, J., Willoughby, J. O., Brazeau, P., and Martin, J. B. (1977): Physiologic secretion of growth hormone and prolactin in male and female rats. *Clin. Endocrinol.,* 6:19s–28s.

65. Vernikos-Danellis, J., Berger, P., and Barchas, J. D. (1973): Brain serotonin and pituitary-adrenal function. *Prog. Brain Res.,* 39:301–309.

66. Voogt, J. L., and Carr, L. A. (1975): Potentiation of suckling-induced release of prolactin by inhibition of brain catecholamine synthesis. *Endocrinology,* 97:891–895.

67. Zanoboni, A., and Zanoboni-Muciaccia, W. (1977): Elevated basal growth hormone levels and growth hormone response to TRH in alcoholic patients with cirrhosis. *J. Clin. Endocrinol. Metab.,* 45:576–578.

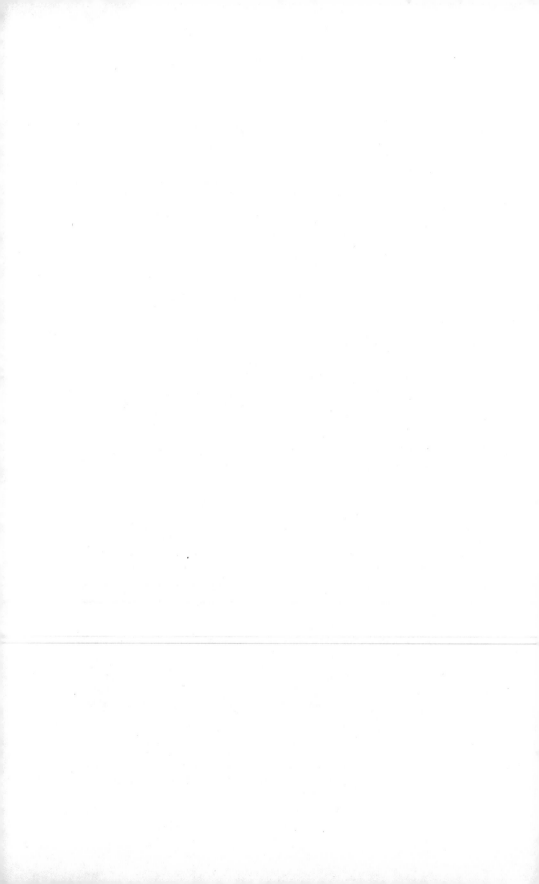

Central Nervous System Effects of Hypothalamic Hormones and Other Peptides, edited by Collu et al.
Raven Press, New York © 1979.

Thyrotropin-Releasing Hormone Influences on Behavior: Possible Involvement of Brain Monoaminergic Systems

Ram B. Rastogi

Division of Pharmacology, Bio-Research Laboratories, Connlab Holdings Limited, Montreal, Canada

Thyrotropin-releasing hormone (TRH) is a tripeptide (L-pyroglutamyl-L-histidyl-L-proline-amide) found in the hypothalamus that functions as a hypophysiotropic hormone. It stimulates the secretion of thyrotropin (TSH) from the anterior pituitary. TSH thus released subsequently stimulates the release of L-triiodothyronine (T_3) and thyroxine (T_4) from the thyroid gland. Recently extrahypothalamic locations of TRH have been reported in the brain of rats (105) as well as humans (63). It has been estimated that as much as 70% of total TRH is present outside the hypothalamus in the central nervous system (CNS) and spinal cord. These findings have also been confirmed by immunohistochemical studies (48), which have shown the presence of TRH-containing nerve terminals in the nucleus accumbens, lateral septal nucleus, and several motor nuclei of the brainstem. It is rather intriguing to note that the extrahypothalamic TRH is synthesized *in situ* and is independent of hypothalamic secretion (13,56). Furthermore, high-affinity binding sites for TRH have been reported in brain as well as pituitary (16).

A series of psychopharmacological studies also support the concept of an extrathyroidal role of TRH. This tripeptide has been shown to produce behavioral excitation (49) and to antagonize pentobarbital-induced sleep and hypothermia as well as the narcosis and hypothermia induced by ethanol (8,78). Clinically, TRH has been found to produce a rapid but transient change in mood and behavior of patients with unipolar depression, although currently controversy surrounds this issue. Moreover, preliminary experiments in spinal cats have demonstrated that, like tricyclic antidepressants, TRH (100 μg/kg i.v.) slightly but significantly potentiated the blood pressure response as determined by norepinephrine (NE) (29).

ARE THE BRAIN MONOAMINERGIC NEURONS INVOLVED IN MEDIATING THE BEHAVIORAL STIMULANT EFFECTS OF TRH?

A functional defect in biogenic amines in the etiology of affective disorder was first hypothesized by Schildkraut (91) in 1965, and now it is generally believed that antidepressant drugs elicit the beneficial effects by altering the disposition and metabolism of brain monoamines. The findings that TRH potentiated the behavioral excitement caused by pargyline-L-DOPA (72) and produced a rapid relief of depressive illness resulted in a flush of enthusiasm among the neurochemists, neuropharmacologists, and psychoneuroendocrinologists to delineate the neuronal mechanisms underlying the pychotropic action of TRH.

Administration of TRH (10 mg/kg i.p.) was found to produce no effect on endogenous levels of NE and dopamine (DA) in several brain areas examined, but increased the behavioral activity, consisting of frequent ambulation, rearing, sniffing, and head shaking. The activity of rate-limiting enzyme tyrosine hydroxylase (TH) in the soluble fraction of striatum tended to increase by 12% in TRH-treated rats; however, the change was statistically nonsignificant. This tripeptide increased the release of NE and DA as evidenced by higher concentrations of their metabolites 4-hydroxy-3-methoxyphenylglycol (MOPEG) and homovanillic acid (HVA), respectively (Table 1). These data are in line with the report of Horst and Spirt (52) who found that TRH produced no effect on NE uptake by the brain tissue but that incubation of rat brain synaptosomes *in vitro* in the presence of TRH resulted in increased release of ^{3}H-NE and ^{3}H-DA. This has also been confirmed by histochemical studies of Constantinidis et al. (23). Reigle and co-workers (88) found no change in NE and DA levels after TRH treatment but a significant increase (16%) in ^{3}H-normetanephrine level (the extraneuronal metabolite) was reported in rats pretreated intracisternally with ^{3}H-NE.

TABLE 1. *Effect of acute TRH on spontaneous locomotor activity as well as soluble form of TH and HVA in striatum and MOPEG in rat brain*

Treatment	Spontaneous locomotor counts/25 min	TH (nmoles DOPA/ mg/hr)	HVA (µg/g)	MOPEG (µg/g)
Con' ol	241 ± 30[a]	17.38 ± 1.26	0.89 ± 0.06	0.43 ± 0.02
TRH	526 ± 54[b]	20.36 ± 1.99	1.09 ± 0.05[b]	0.56 ± 0.02[b]

Rats weighing 115 to 125 g received a single injection of TRH (10 mg/kg i.p.), and the locomotor activity was recorded for 25 min, immediately after TRH treatment. Two hours after TRH treatment, animals were sacrificed for the biochemical assays. Control animals received an equal volume of physiological saline.

[a] Mean ± SEM of six rats in each group.
[b] Significantly different from controls (p < 0.05).

Observations that TRH enhanced the reduction of brain NE by α-methyl-p-tyrosine (α-MPT) and increased the content of metabolite MOPEG (59) and normetanephrine (88) in brain are in accordance with the view that this tripeptide accelerates the release of NE in brain. Additionally, our data demonstrate that TRH increased the lowering of hypothalamic and striatal DA by α-MPT and elevated the level of HVA in striatum (Table 2). In contrast to chronic TRH treatment (84), single TRH injection produced no statistically significant change in the activity of the soluble form of TH in striatum. However, Keller et al. (59) reported an increased conversion of ^{14}C-L-tyrosine into ^{14}C-norepinephrine in rats treated acutely with TRH (68,76). This indicates an increased synthesis of cerebral NE and DA (68,76), which probably compensated for their enhanced release since the steady-state levels after TRH treatment remained unchanged. The fluorescent histochemical studies of Constantinidis et al. (23) showed that TRH by itself produced no change in NE fluorescence but accentuated the decrease of green fluorescence in NE terminals of α-MPT-treated rats. These findings provide additional support to our view that TRH accelerates the turnover of this monoamine in brain, and that the effect might at least in part be associated with the antidepressant action of TRH in man.

A wealth of literature has produced substantial evidence to suggest that stereotypy and locomotor stimulation induced by certain drugs are mediated via the nigrostriatal DA and the mesolimbic DA system, respectively (4,35,60). The most significant sites of the mesolimbic DA system are the nucleus accumbens and tuberculum olfactorium. We observed that the intra-peritoneal injection of TRH resulted in marked locomotor hyperactivity consisting of frequent ambulation, rearing, sniffing, and grooming. Further-more, Segal and Mandell (94) reported that chronic infusion of TRH into the lateral ventricle produced hyperactivity. The findings that animals pre-treated with large doses of Fla 63, a dopamine β-hydroxylase inhibitor and subsequently used in the L-DOPA test still responded to TRH, suggest that TRH may be acting through dopaminergic systems (74). We speculate that mesolimbic dopaminergic neurons are involved in mediating this effect of TRH. This assumption is supported by the fact that the behavioral effects seen after systemic injection of TRH were reproduced by bilateral intra-accumbens injection of DA and TRH. By contrast, no locomotor hyper-activity was observed after bilateral injection of TRH into the caudate nucleus (70). Furthermore, the locomotor stimulation induced by TRH injected peripherally or into the nucleus accumbens was markedly inhibited by the DA receptor blockers haloperidol and pimozide administered either peripherally or into the nucleus accumbens. The presence of substantial amounts of TRH in the nucleus accumbens (48) further supports the above observations. On a molar basis, TRH was found to be about five times as potent as DA in the locomotor stimulation induced by intraaccumbens injec-tion (70), suggesting that TRH may act in some way on the DA system

TABLE 2. *Effect of acute TRH on NE, DA, HVA, and MOPEG levels in brain of α-MPT-treated rats*

Treatment	NE (µg/g)			DA (µg/g)			HVA (µg/g) in striatum	MOPEG (µg/g) in whole brain striatum
	Cortex	Hypothalamus	Midbrain	Hypothalamus	Midbrain	Striatum		
Control	0.32 ± 0.01[a]	2.04 ± 0.13	0.49 ± 0.02	0.20 ± 0.01	0.46 ± 0.03	8.29 ± 0.47	0.89 ± 0.06	0.43 ± 0.02
α-MPT	0.28 ± 0.02	1.14 ± 0.07[b]	0.21 ± 0.01[b]	0.11 ± 0.01[b]	0.32 ± 0.01[b]	5.72 ± 0.36[b]	0.59 ± 0.03[b]	0.25 ± 0.01[b]
α-MPT + TRH	0.25 ± 0.00[b]	0.69 ± 0.03[b,c]	0.16 ± 0.00[b,c]	0.08 ± 0.00[b,c]	0.33 ± 0.01[b]	4.44 ± 0.29[b,c]	0.75 ± 0.05[c]	0.37 ± 0.03[c]

Rats received three injections of α-MPT (100 mg/kg i.p.) at 2-hr intervals and were sacrificed 2 hr after the third injection. A group of α-MPT-treated rats received a single injection of TRH (10 mg/kg i.p.) 4 hr after the first injection of α-MPT and were sacrificed 2 hr after TRH treatment.

[a] Mean ± SEM of six rats in each group.

[b] Significantly different from controls (p < 0.05).

[c] Significantly different from α-MPT-treated rats (p < 0.05).

other than as a direct receptor stimulant. Behavioral (21) and biochemical tests indicate that TRH does not alter postsynaptic DA receptor sensitivity but enhances the release and synthesis of DA (1,59,84). This view was strengthened by the observation that the adenyl cyclase activity and the response of this enzyme to DA were unaltered in the caudate nucleus of animals pretreated with TRH (42).

There is also evidence that the central NE system, in part, contributes to the development of hyperactivity (11,85). Using specific pharmacological tools, Miyamato and Nagawa (70) demonstrated that TRH-induced hyperactivity is not mediated via NE neurons of nucleus accumbens. Further research is obviously needed to implicate the role of noradrenergic neurons of other brain regions in mediation of behavioral activity seen after TRH injection. Horita et al. (50) suggested that analeptic action of TRH may be mediated through NE neurons in the reticular formation.

Neuronal connections exist between the nucleus accumbens and the amygdala, septum, cingulate gyrus, and other areas closely related to emotional activity (77). Many clinicians have suggested that intravenous injection of TRH can alter the symptoms of certain mental disorders. For instance, TRH has been claimed to be an effective antipsychotic agent (104). This finding has been replicated by some (54) but not by others (7,31). In fact, TRH was found to exacerbate some forms of schizophrenia. The electroencephalographic (EEG) recordings after intravenous TRH are similar to those seen after certain psychostimulants (e.g., amphetamine and methylphenidate) (55). It is therefore reasonable to believe that aggravation of certain forms of schizophrenia by TRH might be due to its amphetamine-like action.

A transient antidepressant action of TRH during the alcohol withdrawal syndrome was recently reported (65). Studies of Koranyi et al. (61) revealed that following a few systemic injections of TRH changes that occurred in multiple unit activity were similar to those induced by a single injection of imipramine. Moreover, TRH was found to produce a subtle change in mood and behavior of depressed patients (58,66,80), although other workers have failed to replicate these findings (25,71). Psychophysiological studies of Itil et al. (55) demonstrated that TRH may be effective in patients with psychomotor depression where the affective disorder is the result of a decrease or inhibition of some "instinctive" functions, e.g., interest, desire, and drive for work, food, and sex.

DOES TRH INFLUENCE DOPAMINERGIC NEURONS DIRECTLY?

In view of animal findings discussed in an earlier section, it may well be speculated that TRH modulates the activity of the DA system and possibly NE neurons to control emotional and mental functions. However, the question of whether TRH exerts its primary effects on the dopaminergic system or a "second neuronal" system which indirectly regulates the functioning of DA-containing neurons and, in turn, behavior remains unclear. Evidence suggests that γ-aminobutyric acid (GABA) is a powerful inhibitory transmitter which acts pre- and postsynaptically in the CNS (30). Furthermore, several workers have demonstrated that pretreatment of animals with agents which are thought to mimic at least some of the effects of GABA [e.g., baclophen (3,26,38,39) and GHBA (89,90)] abolish the sleep-reducing effects of TRH in ethanol-treated mice. In addition, the transaminase (GABA-T) inhibitor AOAA, which has been found to elevate brain GABA levels, also antagonized the ability of TRH to reduce ethanol-induced sleep (28). These data suggest that agents which are thought to activate GABA neuronal systems in brain may reduce or eliminate the behavioral effects of TRH. GABA-containing neurons originating in the caudate are presumed to exert an inhibitory influence on nigrostriatal DA neurons (17,33,51). Therefore inhibition of the striatonigral GABA neurons by TRH might in turn result in an enhanced release of DA (as evidenced by an increased level of striatal HVA in the present investigation) and enhanced release of ^{3}H-DA from striatal synaptosomes (52). Furthermore, the only other compound found to mimic the characteristic behavioral effects of TRH is tubocurarine administered either intracisternally (27) or intraventricularly (6). It has been concluded that the underlying mechanisms of the behavioral stimulant effects of intraventricularly injected tubocurarine are due to antagonism of GABA at the GABA receptor sites (46,69). It is therefore likely that TRH primarily affects the GABA-ergic neuron, which, due to disinhibition, results in increased functioning of DA-containing neurons, particularly those comprising the nigrostriatal system of the brain.

EFFECT OF TRH ON TRYPTAMINERGIC NEURONS

The hypothesis of a central 5-hydroxytryptamine (5-HT) deficiency playing a role in the pathogenesis of certain depressive symptoms has been examined by several techniques. The results are far from unequivocal but are more in favor of the view than against it. A decreased 5-hydroxyindoleacetic acid (5-HIAA) accumulation has been observed particularly within the group of vital depressions. Recent findings of van Praag and Korf (101) indicated decreased activity of synthesizing enzyme tryptophan hydroxylase (TPH) and/or inefficient uptake mechanism for precursor tryptophan (TP) in the brain of depressive patients. Successful treatment of depression with pharmacological agents [e.g., monoamineoxidase (MAO) inhibitors, tricyclic antidepressants], which alter the metabolism and disposition of 5-HT in brain, led investigators to speculate that derangement in 5-HT neuronal systems was the basis for certain types of depression. It is now believed that reduced 5-hydroxytryptaminergic activity, whatever its cause may be, is related to instability of mood regulation, and diminished catecholaminergic activity to inhibition of drive.

TRH potentiated the behavioral excitement caused by 5-hydroxytryptophan (41,53) and increased the turnover of 5-HT, as evidenced by increased TPH activity in midbrain and elevated levels of 5-HIAA in hypothalamus of the rat (84). Chronic L-triiodothyronine treatment produced a similar type of effect on 5-HT synthesis and turnover in brain of developing rats (95).

EFFECT OF TRH ON CHOLINERGIC NEURONS

Previous studies demonstrating that the antagonism of barbiturate-induced sleeping time in mice by TRH can be inhibited or reduced by atropine suggest that cholinergic mechanisms may contribute to some of the behavioral effects of TRH (9). The view gains support from a report in which TRH selectively enhanced the excitatory effect of acetylcholine and carbachol on single cortical neurons (106). This is in line with the findings that general anesthetics (particularly barbiturates) selectively reduce the sensitivity of cerebral cortical neurons to the excitatory actions of iontophoretically applied acetylcholine (20). Thus one important action of this neuropeptide is to facilitate cholinergic activity. The finding that scopolamine completely blocked the EEG effect of TRH whereas chlorpromazine did not (5) is also consistent with this view. Repeated administraton of L-triiodothyronine in developing rats was also found to increase significantly the synthesis and release of acetylcholine in brain (83). In view of these considerations, it remains to be seen whether the effect of TRH on brain cholinergic neurons is independent of the pituitary-thyroidal axis.

DEPRESSIVE ILLNESS VERSUS HYPOTHYROIDISM

Evidence from clinical as well as animal studies indicate that a number of metabolic and psychic disturbances may be common to thyroid deficiency and affective illness. A diminished response to infused norepinephrine (79,93) has been observed in hypothyroid and depressed patients. Disturbances in sodium, potassium, and calcium metabolism have also been found in affective illness (24) as well as thyroid dysfunction (37,87). Furthermore, psychological studies suggest that the symptoms of myxedema, a severe form of hypothyroidism, make an insidious appearance and are generally characterized by listlessness, lack of energy, slowness of speech, reduced sensory capacity, memory impairment, somnolence, social withdrawal, and an altered sleep pattern (34,57). Several of these psychological symptoms (e.g., somnolence, slowness of speech, reduced sensory capacity, lack of energy, social withdrawal, and altered sleep pattern) are commonly seen in depressed patients (64,102,103). Although hypothyroidism in man was found to produce no significant differences in rapid eye movement (REM) sleep or total sleep time, the duration of time spent in stages 3 and 4 were consistently decreased (98). Observed changes in sleep pattern seemed to be thyroid hormone-specific since treatment with desiccated thyroid increased these sleep phases in hypothyroid patients. There is indirect evidence suggesting that depressed patients may actually have lower thyroid hormone levels than are normally present. Indeed, Dewhurst et al. (32) reported abnormally high levels of thyrotropic hormone in the blood of depressed patients, although it was suggested that the emotional stress associated with psychiatric illness might have been the cause of this hormonal increase. More recently, Hatotani et al. (45) suggested that a number of persistently depressed patients show a latent hypothyroidism possibly due to hypothalamo-pituitary dysfunction.

Our neurochemical studies demonstrated that radiothyroidectomy at birth was accompanied by suppressed behavioral activity as well as decreased synthesis and metabolism of brain NE and DA (96). We therefore employed neonatally hypothyroid animals as a model for depression and to investigate the antidepressant action of TRH. Repeated administration of TRH (4 mg/kg twice a day) for 10 days in hypothyroid rats not only increased the spontaneous locomotor activity but also increased the rate of synthesis of catecholamines. The latter effect is evidenced by increased TH activity (1). This action is apparently independent of any effect of TRH on thyroid gland.

POTENTIATION OF ANTIDEPRESSANT EFFECT OF IMIPRAMINE BY TRH: NEUROCHEMICAL EVIDENCE

Unlike classic tricyclic antidepressive drugs, which enhance the effective levels of neurotransmitters at the receptor sites by blocking their reuptake, TRH exerts mood-elevating effects in man by augmenting the synthesis and turnover of NE, DA, and 5-HT in brain (86). Tricyclic antidepressant drugs, when administered to rats in a single dose, cause a reduction in the rate of synthesis of NE and lower the formation of MOPEG (72). However, when these compounds are given chronically to rats, they stimulate the turnover rate of NE (92). The delay in the onset of increase in catecholamine turnover induced by tricyclic compounds correlates well with the delay (2 to 3 weeks) in onset of antidepressive action in patients. The fact that TRH augments the turnover rate of catecholamines after acute treatment (59) may explain its immediate therapeutic effect in depressed patients, which becomes apparent 2 hr after treatment (80). Since the omnipresent danger of suicide in depressed patients makes speed of treatment a prime consideration, an empirical treatment for the affective disorder that is faster in onset of action than the tricyclics is of considerable value in clinical psychiatry.

Evidence also indicates that tricyclic antidepressants produce a number of side effects on the cardiovascular system (e.g., arrhythmias, postural hypotension, electrocardiographic changes, hypokalemia, and decreased myocardial contractility) (15,82), as well as on the CNS (12,40), including the suppression of REM sleep (44,47). On the other hand, TRH possesses a rapid antidepressant action, and this tripeptide does not suppress REM sleep (61). The finding that TRH potentiated the antidepressant effects of imipramine in patients resistant to imipramine alone (74) prompted us to investigate the neurochemical mechanisms underlying this action.

Administration of TRH (20 mg/kg/day in two equally divided doses) for 10 days significantly increased the soluble form of TH in striatum. However, in contrast to our results, Nemeroff et al. (73) reported no change in TH activity of hypothalamus, midbrain, pons-medulla, and forebrain. This discrepancy may be explained by the fact that a smaller dose of TRH (10 mg/kg) was used by these investigators. Furthermore, chronic TRH treatment increased the synthesis and release of 5-HT in the brain but produced no effect on the synaptosomal uptake of ^{3}H-5-HT (86).

Chronic imipramine (10 mg/kg) treatment for 10 days blocked the uptake of ^{3}H-NE and possibly of DA. This is evidenced by low levels of endogenous NE and DA and high levels of MOPEG, normetanephrine, and HVA (Table 3). Neilsen et al. (72) reported a 22% increase in ^{3}H-HVA levels following acute imipramine treatment in rats pretreated with ^{3}H-L-DOPA. The decrease in the activity of the soluble form of TH in striatum of imipramine-treated rats is consistent with the findings of Mandell (67). This is most likely an adaptive change in response to postulated high levels of catecholamines in synaptic clefts, which by receptor-mediated feedback mechanism decreased TH activity.

Chronic imipramine treatment decreased 5-HT and 5-HIAA levels. This is consistent with the findings of Alpers and Himwich (2). The decrease in

TABLE 3. *Effect of chronic imipramine alone and in combination with TRH on striatal HVA and whole brain MOPEG*

Treatment	HVA (μg/g)	MOPEG (μg/g)
Control	0.61 ± 0.02[a]	0.39 ± 0.02
TRH (20 mg/kg)	0.72 ± 0.03[b]	0.57 ± 0.03[b]
Imipramine (10 mg/kg)	0.81 ± 0.05[b]	0.50 ± 0.04[b]
Imipramine (10 mg/kg) + TRH (20 mg/kg)	0.97 ± 0.05[b,c]	0.71 ± 0.06[b,c]
Imipramine (5 mg/kg) + TRH (20 mg/kg)	0.84 ± 0.06[b]	0.53 ± 0.04[b]

Rats weighing 115 to 125 g were injected daily with TRH in a dose of 20 mg/kg (in two equally divided doses at 8 a.m. and 5 p.m.) for 10 days. Imipramine was given in doses of either 10 or 5 mg/kg i.p. for 10 days. Appropriate controls received an equal volume of physiological saline.
[a] Mean $\pm$ SEM of at least six rats in each group.
[b] Significantly different from controls (p < 0.05).
[c] Significantly different from imipramine-treated rats (p < 0.05).

5-HT levels was much more pronounced than the reduction in NE level. This might be related to a more pronounced blockade of synaptosomal up-take of ^{3}H-5-HT, which was decreased by 53% compared to ^{3}H-NE uptake, which was lowered by only 27% (Fig. 1). There is also histochemical and *in vitro* evidence (18,19) to suggest that extraneuronal 5-HT concentration rises as a result of imipramine or chlorimipramine treatment. The low 5-HIAA levels may be due to reduced 5-HT deamination. It is possible that, owing to slowed uptake, 5-HT is prevented from reaching MAO, whose activity remained unchanged after 10 days of imipramine treatment. In line with our data, Bruinvels (14) reported decreased formation of 5-HT from its precursor tryptophan in rats pretreated with imipramine. However, ad-ministration of 5-hydroxytryptophan in imipramine-pretreated rats failed to decrease the synthesis of 5-HT (14). This is also supported by our recent work in which imipramine failed to produce any change in the activity 5-hydroxytryptophan-decarboxylase enzyme (*unpublished data*). This para-digm seems consistent with the notion of receptor-mediated feedback action on the rate-limiting enzyme TPH.

One intriguing aspect of our present investigation is the finding that chronic administration of TRH—which failed to produce any change in synaptosomal uptake of NE or 5-HT when injected alone (88)—potentiated the effect of imipramine, particularly on ^{3}H-5-HT uptake and TPH activity (Fig. 1). Similarly, more pronounced decreases were noted in the concen-trations of NE, DA, 5-HT, and 5-HIAA when imipramine was injected in conjunction with TRH. The synergistic effects of TRH and imipramine on HVA and MOPEG levels also suggests that both of these pharmacological agents probably increase the effective levels of NE and DA in the synaptic

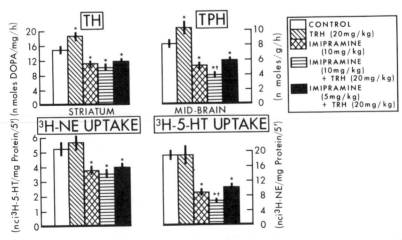

FIG. 1. Effect of chronic imipramine alone and in combination with TRH on TH, TPH, and uptake of ^{3}H-NE and ^{3}H-5-HT in crude synaptosomal (P$_2$ pellet) fraction. For experimental details, see Table 3. *Significantly different from controls ($p < 0.05$). †Significantly different from imipramine-treated rats ($p < 0.05$).

clefts. It is speculated that TRH increases the release of catecholamines, whereas imipramine blocks their reuptake in the presynaptic membrane. In line with these neurochemical results, it was reported earlier that TRH potentiated the antidepressant effects of imipramine in patients resistant to imipramine (74). Thus TRH may perhaps be found useful as an adjunct to tricyclic antidepressants.

Our data indicating that injection of imipramine in a smaller dose (5 mg/kg) along with TRH produced effects on various neuronal components of the monoaminergic system that were virtually similar to those observed after a larger dose (10 mg/kg) of imipramine alone may have clinical importance. Several possible interpretations can be offered for the observed potentiation of imipramine effects by TRH. It is probable that imipramine possesses some antithyroid property, and TRH, by acting on the pituitary, may rectify it. Fischetti (36) reported that in the rabbit small doses of imipramine increased thyroid secretion and larger doses decreased it. However, Prange et al. (81) found no change in the protein-bound iodine value in patients treated with imipramine for 27 days. The possibility also exists that TRH alters imipramine levels in the brain by influencing its metabolism centrally and/or peripherally. Breese et al. (10) reported that T_3 treatment failed to change the levels of radioactive imipramine in brain. However, since TRH is known to elicit its effects on the brain independent of the thyroid axis, further work on the influence of TRH on imipramine distribution and metabolism is required. Finally, it is also possible that TRH hastens the demethylation of imipramine into desmethylimipramine, which is believed to be a more potent tricyclic antidepressant than imipramine. Thus the present study shows that TRH can accelerate the action of imipramine on central amine disposition and metabolism. Our data raise the possibility that, by the inclusion of TRH in the therapeutic regimen, the doses of imipramine required to produce beneficial effects can be significantly reduced.

CONCLUSIONS

It is evident that over the past decade a considerable amount of work has been carried out to investigate the neurotransmitter abnormalities in affective disorders, neurotransmitter regulation of the hypothalamic-pituitary axis, and pituitary function in these kinds of psychiatric illness. The clinical features of depression (e.g., the characteristic and lasting mood changes; the disturbance in vital functions such as sleep, loss of appetite, and energy; and changes in sexual drive as well as cognitive alterations) suggest that a neurotransmitter abnormality would involve the limbic system, the reticular formation, the hypothalamus, and cortical areas. The abnormal neurotransmitter activity may result in changes in behavior patterns (e.g., altered mood, changes in aggressive drive and libido, altered appetite, sleep patterns, and autonomic functions). In addition, neurotransmitter derangements may result in altered hypothalamic and pituitary function. This in turn leads to abnormal secretion of TRH from hypothalamus and TSH from pituitary. In point of fact, it has been suggested that TRH-secreting cells in hypothalamus are regulated by an adrenergic and a 5-hydroxytryptaminergic neuronal system, the former being excitatory and the latter inhibitory (Fig. 2). In line with this suggestion, Grimm and Reichlin (43) demonstrated that 5-HT inhibited the release of radiolabeled TRH from mouse hypothalamic slices. Additionally, Tuomisto et al. (100) found that administration of 5-hydroxytryptophan (5-HTP), a 5-HT precursor capable of increasing 5-hydroxytryptaminergic tonus, significantly reduced the response of TSH to cold. It is therefore plausible that an increase in functioning of 5-HT-containing neurons after exogenous TRH administration may in part be due to a negative feedback effect of high TRH level at target organs. Dopaminergic neurons have been shown to inhibit growth hormone secretion (22), and it is likely that there may be another TRH inhibitory mechanism under the control of dopaminergic neurons; however, evidence to support this consideration is sparse and inconclusive (97,100). The results of Kotani et al. (62) suggested that acetylcholine may have a positive transmitter role in the regulation of TSH release, although others question this conclusion (100).

Many lines of evidence now suggest that this tripeptide may modulate the synthesis and turnover of catecholamines and possibly 5-HT in the brain and, in turn, control emotional behavior and mental function. In contrast to tricyclic antidepressants, TRH is ineffective in inhibiting the *in vitro* uptake of NE, DA, and 5-HT by rat brain synaptosomes or rabbit blood platelets (99). The fact that TRH enhances the turnover rate of catecholamines and possibly 5-HT may explain its immediate therapeutic effect in some types of depressed patients, in contrast to delayed onset of action of

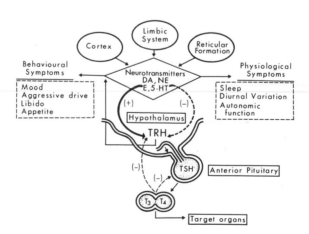

FIG. 2. Hypothetical model illustrating the mechanism of action of TRH.

tricyclic compounds. TRH is not an effective antidepressant agent in all types of depressive disorders. Nevertheless, it appears that some patients exhibit pronounced improvement in certain components of behavior, e.g., motivation and interest. Our finding that TRH potentiated the effects of imipramine on the disposition and metabolism of brain monoamines is intriguing, and it is likely that TRH may prove to be an adjunct to tricyclic antidepressant therapy. Whether such effects hold promise for TRH to be a clinical and therapeutic agent in the treatment of psychiatric and neurological disorders depends on new developments of a series of chemically related hypothalamic peptides, which probably will have more specific clinical effects with therapeutic utility, longer half-life than TRH, and easily cross the blood-brain barrier.

ACKNOWLEDGMENTS

This work was supported by grant 70–296 from the Ontario Mental Health Foundation.

REFERENCES

1. Agarwal, R. A., Rastogi, R. B., and Singhal, R. L. (1977): Enhancment of locomotor activity and catecholamine and 5-hydroxytryptamine metabolism by thyrotropin-releasing hormone. *Neuroendocrinology,* 23:236–247.
2. Alpers, H. S., and Himwich, H. E. (1972): The effects of chronic imipramine administration on rat brain levels of serotonin, 5-hydroxyindoleacetic acid, norepinephrine, and dopamine. *J. Pharmacol. Exp. Ther.,* 180:531–538.
3. Andén, N. E., and Wachtel, H. (1977): Biochemical effects of baclofen (β-parachlorophenyl GABA) on the dopamine and noradrenaline in the rat brain. *Acta Pharmacol. (Kbh),* 40:310–320.
4. Asher, I. M., and Aghjanian, G. K. (1974): 6-Hydroxydopamine lesions of olfactory tubercles and caudate nuclei: Effect on amphetamine-induced stereotyped behaviour in rats. *Brain Res.,* 82:1–8.
5. Beale, J. S., White, R. P., and Huang, S. P. (1977): EEG and blood pressure effects of TRH in rabbits. *Neuropharmacology,* 16:499–506.
6. Beleslin, D. B., and Samardzic, R. (1976): Failure of autonomic and central nervous system blocking agents to antagonize the gross behavioural effects of tubocurarine injected intraventricularly in conscious cats. *J. Pharm. Pharmacol.,* 28:519–522.
7. Bigelow, L. G., Gillin, J. C., Semal, C., and Wyatt, R. J. (1975): Thyrotropin-releasing hormone in chronic schizophrenia. *Lancet,* 2:869–870.
8. Breese, G. R., Cooper, B. R., Prange, A. J., Cott, J. M., and Lipton, M. A. (1974): Interactions of thyrotropin-releasing hormone with centrally acting drugs. In: *The Thyroid Axis, Drugs and Behaviour,* edited by A. J. Prange, Jr., pp. 115–127. Raven Press, New York.
9. Breese, G. R., Cott, J. M., Cooper, B. R., Prange, A. J., Jr., Lipton, M. A., and Plotnikoff, N. P. (1975): Effects of thyrotropin-releasing hormone (TRH) on the actions of pentobarbital and other centrally acting drugs. *J. Pharmacol. Exp. Ther.,* 193:11–22.
10. Breese, G. R., Traylor, T. D., and Prange, A. J., Jr. (1972): The effect of triiodothyronine on the disposition and actions of imipramine. *Psychopharmacology,* 25:101–111.
11. Broitman, S. T., and Donoso, A. O. (1971): Locomotor activity and regional

brain NE levels in rats treated with phenylamine. *Experientia,* 27:1308–1309.
12. Brown, T. C. K., Dwyner, M. E., and Stocks, J. G. (1971): Antidepressant overdosage in children—a new menace. *Med. J. Aust.,* 2:848–851.
13. Brownstein, M. J., Palkovits, M., and Saavedra, J. M. (1974): Thyrotropin-releasing hormone in specific nuclei of rat brain. *Science,* 185:267–269.
14. Bruinvels, J. (1972): Inhibition of the biosynthesis of 5-hydroxytryptamine in rat brain by imipramine. *Eur. J. Pharmacol.,* 20:231–237.
15. Burckhardt, D., Raeder, E., Muller, V., Imhof, P., and Naubauer, H. (1978): Cardiovascular effects of tricyclic and tetracyclic antidepressants. *JAMA,* 239:213–216.
16. Burt, D. R., and Snyder, S. H. (1975): Thyrotropin-releasing hormone: Apparent receptor binding in rat brain membranes. *Brain Res.,* 93:309–328.
17. Carlsson, A. (1974): Pharmacological approach to schizophrenia. In: *Schizophrenia: Biological and Physiological Perspectives,* edited by E. Usdin, pp. 102–124. Brunner/Mazerl, New York.
18. Carlsson, A., Corrodi, H., Fuxe, K., and Hökfelt, T. (1969): Effects of some antidepressant drugs on the depletion of intraneuronal brain catecholamine stores caused by 4, α-dimethyl-metatyramine. *Eur. J. Pharmacol.,* 5:367–373.
19. Carlsson, A., Jonason, J., Lindquvist, M., and Fuxe, K. (1969): Demonstration of extraneuronal 5-hydroxytryptamine accumulation in brain following membrane-pump blockade by chlorimipramine. *Brain Res.,* 12:456–460.
20. Catchlove, R. R. H., Krnjevik, K., and Maretic, H. (1972): Similarity between effects of general anaesthetics and dinitrophenol on cortical neurones. *Can. J. Physiol. Pharmacol.,* 50:1111–1114.
21. Cohn, M. L., Cohn, M., and Taylor, F. H. (1975): Thyrotropin releasing factor (TRF) regulation of rotation in the non-lesioned rat. *Brain Res.,* 96:134–145.
22. Collu, R., Fraschini, F., Visconti, P., and Martini, L. (1972): Adrenergic and serotonergic control of growth hormone secretion in adult male rats. *Endocrinology,* 90:1231–1240.
23. Constantinidis, J., Geissbuhler, F., Gaillard, J. M., Hovaguimian, Th., and Tissot, R. (1974): Enhancement of cerebral noradrenaline turnover by thyrotropin releasing hormone: Evidence by fluorescence histochemistry. *Experientia,* 30:1182–1183.
24. Coppen, A. (1965): Mineral metabolism in affective disorders. *Br. J. Psychiatry,* 111:1133–1142.
25. Coppen, A., Montgomery, S., Peet, M., and Bailey, J. (1974): Thyrotropin-releasing hormone in the treatment of depression. Lancet, 2:433–434.
26. Cott, J. M., Breese, G. R., Cooper, B. R., Barlow, T. S., and Prange, A. J., Jr. (1976): Investigation into the mechanism of reduction of ethanol sleep by thyrotropin-releasing hormone (TRH). *J. Pharmacol. Exp. Ther.,* 196:594–604.
27. Cott, J. M., Carlsson, A., Engel, J., and Lindquist, M. (1976): Suppression of ethanol-induced locomotor stimulation by GABA-like drugs. *Naunyn Schmiedebergs Arch. Pharmacol.,* 295:203–209.
28. Cott, J., and Engel, J. (1977): Antagonism of the analeptic activity of thyrotropin-releasing hormone (TRH) by agents which enhance GABA transmission. *Psychopharmacology,* 52:145–149.
29. Cuenca, E., Serrano, M. I., Gibert-Rahola, J., and Galiana, J. (1975): Enhancement of noradrenaline responses by thyrotropin-releasing hormone. *J. Pharm. Pharmacol.,* 27:199–200.
30. Curtis, D. R., and Johnson, G. A. R. (1974): Amino acid transmitters in mammalian central nervous system. *Rev. Physiol. Biochem. Exp. Pharmacol.,* 69:97–188.
31. Davis, K. L., Hollister, L. E., and Berger, P. A. (1974): Thyropin-releasing hormone in schizophrenia. *Am. J. Psychiatry,* 132:951–953.
32. Dewhurst, K. E., El kabir, D. J., and Harris, G. W. (1969): Observation on the blood concentration of thyrotropic hormone (TSH) in schizophrenia and affective states. *Br. J. Psychiatry,* 115:1003–1011.

33. Dray, A., and Straughan, D. W. (1976): Synaptic mechanisms in the substantia nigra. *J. Pharm. Pharmacol.*, 28:400–405.
34. Eayrs, J. T. (1960): Influence of the thyroid on the central nervous system. *Br. Med. Bull.*, 16:122–127.
35. Ernst, A. M., and Smelik, P. G. (1966): Site of action of dopamine and apomorphine on compulsive gnawing behaviour in rats. *Experientia*, 22:837–840.
36. Fischetti, B. (1962): Pharmacological influences on thyroid activity. *Arch. Ital. Sci. Farmacol.*, 12:33–109.
37. Frizel, D., Malleson, A., and Marks, V. (1967): Plasma levels of ionized calcium and magnesium in thyroid disease. *Lancet*, 1:1360–1361.
38. Fuxe, K., Agnati, L. F., Hökfelt, T., Johnson, G., Lidbrink, P., and Ljungdahl, A. (1975): The effect of dopamine receptor stimulating and blocking agents on the activity of supersensitive dopamine receptors and on the amine turnover in various nerve terminal systems in the rat brain. *J. Pharmacol.*, 6:117–129.
39. Fuxe, K., Hökfelt, T., Ljungdahl, A., Agnati, L., Johansson, O., and Perez de la Mora, M. (1975): Evidence for an inhibitory gabergic control of the mesolimbic dopamine neurons: Possibility of improving treatment of schizophrenia by combined treatment with neuroleptics and gabergic drugs. *Med. Biol.*, 53:117–183.
40. Giles, H. McC. (1963): Imipramine poisoning in childhood. *Br. Med. J.*, 2:844–846.
41. Green, A. R., and Grahame-Smith, D. G. (1974): TRH potentiates behavioural changes following increased brain 5-hydroxytryptamine accumulation in rats. *Nature (Lond)*, 251:524–526.
42. Green, A. R., Heal, D. J., Grahame-Smith, D. G., and Kelly, P. H. (1976): The contrasting action of TRH and cycloheximide in altering the effects of centrally acting drugs: Evidence for the non-involvement of dopamine sensitive adenylate cyclase. *Neuropharmacology*, 15:591–599.
43. Grimm, Y., and Reichlin, S. (1973): Thyrotropin releasing hormone: Neurotransmitter regulation of secretion by mouse hypothalamic tissues in vitro. *Endocrinology*, 93:626–631.
44. Hartmann, E. (1968): The effect of four drugs on sleep patterns in man. *Psychopharmacologia*, 12:346–353.
45. Hatotani, N., Nomura, J., Yamaguchi, T., and Kitayama, I. (1977): Clinical and experimental studies on the pathogenesis of depression. *Psychoneuroendocrinology*, 2:115–130.
46. Hill, R. G., Simmonds, M. A., and Straughan, D. E. (1973): A comparative study of some convulsant substances as γ-aminobutyric acid antagonists in the feline cerebral cortex. *Br. J. Pharmacol.*, 49:37–51.
47. Hishikawa, Y., Nakai, K., Ida, H., and Kaneko, Z. (1965): The effect of imipramine, desmethylimipramine and chlorpromazine on the sleep-wakefulness cycle on the cat. *Electroencephalogr. Clin. Neurophysiol.*, 19:518–521.
48. Hökfelt, T., Fuxe, K., Johansson, O., Jeffcoate, S., and White, N. (1975): Distribution of thyrotropin-releasing hormone (TRH) in the central nervous system as revealed with immunohistochemistry. *Eur. J. Pharmacol.*, 34:389–396.
49. Horita, A., and Carino, M. A. (1975): Thyrotropin-releasing hormone (TRH)-induced hyperthermia and behavioural excitation in rabbits. *Psychopharmacol. Commun.*, 1:403–414.
50. Horita, A., Carino, M. A., and Lai, H. (1977): Influence of catecholamine antagonists and depletors on the CNS effects of TRH in rabbits. *Prog. Neuropsychopharmacol.*, 1:107–113.
51. Hornykiewicz, O., Lloyd, K. G., and Davidson, L. (1976): The GABA system function of the basal ganglia, and Parkinson's disease. In: *GABA in Nervous System Function*, edited by E. Roberts, T. N. Chase, and D. B. Tower, pp. 479–485. Raven Press, New York.
52. Horst, W. D., and Spirt, N. (1974). A possible mechanism for the antidepressant activity of thyrotropin-releasing hormone. *Life Sci.*, 15:1073–1082.
53. Huidobro-Toro, J. P., Scotti de Carolis, A., and Longo, V. G. (1975): Intensification of central catecholaminergic and serotonergic processes by the hypo-

thalamic factors MIF and TRH and by angiotensin II. *Pharmacol. Biochem. Behav.*, 3:235–242.

54. Inanaga, K., Nakano, Nagata, T., and Tanaka, M. (1975): Effects of thyrotropin-releasing hormone in schizophrenia. *Kurume Med. J.*, 22:159–168.

55. Itil, T. M., Patterson, C. D., Polvan, N., Bigelow, A., and Bergey, B. (1975): Clinical and CNS effects of oral and i.v. thyrotropin-releasing hormone in depressed patients. *Dis. Nerv. Syst.*, 36:529–536.

56. Jackson, I. M. D., and Reichlin, S. (1977): Brain thyrotropin-releasing hormone is independent of the hypothalamus. *Nature (Lond)*, 267:853–854.

57. Kales, A., Heuser, G., Jacobsen, A., Kales, J. D., Hanley, J., Zweizig, J. R., and Paulson, M. J. (1967): All night sleep studies in hypothyroid patients before and after treatment. *J. Clin. Endocrinol.*, 27:1593–1599.

58. Kastin, A. J., Ehrensing, R. H., Schlach, D. S., and Anderson, M. S. (1972): Improvement in mental depression with decreased thyrotropin response after administration of thyrotropin-releasing hormone. *Lancet*, 2:740–742.

59. Keller, H. H., Bartholini, G., and Pletscher, A. (1974): Enhancement of cerebral noradrenaline turnover by thyrotropin-releasing hormone. *Nature (Lond)*, 248:528–529.

60. Kelly, P. H., Seviour, P. W., and Iversen, S. D. (1975): Amphetamine and apomorphine response in the rat following 6-OHDA lesions of the nucleus accumbens septi and corpus striatum. *Brain Res.*, 94:507–516.

61. Koranyi, L., Tamasy, V., Lissak, K., Kiraly, I., and Borsy, J. (1976): Effect of thyrotropin-releasing hormone and antidepressant agents on brain stem and hypothalamic multiple unit activity in the cat. *Psychopharmacology*, 49:197–200.

62. Kotani, M., Onaya, T., and Yamada, T. (1973): Acute increase of thyroid hormone secretion in response to cold and its inhibition by drugs which act on the autonomic and central nervous system. *Endocrinology*, 92:288–294.

63. Kubek, M. J., Lorincz, M. A., and Wilber, J. F. (1977): The identification of thyrotropin-releasing hormone (TRH) in hypothalamic and extrahypothalamic loci of the human nervous system. *Brain Res.*, 126:196–200.

64. Libow, L. S., and Durrell, J. (1965): Clinical studies on the relationship between psychosis and the regulation of thyroid gland activity. *Psychosom. Med.*, 27:377–382.

65. Loosen, P. T., Wilson, I. C., Lara, P. P., Prange, A. J., Jr., and Pettus, C. (1976): Beoinflussung depressiver Zustaende in Alkoholentzugsyndrom mit TRH (Thyrotropin-releasing hormone). *Arzneim. Forsch.*, 26:1164–1166.

66. Maggini, C. M., Guazzelli, M., Mauri, S., Carrara, P., Farnaro, E., Martino, E., MacChia, E., and Baschieri, L. (1978): Sleep, clinical and endocrine studies in depressive patients treated with thyrotropin-releasing hormone. In: *Second European Congress on Sleep*, edited by W. P. Koella, P. Levin, and M. Bertini. Karger, Basel (*in press*).

67. Mandell, A. J. (1975): Neurobiological mechanisms of presynaptic metabolic adaptation and their organization: Implications for a pathophysiology of the affective disorders. In: *Neurobiological Mechanisms of Adaptation and Behaviour*, edited by A. J. Mandell, pp. 17–19. Raven Press, New York.

68. Marek, K., and Haubrich, D. R. (1977): Thyrotropin-releasing hormone-increased catabolism of catecholamines in brains of thyroidectomized rats. *Biochem. Pharmacol.*, 26:1817–1818.

69. McKenzie, G. M., and Viik, K. (1975): Chemically induced choreiform activity: Antagonism by GABA and EEG patterns. *Exp. Neurol.*, 46:229–243.

70. Miyamoto, M., and Nagawa, Y. (1977): Mesolimbic involvement in the locomotor stimulant action of thyrotropin-releasing hormone (TRH) in rats. *Eur. J. Pharmacol.*, 44:143–152.

71. Mountjoy, C. Q. (1976): The possible role of thyroid and thyrotropic hormones in depressive illness. *Postgrad. Med. J.*, 52:103–107.

72. Nielsen, M., Eplov, L., and Scheel-Kruger, J. (1975): The effect of amitriptyline, desipramine and imipramine on the in vitro brain synthesis of ^{3}H-noradrenaline from ^{3}H-L-DOPA in the rat. *Psychopharmacology*, 41:249–254.

73. Nemeroff, C. B., Diez, J. A., Bissette, G., Prange, A. J., Jr., Harrell, L. E., and Lipton, M. A. (1977): Lack of effect of chronically administered thyrotropin-releasing hormone (TRH) on regional rat brain tyrosine hydroxylase activity. *Pharmacol. Biochem. Behav.,* 6:467–469.
74. Plotnikoff, N. P., and Kastin, A. J. (1976): Neuropharmacology of hypothalamic releasing factors. *Biochem. Pharmacol.,* 25:363–365.
75. Plotnikoff, N. P., Prange, A. J., Jr., Breese, G. R., Anderson, M. S., and Wilson, I. C. (1972): Thyrotropin-releasing hormone: Enhancement of L-DOPA activity by a hypothalamic hormone. *Science,* 178:417–418.
76. Plotnikoff, N. P., Prange, A. J., Jr., Breese, G. R., Anderson, M. S., and Wilson, I. C. (1974). The effects of thyrotropin-releasing hormone in normal, hypophysectomized and thyroidectoctomized animals. In: *The Thyroid Axis, Drugs and Behaviour,* edited by A. J. Prange, Jr., pp. 103–113. Raven Press, New York.
77. Powell, E. W., and Leman, R. B. (1976): Connections of the nucleus accumbens. *Brain Res.,* 105:389–394.
78. Prange, A. J., Jr., Breese, G. R., Cott, J. M., Martin, B. R., Cooper, B. R., Wilson, I. C., and Plotnikoff, N. P. (1974): Thyrotropin-releasing hormone: Antagonism of pentobarbital in rodents. *Life Sci.,* 14:447–455.
79. Prange, A. J., Jr., McCurdy, R. L., and Cochrane, C. M. (1967): The systolic blood pressure response of depressed patients to infused norepinephrine. *J. Psychiatr. Res.,* 5:1–13.
80. Prange, A. J., Jr., and Wilson, I. C. (1972): Thyrotropin-releasing hormone for the immediate relief of depression: A preliminary report. *Psychopharmacology (Suppl.),* 28:82–87.
81. Prange, A. J., Jr., Wilson, I. C., and Rabon, M. (1969): Enhancement of imipramine antidepressant activity by thyroid hormone. *Am. J. Psychiatry,* 126:457–469.
82. Raisfeld, I. H. (1972): Cardiovascular complications of antidepressant therapy. *Am. Heart J.,* 83:129–133.
83. Rastogi, R. B., Hrdina, P. D., Dubas, T., and Singhal, R. L. (1977): Alterations of brain acetylcholine metabolism during neonatal hyperthyroidism. *Brain Res.,* 123:188–192.
84. Rastogi, R. B., and Singhal, R. L. (1977): Thyrotropin-releasing hormone (TRH): Potentiation of imipramine effects on the metabolism and the uptake of brain monoamines. *Fed. Proc.,* 36:951.
85. Rastogi, R. B., and Singhal, R. L. (1977): Lithium: Modification of behavioural activity and brain biogenic amines in developing hyperthyroid rats. *J. Pharmacol. Exp. Ther.,* 201:92–102.
86. Rastogi, R. B., Singhal, R. L., and Lapierre, Y. D. (1978): Thyrotropin-releasing hormone: Neurochemical evidence for the potentiation of imipramine effects on the metabolism and uptake of brain norepinephrine and 5-hydroxytryptamine. *(Submitted for publication)*
87. Rawson, R. W. (1953): L-Triiodothyromine versus L-thyroxine: A comparison of their metabolic effects in human myxedema. *Am. J. Med. Sci.,* 226:405–411.
88. Reigle, T. G., Avni, J., Platz, P. A., Schildkraut, J. J., and Plotnikoff, N. P. (1974): Norepinephrine metabolism in the rat brain following acute and chronic administration of thyrotropin-releasing hormone. *Psychopharmacology,* 37:1–6.
89. Roth, R. H., and Suhr, Y. (1970): Mechanism of the γ-hydroxybutyrate-induced increase in brain dopamine and its relationship to "sleep." *Biochem. Pharmacol.,* 19:3001–3012.
90. Roth, R. H., Walters, J. R., and Aghajanian, G. K. (1973): Effects of impulse flow on the release and synthesis of dopamine in the rat striatum. In: *Frontiers of Catecholamine Research,* edited by E. Usdin and S. Snyder, pp. 567–574. Pergamon Press, New York.
91. Schildkraut, J. J. (1965): The catecholamine hypothesis of affective disorders: A review of supporting evidence. *Am. J. Psychiatry,* 122:509–522.
92. Schildkraut, J. J. (1975): Norepinephrine metabolism after short and long-term administration of tricyclic antidepressant drugs and electroconvulsive shock. In:

Neurobiological Mechanisms of Adaptation and Behaviour, edited by A. J. Mandell, pp. 137–153. Raven Press, New York.

93. Schneckloth, R. E., Kurland, G. S., and Freedberg, A. S. (1953): Effect of variation in thyroid function on pressor response to norepinephrine in man. *Metabolism,* 2:546–555.

94. Segal, D. S., and Mandell, A. J. (1974): Differential behavioural effects of hypothalamic polypeptides. In: *The Thyroid Axis, Drugs and Behaviour,* pp. 129–134. Raven Press, New York.

95. Singhal, R. L., Rastogi, R. B., and Agarwal, R. A. (1978): Brain biogenic amines in mental dysfunction attributable to thyroid hormone abnormalities. In: *Hormones and Developing Brain,* edited by S. Kumar. Pergamon Press, New York (*in press*).

96. Singhal, R. L., and Rastogi, R. B. (1978): Neurotransmitter mechanisms during mental illness induced by alterations in thyroid function. *Adv. Pharmacol. Chemother.* 15:204–263.

97. Spaulding, S. W., Burrow, G. N., Donabedian, R., and Van Woert, M. (1972): L-DOPA suppression of thyrotropin releasing hormone response in man. *J. Clin. Endocrinol. Metab.,* 35:182–189.

98. Taber, E. (1963): Histogenesis of brain stem neurons studied autoradiographically with thymidine-H^3 in the mouse. *Anat. Rec.,* 145:291–297.

99. Tuomisto, J., and Mannisto, P. (1973): Amine uptake and thyrotropin-releasing hormone. *Lancet,* 1:836–838.

100. Tuomisto, J., Ranta, T., Mannisto, P., Saarinen, A., and Leppaluoto, J. (1975): Neurotransmitter control of thyrotropin secretion in the rat. *Eur. J. Pharmacol.,* 30:221–229.

101. Van Praag, H. M., and Korf, J. (1975): Central monomaine deficiency in depression: Causative or secondary phenomenon. *Pharmacopsychiatry,* 8:322–326.

102. Whybrow, P. C., and Ferrell, R. (1974): Thyroid state and human behaviour: Contributions from a clinical perspective. In: *The Thyroid Axis, Drugs and Behaviour,* edited by A. J. Prange, Jr., pp. 5–28. Raven Press, New York.

103. Whybrow, P. C., Prange, A. J., Jr., and Treadway, C. R. (1969): Mental changes accompanying thyroid gland dysfunction. *Arch. Gen. Psychiatry,* 20:48–63.

104. Wilson, I. C., Lara, P. P., and Prange, A. J., Jr. (1973): Thyrotropin-releasing hormone in schizophrenia. *Lancet,* 2:43–44.

105. Winokur, A., and Utiger, R. D. (1974): Thyrotropin-releasing hormone, regional distribution in rat brain. *Science,* 185:265–266.

106. Yarbrough, G. G. (1976): TRH potentiates excitatory actions of acetylcholine on cerebral cortical neurones. *Nature (Lond),* 263:523–524.

Central Nervous System Effects of Hypothalamic
Hormones and Other Peptides, edited by Collu et al.
Raven Press, New York © 1979.

Influence of Thyrotropin-Releasing Hormone on the Synaptic Availability of Catecholamines in Brain

W. Dale Horst, Nena Spirt, and Gordon Bautz

Department of Pharmacology, Hoffmann-La Roche Inc., Nutley, New Jersey 07110

Thyrotropin-releasing hormone (TRH; L-pyroglutamyl-L-histidyl-L-proline-amide) has been reported to influence several central nervous system (CNS) responses in animals and humans. Accordingly, TRH has been described as an antidepressant (9,10), an antagonist of the behavioral effects of pentobarbital (11), and a potentiator of the behavioral effects of L-DOPA (8). Since these influences of TRH on the CNS may be classified as "arousal" responses, investigations on the mode of TRH action have focused on brain catecholaminergic systems.

Unlike most known psychostimulants or antidepressants, TRH does not inhibit either amine reuptake into presynaptic nerve endings or monoamine oxidase (1,5). However, several studies indicate that TRH may potentiate norepinephrine CNS response by stimulating norepinephrine turnover or release. Constantinidis et al. (4) and Horst and Spirt (5) showed that TRH at doses of 10 to 40 mg/kg increases the rate of α-methyl-p-tyrosine-induced norepinephrine disappearance from various areas of rat brain. Keller et al. (6) found that TRH (10 mg/kg) increases brain concentrations of the norepinephrine metabolite 3-methoxy-4-hydroxyphenylethyleneglycol (MOPEG) in rats, a phenomenon also associated with increased norepinephrine turnover. In addition, TRH (10 mg/kg) hastens the disappearance of ^{3}H-norepinephrine from brain and increases brain concentrations of ^{3}H-normetanephrine following the intracisternal injection of ^{3}H-norepinephrine (5).

TRH appears to have a selective influence on norepinephrine synapses. Although Marek and Haubrich (7) demonstrated that TRH (15 mg/kg) increases the rate of dopamine turnover in rat brain, several other investigators failed to observe this effect *in vivo* (4–6).

The fact that TRH administration does not diminish endogenous levels of norepinephrine (4–6) suggests that synthesis rates increase to compensate for the increased utilization. Keller et al. (6) demonstrated a TRH-induced increase in the conversion of ^{14}C-L-tyrosine to ^{14}C-norepinephrine in rat brain.

The TRH-induced influences on norepinephrine turnover, like many behavioral influences (2,8,11), are not mediated through pituitary or thyroid

TABLE 1. *Influence of TRH on the release of* ^{3}*H-norepinephrine from superfused brain synaptosomes*

Time	Control[a]	TRH[a]
Hypothalamus		
0 to 1 min	23.15 ± 0.77	25.20 ± 1.94
1 to 4 min	38.47 ± 1.80	39.42 ± 1.66
Cortex		
0 to 1 min	18.84 ± 0.96	21.50 ± 0.86
1 to 4 min	32.26 ± 1.48	29.49 ± 1.77

Brain synaptosomes were prepared as before (5), preincubated with ^{3}H-norepinephrine (0.2 μM) for 20 min and TRH (1×10^{-4} M) for 60 min, then superfused as described by Raiteri et al. (12). The superfusates for the TRH-treated synaptosomes also contained TRH (10^{-4} M).

[a] Results are the means ± SEM of at least five determinations and are expressed as the percent of the total ^{3}H-norepinephrine released. None of the values obtained with TRH are significantly different from their respective control values.

hormones since TRH (10^{-4} M) was found to increase the release or turnover of ^{3}H-catecholamines from incubated, suspended brain synaptosomes (5). These *in vitro* effects also indicate that TRH influences norepinephrine fibers directly and that the *in vivo* alterations in norepinephrine turnover are not mediated by influences on other neuronal types which impinge on norepinephrine neurons.

Recently we investigated the influence of TRH on the release of ^{3}H-norepinephrine from superfused brain synaptosomes. As seen in Table 1, TRH has no influence on ^{3}H-norepinephrine release from hypothalamic or cerebral cortical synaptosomes in this preparation. The discrepancy between TRH effects on ^{3}H-norepinephrine release from suspended and superfused brain synaptosomes suggests a hypothesis for a TRH mechanism of action.

Receptor sites, located on the presynaptic nerve terminals and sensitive to the neurotransmitter of the neuron on which they are localized, have been described for many neurotransmitters in brain, including norepinephrine (3). These "autoreceptors" are believed to play an important role in regulating the rate of neurotransmitter release or turnover.

One major difference between neurotransmitter release from suspended and from superfused synaptosomes is the availability of neurotransmitter for interaction at presynaptic autoreceptor sites. In the case of incubated, suspended synaptosomes, released norepinephrine in the incubation medium is available for interaction at extraneuronal uptake and autoreceptor sites, and presumably drugs could alter norepinephrine fluxes by altering autoreceptor sensitivity. On the other hand, norepinephrine released from superfused synaptosomes is removed rapidly (12) and would have little or no opportunity to interact at these extraneuronal sites; therefore drug-induced alterations in autoreceptor sensitivity would not be expected to be expressed under these conditions. Thus TRH may increase norepinephrine turnover by decreasing the sensitivity of a presynaptic, negative feedback regulatory mechanism. Whether this is true remains to be determined.

Since substantial endogenous levels of TRH have been found in several brain areas, this tripeptide may play an important role in the regulation of norepinephrine release from nerve terminals.

ACKNOWLEDGMENT

The authors thank Mr. Jonathan Jantz of Bethel College (North Newton, Kansas) and Miss Kristin Isaak of Bluffton College (Bluffton, Ohio) for their help in conducting the experiments on norepinephrine release from superfused synaptosomes.

REFERENCES

1. Breese, G. R., Cooper, B. R., Prange, A. J., Jr., Cott, J. M., and Lipton, M. A. (1974): Interactions of thyrotropin-releasing hormone with centrally acting drugs. In: *The Thyroid Axis, Drugs, and Behavior,* edited by A. J. Prange, Jr., pp. 115–127. Raven Press, New York.
2. Breese, G. R., Cott, J. M., Cooper, B. R., and Prange, A. J., Jr. (1974): Antagonism of ethanol narcosis by thyrotropin releasing hormone. *Life Sci.,* 14:1053–1063.
3. Bunney, B. S., and Aghajanian, G. K. (1975): Evidence for drug actions on both pre- and post-synaptic catecholamine receptors in the CNS. In: *Pre- and Post-Synaptic Receptors,* edited by E. Usdin and W. E. Bunney, Jr., pp. 89–120. Marcel Dekker, New York.
4. Constantinidis, J., Geissbühler, F., Gaillard, J. M., Hovaguimian, Th., and Tissot, R. (1974): Enhancement of cerebral noradrenaline turnover by thyrotropin-releasing hormone: Evidence by fluorescence histochemistry. *Experientia,* 30:1182.
5. Horst, W. D., and Spirt, N. (1974): A possible mechanism for the antidepressant activity of thyrotropin releasing hormone. *Life Sci.,* 15:1073–1082.
6. Keller, H. H., Bartholini, G., and Pletscher, A. (1974): Enhancement of cerebral noradrenaline turnover by thyrotropin-releasing hormone. *Nature (Lond),* 248:528–529.
7. Marek, K., and Haubrich, D. R. (1977): Thyrotropin-releasing hormone—increased catabolism of catecholamines in brains of thyroidectomized rats. *Biochem. Pharmacol.,* 26:1817–1818.
8. Plotnikoff, N. P., Prange, A. J., Jr., Breese, G. R., Anderson, M. S., and Wilson, I. C. (1972): Thyrotropin releasing hormone: Enhancement of DOPA activity by a hypothalamic hormone. *Science,* 178:417–418.
9. Prange, A. J., Jr., and Wilson, I. C. (1972): Thyrotropin releasing hormone (TRH) for the immediate relief of depression: A preliminary report. *Psychopharmacologia (Suppl. 82),* 26.
10. Prange, A. J., Jr., Wilson, I. C., Lara, P. P., and Alltop, L. B. (1974): Effect of thyrotropin-releasing hormone in depression. In: *The Thyroid Axis, Drugs, and Behavior,* edited by A. J. Prange, Jr., pp. 135–145. Raven Press, New York.
11. Prange, A. J., Jr., Breese, G. R., Cott, J. M., Martin, B. R., Cooper, B. R., Wilson, I. C., and Plotnikoff, N. P. (1974): Thyrotropin releasing hormone: Antagonism of pentobarbital in rodents. *Life Sci.,* 14:447–455.
12. Raiteri, M., Angelini, F., and Levi, G. (1974): A simple apparatus for studying the release of neurotransmitters from synaptosomes. *Eur. J. Pharmacol.,* 25:411–414.

CRF–ACTH–Catecholamines

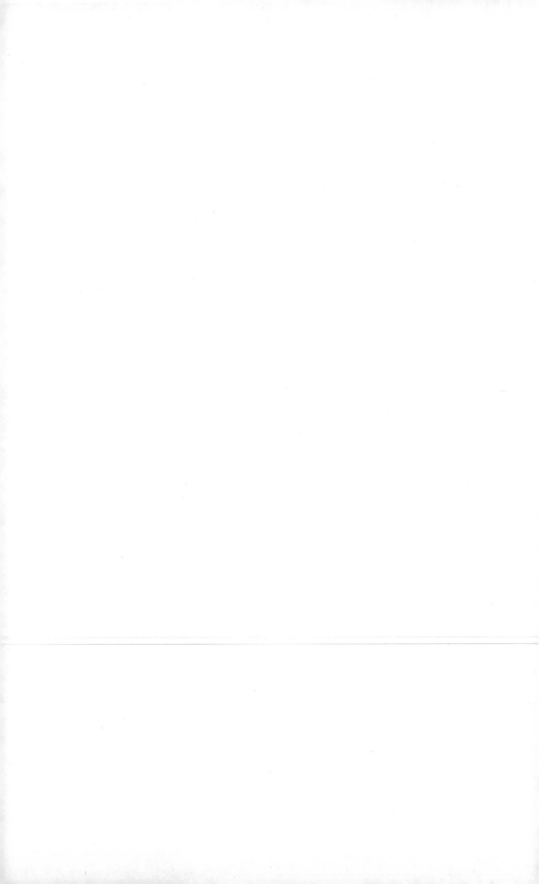

Central Nervous System Effects of Hypothalamic Hormones and Other Peptides, edited by Collu et al. Raven Press, New York © 1979.

Effects of Peptides on Central Neuronal Excitability

Leo P. Renaud, Quentin J. Pittman, Howard W. Blume, Yvon Lamour, and Elisabeth Arnauld

Division of Neurology, Montreal General Hospital, Montreal, Quebec, Canada H3G 1A4

Electrophysiology has significantly enhanced our understanding of synaptic transmission and central nervous system (CNS) pharmacology. The actions of several substances endogenous to brain tissue have been tentatively identified as neurotransmitter agents following electrophysiological measurement of their effects on neural tissue. Recent progress in the isolation and structural characterization of endogenous peptides has permitted their distribution to be verified quantitatively by radioimmunoassay and immunohistochemistry. The synthesis of these peptides and their analogs has made possible electrophysiological measurement of their effects on a variety of neural tissues. This chapter reviews some of the evidence from these investigations indicating the potential importance of several endogenous brain peptides in neural function and interneuronal communication (see also refs. 2,45,46, 50,60,74,79).

ELECTROPHYSIOLOGICAL TECHNIQUES FOR THE STUDY OF PEPTIDE ACTIONS IN NEURAL TISSUE

Two basic methodologies have been utilized to study the effects of peptide actions in neural tissue. The *in vitro* technique allows for the recording of electrical activity during perfusion of an isolated but relatively intact nervous system with known concentrations of peptides. With the *in vivo* technique, a combination of microiontophoresis (37) and extra- or intracellular recordings provides the most definitive observations. The relative advantages and disadvantages of each approach were recently reviewed (79). The following sections summarize these electrophysiological observations using both techniques and explore the neural circuitry of the hypothalamic peptidergic neurons.

STUDIES WITH SUBSTANCE P

In 1931 von Euler and Gaddum reported the isolation from gut and brain of a preparation "P" containing a low-molecular-weight polypeptide with potent contractile and hypotensive properties (89). This material, eventually referred to as substance P, was later detected in high concentrations in specific regions of the CNS, notably the hypothalamus and spinal dorsal root fibers (42,87). This distribution in the CNS led to the proposal that substance P might have a neurotransmitter function, especially in primary afferent fibers (42,55). Recent studies tend to support this postulate. This evidence is reviewed briefly since it provides worthwhile guidelines for the assessment of other endogenous CNS peptides.

Otsuka and his colleagues reported that a peptide extracted from bovine dorsal root fibers exerted a potent depolarizing action on motoneurons of the isolated frog and rat spinal cord (36,54,57). Subsequently this endogenous peptide was identified as the undecapeptide substance P isolated from bovine hypothalamus and structurally characterized by Leeman and her colleagues (41,86). Related compounds with common C-terminal sequences (e.g., physalaemin and eledoisin) also exerted a potent and prolonged direct excitation of motoneurons (35,55). This action was considerably more potent on an equimolar basis than that of other putative neurotransmitter agents, including L-glutamate (Fig. 1) and L-aspartate (55). Substance P-induced depolarization appeared to be independent of the action of other putative neurotransmitter substances and was associated with an increase in membrane conductance presumably for sodium ions (50).

A variety of other studies tend to support the possible role for substance P as a neurotransmitter in primary afferent fibers. With dorsal root stimulation, calcium-dependent release of substance P can be detected from isolated neural tissue (31,49,56). These findings are in accord with the immunohistochemical evidence of substance P-like material in neurons in the dorsal root ganglia and nerve terminals in the dorsal horn of the spinal cord (7,15,24–26). At the ultrastructural level, substance P-like immunoreactivity is con-

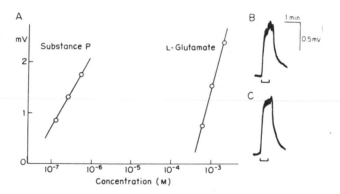

FIG. 1. Comparison of the effect of substance P and L-glutamate on rat spinal motoneurons obtained by extracellular recordings. (A): Dose-response curves of substance P and L-glutamate illustrate the greater equimolar potency of substance P. (B, C): Actual depolarizing responses to substance P (2×10^{-7} M) and L-glutamate (7×10^{-4} M) recorded from an L3 ventral root during the period of drug application marked under the records. (From ref. 55.)

centrated in synaptic vesicles in the nerve terminals of the rat spinal cord (6,63) and in vesicular subcellular fractions in rat brain (8).

The use of microiontophoresis during *in vivo* studies led to further characterization of the action of substance P on neural tissue. Application of substance P on neurons in the mammalian spinal cord, brainstem, and subcortical and cortical regions is frequently associated with an enhancement of neuronal excitability in a characteristic manner (10,19,20,22,40,44,61,62). The response is usually delayed by 10 to 30 sec after the onset of application and outlasts the application period by several tens of seconds (Fig. 2). The slow excitatory action of substance P contrasts with the brisk onset of excitation evoked by other putative neurotransmitter substances, including L-glutamate (Fig. 2). This delayed action of substance P also contrasts sharply with the responses of substance P-sensitive neurons to proprioceptive stimuli (Fig. 2). These observations argue against a neurotransmitter function for substance P. However, substance P is present in the *smaller* neurons of dorsal root ganglia (26), usually associated with smaller slower-conducting primary afferent fibers involved in nociception. There are now several indications that substance P is in fact associated with pain pathways (16,21, 25,30,66,67).

Substance P also affects the excitability of neurons in other areas of the CNS unlikely to be involved in nociception. Throughout these areas only certain cells are sensitive to substance P, and the effect depends specifically on the nature of the cell tested. For example, although the most commonly observed effect is enhancement of excitability, substance P applied to spinal cord Renshaw neurons is associated with a selective decrease in their response to acetylcholine and synaptic activation of nicotinic receptors (4,39). It is not yet certain whether the latter observation results from a pre- or a postsynaptic site of action, although both are possible (38,82,83).

In summary, the presence of substance P within neural tissue, its release at nerve terminals, and its effects on the excitability of central neurons suggest an important role in interneuronal communication, possibly as a

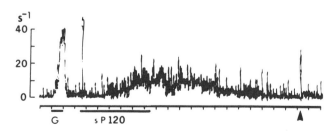

FIG. 2. Ratemeter record of the spike discharge frequency of a cat spinal cord dorsal horn neuron, demonstrating the contrasting activation patterns obtained by microiontophoretic application of L-glutamate (G, 60 nA), substance P (sP, 120 nA), and a jet of air applied to the peripheral receptive field (*arrowhead*). Note the very brief response to the latter stimulus, the relatively brisk response to glutamate, and the slowly developing response to substance P. (From ref. 22.)

neurotransmitter or a neuromodulatory agent. Substance P is one example of a peptide waiting for its specific function in the hypothalamic area to be discovered, although there is already evidence of a functional role in other areas of the nervous system.

STUDIES ON PEPTIDERGIC PATHWAYS

The neurophysiology of peptidergic neurons was first described in detail by Kandel (32), who examined the electrical properties of putative neurosecretory neurons in the goldfish preoptic area. Intracellular studies clearly illustrated the neuronal characteristics of these neurosecretory neurohypophysial neurons and their ability to display antidromic and orthodromic responses. Kandel also noted that antidromic activation of neurosecretory neurons was followed by a prominent inhibitory postsynaptic potential considered to arise from axon collaterals of neurohypophysial fibers that either synapsed directly on the parent neuron or onto inhibitory interneurons which then projected to the neurosecretory neuron. Similar observations indicative of axon collaterals in neurohypophysial fibers have been obtained from studies in higher vertebrates (for review see refs. 2,73). Anatomical and functional evidence for axon collaterals in peptidergic pathways has raised important conceptual issues (2,50,52,73). In accordance with Dale's postulate (9) that the same substance should be released from all branches of the same axon, activity in the neurohypophysial system with release of peptides into the circulation of the posterior pituitary should be accompanied by the release of the same substance from central terminals of these axons. Thus oxytocin and/or vasopressin might be the neurotransmitter agents in a recurrent inhibitory pathway of the neurohypophysial system. Although the microiontophoretic application of both peptides modifies the excitability of both neurosecretory and nonneurosecretory central neurons (47,52) (Fig. 3), clear experimental evidence supporting a role for these peptides in the recurrent inhibitory pathway has not yet been presented. For example, the neurohypophysial tract of the vasopressin-deficient homozygous Brattleboro rat continues to demonstrate evidence of a functional recurrent inhibitory pathway (13). Nevertheless, the notion that vasopressin and/or oxytocin are engaged in neuronal intercommunication deserves serious consideration in view of recent immunohistochemical data illustrating central neurophysin, oxytocin, and vasopressin pathways (1,15,24,81,84)

The parvicellular neurons that project to the portal capillaries of the median eminence and are engaged in the release of peptide factors into the pituitary portal circulation have been collectively described as components of the tuberoinfundibular system (85). Immunohistochemical procedures have now successfully stained somata and axons immunoreactive for TRH, LH-RH, and somatostatin (15,23,24). Those neurons with fibers projecting to the median eminence are most likely involved as part of the tuberoin-

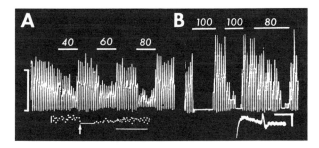

FIG. 3. Records from cat supraoptic neurosecretory neurons that displayed evidence of antidromic activation (*lower right*) and a silent interval in the poststimulus histogram (*lower left*) following stimulation of the neurohypophysis. The upper parts of A and B represent ratemeter discharge frequency records that display a dose-dependent decrease in excitability during the microiontophoretic application of lysine vasopressin. (From ref. 52.)

fundibular system. Tuberoinfundibular neurons can also be identified according to electrophysiological criteria (34,43,45,70,75,80) and have been located throughout the medial hypothalamus and medial preoptic area (Fig. 4). Unlike the neurohypophysial system, where cells are tentatively characterized as vasopressin or oxytocin neurons according to their activity patterns (65), tuberoinfundibular neurons cannot be associated with a particular peptide and can be only tentatively considered as peptidergic in na-

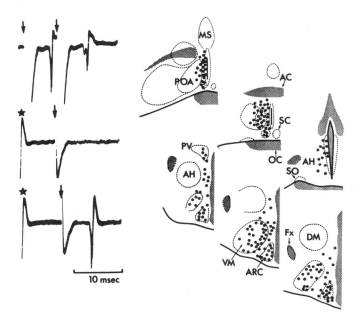

FIG. 4. Electrophysiological identification of tuberoinfundibular neurons requires evidence for antidromic activation (series of oscilloscope traces shown on the left) following median eminence stimulation (*arrows*). The locations of tuberoinfundibular neurons in the medial hypothalamus and preoptic area are shown on the series of schematic coronal sections on the right.

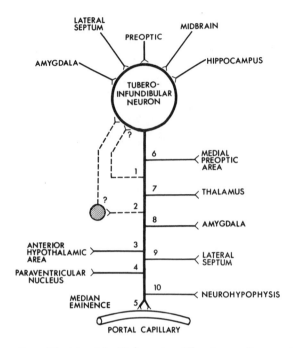

FIG. 5. Known connections of the tuberoinfundibular system. Efferent connections are shown in the lower half of the diagram. The heavy vertical line represents the axon connecting this peptidergic or dopaminergic tuberoinfundibular cell to the portal capillary. Intrahypothalamic axon collaterals are referred to by the numbers 1 through 5: (1 and 2) Direct or indirect recurrent inhibitory or excitatory pathways whose transmitter agent is unknown (?), as are those released from the other central axon collaterals. (3 and 4) Axon collaterals to the anterior hypothalamic area and paraventricular nucleus. (5) Terminal branches seen in the vicinity of the portal plexus. Extrahypothalamic axon collaterals are depicted as numbers 6 through 10 on the right side of the diagram, extending to several areas including the neurohypophysis. At the top are the afferent connections of some tuberoinfundibular neurons, connections that are presumably important for the expression of CNS actions on the endocrine system.

ture. However, only electrophysiological studies permit a detailed examination of the extent and nature of connections of these neurons. At the moment, there is evidence for extensive intra- and extrahypothalamic axon collaterals in the tuberoinfundibular system (69,71,72,75) (Fig. 5). By analogy with the neurohypophysial system, suggesting the release of peptides from terminals of central axon collaterals, one is tempted to speculate that releasing factors may also function at central synaptic sites in addition to their role in anterior pituitary regulation (68,75).

EFFECTS OF TRH, LH-RH, AND SOMATOSTATIN ON NEURAL TISSUE

The effects of the three structurally characterized hypothalamic peptides have been examined in a variety of neural tissues.

TRH

TRH exerts a depolarizing action on motoneurons in the isolated frog spinal cord (51). This action differs from depolarization evoked by L-glutamate in that it produces a background facilitatory action rather than a marked enhancement of excitability. The effect is of long duration, often shows tachyphylaxis, and is presumably the result of a direct postsynaptic and an indirect presynaptic action. The depolarizing action is associated with a small increase in membrane conductance, possibly to sodium ions. Studies with TRH analogs indicate that the 1-methyl-His TRH analog, which does not release TSH from the adenohypophysis, is devoid of activity in the isolated spinal cord; the 3-methyl-His TRH analog, which is more potent than TRH in terms of TSH release, is also more potent in its effects on spinal cord motoneurons.

In vivo microiontophoretic studies indicate that TRH can affect the excitability of central neurons in a variety of areas (14,46,76–78). In most instances iontophoresis of TRH is associated with an abrupt and readily reversible change in spontaneous or glutamate-evoked activity, with the predominant response occurring as a depression in excitability (Figs. 6 and 7). The depressant effect appears resistant to antagonism by picrotoxin and bicuculline (76). Microiontophoretic application of TRH on certain brainstem neurons exerts a prolonged enhancement of excitability that greatly outlasts the period of application by several tens of seconds (Briggs, *personal communication*). Although these effects could result from direct synaptic actions of TRH, there are indications that TRH may modify the action of other neurotransmitter substances. For example, Yarbrough (91) presented evidence for selective enhancement of the excitatory actions of

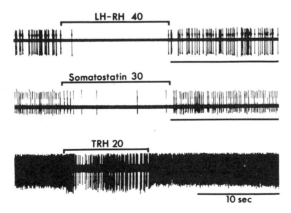

FIG. 6. Sample oscilloscope traces to display the decrease in action potential frequency and excitability of neurons in the hypothalamus (*top*), parietal cortex (*middle*), and cerebellar cortex (*bottom*) during microiontophoretic application of LH-RH, somatostatin, and TRH. Recordings were obtained from glutamate-evoked (*top two traces*) or spontaneously active (*bottom trace*) cells in pentobarbital-anesthetized male Sprague-Dawley rats. The numbers above each bar indicate the iontophoretic current in nanoamperes.

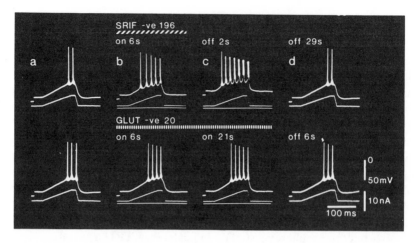

FIG. 7. Intracellular records to illustrate the excitatory action of somatostatin and L-glutamate on a CA1 pyramidal neuron in the rat hippocampal brain slice preparation. In the control records (*left*), depolarizing ramp pulses applied to the intracellular electrode evoke only two or three action potentials, whereas during the iontophoresis of somatostatin or glutamate there is a depolarization and an increase in the number of action potentials evoked by the depolarizing current. The last records indicate full recovery. (From ref. 11.)

acetylcholine, but not glutamate, when TRH is simultaneously applied to sensitive neurons in the cerebral cortex. Although this suggests a possible modulator function for TRH, studies in our laboratory have consistently failed to display similar effects of TRH on cholinoceptive cortical neurons (64).

LH-RH

Luteinizing hormone-releasing hormone (LH-RH) has been shown to influence animal behavior (48,59; Moss et al., *this volume*). Both an increase and a decrease in the excitability of neurons in the hypothalamus have been noted following microiontophoretic application of LH-RH (14,33,45,77,78) (Fig. 6). As with TRH, the observed responses were usually rapid in onset, proportional to the microiontophoretic current, and readily reversible. LH-RH analogs are also effective when applied to central neurons (45,74, 78). Although structure activity relationships are not yet analyzed in detail, preliminary data indicate that potency ratios established for LH-RH activity in the anterior pituitary are only partly similar or analogous to those obtained from studies on central neurons. This raises the possibility that one could dissociate the behavioral and pituitary effects given the appropriate LH-RH analog.

Somatostatin

Somatostatin is present in widespread areas of the CNS, peripheral nervous system, and nonneural tissues (15,23). Neurons containing somatostatin-like immunoreactivity are present in the dorsal root ganglia, are distinct from substance P-containing neurons, and appear to project into the dorsal root entry zone of the spinal cord (26). The release of substance P and somatostatin can be evoked in a calcium-dependent manner from cell cultures of these primary sensory neurons (49). *In vitro* and *in vivo* studies have been conducted in order to delineate the role of somatostatin in neural tissue.

Frog spinal cord contains considerably greater quantities of somatostatin than the mammalian spinal cord (79) with the dorsal quadrant containing approximately 60% more than the ventral quadrant. Somatostatin evokes two responses in the isolated frog spinal cord: First, there is an immediate small hyperpolarization of motoneurons accompanied by a decreased response to ventral and dorsal root responses to glutamate; this is followed by a dose-dependent increase in the size of the ventral root potentials evoked by dorsal root stimulation, a response that begins only 10 to 20 min after the addition of somatostatin and outlasts the application period by 30 to 60 min, with no evidence of desensitization or tachyphylaxis (79). The initial response appears to be a direct (postsynaptic) effect of somatostatin, whereas the later responses probably represent an indirect or presynaptic effect of somatostatin at a location still to be determined.

Dodd and Kelly recently described a depolarizing action of somatostatin in another *in vitro* preparation, the hippocampal brain slice (11). In this preparation, somatostatin evokes a depolarizing action on pyramidal neurons, with effects similar to the action of glutamate (Fig. 7). No further details on the mechanism of action are currently available.

Applied by microiontophoresis to neurons in the cerebral and cerebellar cortex, hypothalamus, and spinal cord, somatostatin has a depressant effect in the anesthetized preparation (44,66,77,78). Somatostatin-evoked responses are usually abrupt in onset, readily reversible (Fig. 6), and resistant to bicuculline and picrotoxin antagonism. The exception to this depressant response has been the report of an excitatory effect of somatostatin in the cerebral cortex of the unanesthetized restrained rabbit (29). Such discrepancies evidently require further investigation and could be related to the presence or absence of anesthesia.

OTHER PEPTIDES OF NEUROBIOLOGICAL SIGNIFICANCE

The brain contains other polypeptides, including angiotensin, neurotensin, some peptides commonly found in the gastrointestinal tract (gastrin, cholecystokinin, and vasoactive intestinal peptide), several hormones of the anterior pituitary (growth hormone, ACTH, gonadotropins, and TSH) and the opioid enkephalin and endorphin peptides (15,18,25,28,58,88). The enkephalins and endorphins are considered important in central pain perception (25,27) and have been examined in detail by electrophysiological methods. One advantage of investigations using opiates and opioid peptides has been the ready availability of specific agonists and antagonists. When applied by microiontophoresis to neurons at various levels of the neural axis, these peptides have a potent but selective action—usually to decrease neuronal excitability (5,12,17,53), although Renshaw cells and neurons in the hippocampus respond with an increase in excitability (53). The action of these peptides seems to be mediated through a postsynaptic mechanism (53); however, a neuromodulatory action functionally distinct from conventional neurotransmitter mechanisms was recently demonstrated (3). For a detailed description of these investigations the reader is referred to the original papers quoted above.

COMMENTARY

The observations presented here indicate that peptides are involved in some aspects of neural function. Peptides appear to modify neuronal activity in a selective manner with respect to their mode and site of action (Fig. 8). Studies with analogs suggest that central receptor sites differ somewhat from those in the pituitary. The short-term action observed following microiontophoretic studies suggests that peptides may be good candidates for

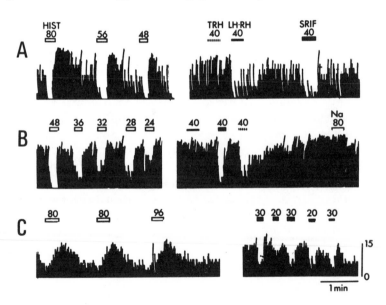

FIG. 8. Examples of the specificity of response of adjacent hypothalamic neurons to different agents. A, B, and C are polygraph records of the action potential frequency of three hypothalamic neurons encountered during a single penetration with the same electrode and tested with histamine, TRH, LH-RH, and somatostatin applied by microiontophoresis. Note that each cell has its own pattern of response to any one of the applied substances. For example, the activity of cell A was initially depressed by histamine, followed by a later, prolonged enhancement of excitability; the activity of cell B was predominantly depressed; and the excitability of cell C was enhanced in a prolonged manner by histamine. Note also that different neurons were sensitive to different peptides.

neurotransmitter agents (90), although their equimolar potency appears to be much higher than for conventional neurotransmitters. The possibility of peptide interactions with other neurotransmitter substances and more prolonged modes of action suggest a neuromodulator function for certain peptides in certain areas, and this aspect deserves further investigation. The hypothalamic peptidergic neurons appear to have more than one function: One is related to control of peptide secretion at the pituitary level, another to central neuronal function. It is possible that an integration of these two functions is required for normal behavioral expression.

ACKNOWLEDGMENTS

The authors are grateful to the Canadian Medical Research Council and the Conseil de la Recherche en Santé du Québec for financial support for the work conducted in this laboratory; to Mr. Brian MacKenzie and Mr. William Ellis for technical assistance; and to Mrs. M. Walker for typing the manuscript.

REFERENCES

1. Antunes, J. L., Carmel, P. W. and Zimmerman, E. A. (1977): Projections from the paraventricular nucleus to the zona externa of the median eminence of the rhesus monkey: An immunohistochemical study. *Brain Res.,* 137:1–10.
2. Barker, J. L. (1977): Physiological roles of peptides in the nervous system. In: *Peptides in Neurobiology,* edited by H. Gainer, pp. 295–343. Plenum Press, New York.
3. Barker, J. L., Neale, J. H., Smith, T. G., Jr., and MacDonald, R. L. (1978): Opiate peptide modulation of amino acid responses suggests novel form of neuronal communication. *Science,* 199:1451–1453.
4. Belcher, G., and Ryall, R. W. (1977): Substance P and Renshaw cells: A new concept of inhibitory synaptic interactions. *J. Physiol. (Lond),* 272:105–119.
5. Bradley, P. B., Briggs, L., Gayton, R. J., and Lambert, L. A. (1976): Effects of microiontophoretically applied methionine-enkephalin on single neurones in rat brainstem. *Nature (Lond),* 261:425–426.
6. Chan-Palay, V., and Palay, S. L. (1977): Ultrastructural identification of substance P cells and their processes in rat sensory ganglia and their terminals in the spinal cord by immunocytochemistry. *Proc. Natl. Acad. Sci. USA,* 74:4050–4054.
7. Cuello, A. C., and Kanazawa, I. (1978): The distribution of substance P immunoreactive fibers in the rat central nervous system. *J. Comp. Neurol.,* 178:129–156.
8. Cuello, A. C., Jessell, T., Kanazawa, I., and Iversen, L. L. (1977): Substance P: Localization in synaptic vesicles in rat central nervous system. *J. Neurochem.,* 29:747–751.
9. Dale, H. A. (1935): Pharmacology and nerve endings. *Proc. R. Soc. Med.,* 28:318–332.
10. Davies, J., and Dray, A. (1976): Substance P in the substantia nigra. *Brain Res.,* 107:623–627.
11. Dodd, J., and Kelly, J. S. (1978): Is somatostatin an excitatory transmitter in the hippocampus? *Nature (Lond),* 273:674–675.
12. Duggan, A. W., Hall, J. G., and Headley, P. M. (1976): Morphine, enkephalin and the substantia gelatinosa. *Nature (Lond),* 264:456–458.
13. Dyball, R. E. J. (1974): Single unit activity in the hypothalamo-neurohypophyseal system of the Brattleboro rat. *J. Endocrinol.,* 60:135–143.

14. Dyer, R. G., and Dyball, R. E. J. (1974): Evidence for a direct effect of LRF and TRF on single unit-activity in rostral hypothalamus. *Nature (Lond)*, 252:486–488.
15. Elde, R., and Hökfelt, T. (1978): Distribution of hypothalamic hormones and other peptides in the brain. In: *Frontiers in Neuroendocrinology*, Vol. 5, edited by W. F. Ganong and L. Martini, pp. 1–33. Raven Press, New York.
16. Frederickson, R. C. A., Burgis, V., Harrell, C. E., and Edwards, J. D. (1978): Dual actions of substance P on nociception: Possible role of endogenous opioids. *Science*, 199:1359–1362.
17. Frederickson, R. C. A., and Norris, F. H. (1976): Enkephalin-induced depression of single neurons in brain areas with opiate receptors—antagonism by naloxone. *Science*, 194:440–442.
18. Goldstein, A. (1976): Opioid peptides (endorphins) in pituitary and brain. *Science*, 193:1081–1086.
19. Henry, J. L. (1975): Substance P excitation of spinal nociceptive neurons. *Neurosci. Abst.*, 1:390.
20. Henry, J. L. (1976): Effects of substance P on functionally identified units in cat spinal cord. *Brain Res.*, 114:439–451.
21. Henry, J. L. (1977): Substance P and pain: A possible relation in afferent transmission. In: *Substance P*, edited by U. S. von Euler and B. Pernow, pp. 231–240. Raven Press, New York.
22. Henry, J. L., Krnjevic, K., and Morris, M. E. (1975): Substance P and spinal neurones. *Can. J. Physiol. Pharmacol.*, 53:423–432.
23. Hökfelt, T., Efendic, S., Hellerstrom, C., Johansson, O., Luft, R., and Arimura, A. (1975): Cellular localization of somatostatin in endocrine-like cells and neurones of the rat with special reference to A_1-cells of the pancreatic islets and to the hypothalamus. *Acta Endocrinol. (Kbh)[Suppl. 200]*, 80:1–40.
24. Hökfelt, T., Elde, R., Fuxe, K., Johansson, O., Ljungdahl, A., Goldstein, M. Luft, R., Efendic, S., Nilsson, G., Terenius, L., Ganten, D., Jeffcoate, S. L., Rehfeld, J., Said, S., Perez de la Mora, M., Possani, L., Tapia, R., Teran, L., and Palacios, R. (1977): Aminergic and peptidergic pathways in the nervous system with special reference to the hypothalamus. In: *The Hypothalamus*, edited by S. Reichlin, R. J. Baldessarini, and J. B. Martin, pp. 69–135. Raven Press, New York.
25. Hökfelt, T., Ljungdahl, A., Terenius, L., Elde, R., and Nilsson, G. (1977): Immunohistochemical analysis of peptide pathways possibly related to pain and analgesia: Enkephalin and substance P. *Proc. Natl. Acad. Sci. USA*, 74:3081–3085.
26. Hökfelt, T., Elde, R., Johansson, O., Luft, R., Nilsson, G., and Arimura, A. (1976): Immunohistochemical evidence for separate populations of somatostatin-containing and substance P-containing primary afferent neurons in the rat. *Neuroscience*, 1:131–136.
27. Hughes, J., and Kosterlitz, H. W. (1977): Opioid peptides. *Br. Med. Bull.*, 33:157–161.
28. Hughes, J., Smith, T. W., Kosterlitz, H. W., Fothergill, L. A., Morgan, B. A., and Morris, H. R. (1975): Identification of two related pentapeptides from the brain with potent opiate agonist activity. *Nature (Lond)*, 258:577–579.
29. Ioffe, S., Havlicek, V., Friesen, H., and Cherniak, V. (1977): The excitatory effect of iontophoretically applied somatostatin (SRIF) on cortical neurons in awake unanaesthetized animals. *Fed. Proc.*, 36:364 (abstract 501).
30. Jessell, T. M., and Iversen, L. L. (1977): Opiate analgesics inhibit substance P release from rat trigeminal nucleus. *Nature (Lond)*, 268:549–551.
31. Jessell, T., Iversen, L. L., and Kanazawa, I. (1976): Release and metabolism of substance P in rat hypothalamus. *Nature (Lond)*, 264:81–83.
32. Kandel, E. R. (1964): Electrical properties of hypothalamic neuroendocrine cells. *J. Gen. Physiol.*, 47:691–717.
33. Kawakami, M., and Sakuma, Y. (1974): Responses of hypothalamic neurons to the microiontophoresis of LH-RH, LH and FSH under various levels of circulating ovarian hormones. *Neuroendocrinology*, 15:290–307.
34. Kawakami, M., and Sakuma, Y. (1976): Electrophysiological evidence for pos-

sible participation of periventricular neurons in anterior pituitary regulation. *Brain Res.*, 101:79–94.

35. Konishi, S., and Otsuka, M. (1974): The effects of substance P and other peptides on spinal neurons of the frog. *Brain Res.*, 65:397–410.
36. Konishi, S., and Otsuka, M. (1974): Excitatory action of hypothalamic substance P on spinal motoneurons of newborn rats. *Nature (Lond)*, 252:734–735.
37. Krnjevic, K. (1971): Microiontophoresis. In: *Methods in Neurochemistry*, edited by R. Fried, pp. 129–172. Marcel Dekker, New York.
38. Krnjevic, K. (1977): Effects of substance P on central neurones in cats. In: *Substance P*, edited by U. S. von Euler and B. Pernow, pp. 217–230. Raven Press, New York.
39. Krnjevic, K., and Lekic, D. (1977): Substance P selectively blocks excitation of Renshaw cell by acetylcholine. *Can. J. Physiol. Pharmacol.*, 55:958–961.
40. Krnjevic, K., and Morris, M. E. (1974): An excitatory action of substance P on cuneate neurones. *Can. J. Physiol. Pharmacol.*, 52:736–744.
41. Leeman, S. E., and Mroz, E. A. (1974): Substance P. *Life Sci.*, 15:2033–2044.
42. Lembeck, F. (1953): Zur Frage der zentralen ubertragung afferenter impulse. III. Das vorkommen und die bedentung substanz P in der dorsalen Wurzelin des Ruchenmarks. *Arch. Exp. Pathol. Pharmakol.*, 219:197–213.
43. Makara, G. B., Harris, M. C., and Spyer, K. M. (1972): Identification and distribution of tuberoinfundibular neurones. *Brain Res.*, 40:283–290.
44. Miletic, V., Kovacs, M. S., and Randic, M. (1977): Effects of substance P and somatostatin on activity of cat dorsal horn neurons activated by noxious stimuli. *Fed. Proc.*, 36:1014 (abstract 2915).
45. Moss, R. L. (1977): Role of hypophysiotropic neurohormones in mediating neural and behavioral events. *Fed. Proc.*, 1978–1983.
46. Moss, R. L., Dudley, C. A., and Kelly, M. J. (1978): Hypothalamic polypeptide releasing hormones: Modifiers of neuronal activity. *Neuropharmacology*, 17:87–93.
47. Moss, R. L., Dyball, R. E. J., and Cross, B. A. (1972): Excitation of antidromically identified neurosecretory cells in the paraventricular nucleus by oxytocin applied iontophoretically. *Exp. Neurol.*, 14:95–102.
48. Moss, R. L., and McCann, S. M. (1973): Induction of mating behavior in rats by luteinizing hormone-releasing factor. *Science*, 181:177–179.
49. Mudge, A. W., Fishback, G. D., and Leeman, S. E. (1977): The release of immunoreactive substance P and somatostatin from sensory neurons in dissociated cell cultures. *Neurosci. Abst.*, 3:410.
50. Nicoll, R. A. (1976): Promising peptides. In: *Neurotransmitters, Hormones and Receptors: Novel Approaches*, edited by J. A. Ferrendelli, B. S. McEwen, and S. H. Snyder. Society for Neuroscience, Bethesda, Md.
51. Nicoll, R. A. (1977): Excitatory action of TRH on spinal motoneurones. *Nature (Lond)*, 265:242–243.
52. Nicoll, R. A., and Barker, J. L. (1971): The pharmacology of recurrent inhibition in the supraoptic neurosecretory system. *Brain Res.*, 35:501–511.
53. Nicoll, R. A., Siggins, G. R., Ling, N., Bloom, F. E., and Guillemin, R. (1977): Neuronal actions of endorphins and enkephalins among brain regions: A comparative microiontophoretic study. *Proc. Natl. Acad. Sci. USA*, 74:2584–2588.
54. Otsuka, M., Konishi, S., and Takahashi, T. (1972): A further study of the motoneuron-depolarizing peptide extracted from dorsal roots of bovine spinal nerves. *Proc. Jpn. Acad.*, 48:747.
55. Otsuka, M., and Konishi, S. (1975): Substance P and excitatory transmitter of primary sensory neurons. *Cold Spring Harbor Symp. Quant. Biol.*, 40:135–143.
56. Otsuka, M., and Konishi, S. (1976): Release of substance P-like immunoreactivity from isolated spinal cord of newborn rat. *Nature (Lond)*, 264:83–84.
57. Otsuka, M., Konishi, S., and Takahashi, T. (1972): The presence of a motoneuron depolarizing peptide in bovine dorsal roots of spinal nerves. *Proc. Jpn. Acad.*, 48:342–346.
58. Pacold, S. T., Kirsteins, L., Hojvat, S., and Lawrence, A. M. (1978): Biologically active pituitary hormones in the rat brain amygdaloid nucleus. *Science*, 199:804–806.

59. Pfaff, D. W. (1973): Luteinizing hormone-releasing factor (LRF) potentiates lordosis behavior in hypophysectomized ovariectomized female rats. *Science*, 182: 1148–1149.

60. Phillis, J. W. (1977): Substance P and related peptides. In: *Approaches to the Cell Biology of Neurons*, edited by W. M. Cowan and J. A. Ferrendelli, pp. 241–264. Society for Neuroscience, Bethesda, Maryland.

61. Phillis, J. W., and Limacher, J. J. (1974): Substance P excitation of cerebral cortical Betz cells. *Brain Res.*, 69:158–163.

62. Phillis, J. W., and Limacher, J. J. (1974): Excitation of cerebral cortical neurons by various polypeptides. *Exp. Neurol.*, 43:414–423.

63. Pickel, V. M., Reis, D. J., and Leeman, S. E. (1977): Ultrastructural localization of substance P in neurons of rat spinal cord. *Brain Res.*, 122:534–540.

64. Pittman, Q. J., Blume, H. W., and Renaud, L. P. (1978): Depressant effect of thyrotropin releasing hormone (TRH) and TRH analogs on central neuronal excitability: *Proc. Can. Fed. Biol. Soc. (in press)*.

65. Poulain, D. A., Wakerley, J. B., and Dyball, R. E. J. (1977): Electrophysiological differentiation of oxytocin- and vasopressin-secreting neurones. *Proc. R. Soc. Lond.* [*Biol*], 196:367–384.

66. Randic, M., and Miletic, V. (1977): Actions of peptides on cat dorsal horn neurones activated by noxious stimuli. In: *Iontophoresis and Transmitter Mechanisms in the Mammalian Central Nervous System*, edited by R. Ryall and J. S. Kelly, pp. 127–130. Elsevier, Amsterdam.

67. Randic, M., and Miletic, V. (1977): Effect of substance P in cat dorsal horn neurones activated by noxious stimuli. *Brain Res.*, 128:164–169.

68. Renaud, L. P. (1975): Electrophysiological evidence to suggest that hypothalamic releasing (inhibiting) peptides may be liberated from nerve terminals in the CNS. *Neurosci. Abst.*, 1:441.

69. Renaud, L. P. (1976): Electrophysiological evidence for axon collaterals in the tuberoinfundibular system of the rat. *J. Physiol. (Lond)*, 254:20P–21P.

70. Renaud, L. P. (1976): Tuberoinfundibular neurons in the basomedial hypothalamus of the rat: Electrophysiological evidence for axon collaterals to hypothalamic and extrahypothalamic areas. *Brain Res.*, 105:59–72.

71. Renaud, L. P. (1976): Influence of amygdala stimulation on the activity of identified tuberoinfundibular neurones in the rat hypothalamus. *J. Physiol. (Lond)*, 260:237–252.

72. Renaud, L. P. (1977): Influence of medial preoptic-anterior hypothalamic area stimulation on the excitability of mediobasal hypothalamic neurones in the rat. *J. Physiol. (Lond)*, 264:541–564.

73. Renaud, L. P. (1977): Neurophysiological organization of the endocrine hypothalamus. In: *The Hypothalamus*, edited by S. Reichlin, R. J. Baldessarini, and J. B. Martin, pp. 269–300. Raven Press, New York.

74. Renaud, L. P. (1977): TRH, LHRH and somatostatin: distribution and physiological action in neural tissue. In: *Approaches to the Cell Biology of Neurones*, edited by W. M. Cowan and J. A. Ferrendelli, pp. 269–290. Society for Neuroscience, Bethesda, Maryland.

75. Renaud, L. P., Blume, H. W., and Pittman, Q. J. (1978): Neurophysiology and neuropharmacology of the hypothalamic tuberoinfundibular system. In: *Frontiers in Neuroendocrinology*, Vol. 5, edited by W. F. Ganong and L. Martini, pp. 135–162. Raven Press, New York.

76. Renaud, L. P., and Martin, J. B. (1975): Thyrotropin releasing hormone (TRH)—depressant action on central neuronal activity. *Brain Res.*, 86:150–154.

77. Renaud, L. P., Martin, J. B., and Brazeau, P. (1975): Depressant action of TRH, LH-RH and somatostatin on activity of central neurones. *Nature (Lond)*, 255: 233–235.

78. Renaud, L. P., Martin, J. B., and Brazeau, P. (1976): Hypothalamic releasing factors: Physiological evidence for a regulatory action on central neurons and

pathways for their distribution in brain. *Pharmacol. Biochem. Behav. (Suppl. I)*, 5:171–178.

79. Renaud, L. P., and Padjen, A. (1977): Electrophysiological analysis of peptide actions in neural tissue. In: *Centrally Acting Peptides*, edited by J. Hughes, pp. 59–84. Macmillan, London.
80. Sawaki, Y., and Yagi, K. (1973): Electrophysiological identification of cell bodies of the tuberoinfundibular neurones in the rat. *J. Physiol. (Lond)*, 230:75–85.
81. Sofroniew, M. V., and Weindl, A. (1978): Extrahypothalamic neurophysin-containing perikarya, fiber pathways and fiber clusters in the rat brain. *Endocrinology*, 102:334–337.
82. Steinacker, A. (1977): Calcium-dependent presynaptic action of substance P at the frog neuromuscular junction. *Nature (Lond)*, 267:268–270.
83. Steinacker, A., and Highstein, S. M. (1976): Pre- and post-synaptic action of substance P at the Mauthner fiber-giant fiber synapse in the hatchetfish. *Brain Res.*, 114:128–133.
84. Swanson, L. W. (1977): Immunohistochemical evidence for a neurophysin-containing autonomic pathway arising in the paraventricular nucleus of the hypothalamus. *Brain Res.*, 128:346–353.
85. Szentagothai, J., Flerko, B., Mess, B., and Halasz, B. (1968): *Hypothalamic Control of the Anterior Pituitary*. Akademiai Kiado, Budapest.
86. Takahashi, T., Konishi, S., Powell, D., Leeman, S. E., and Otsuka, M. (1974): Identification of the motoneuron depolarizing peptide in bovine dorsal root as hypothalamic substance P. *Brain Res.*, 73:59–69.
87. Takahashi, T., and Otsuka, M. (1975): Regional distribution of substance P in the spinal cord and nerve roots of the cat and the effect of dorsal root section. *Brain Res.*, 87:1–11.
88. Uhl, G. R., Kuhar, M. J., and Snyder, S. H. (1977): Neurotensin-immunohistochemical localization in rat central nervous system (amygdala-substantia gelatinoso-pituitary-peptide-hypothalamus). *Proc. Natl. Acad. Sci. USA*, 74:4059.
89. Von Euler, U. S. and Gaddum, J. H. (1931): An unidentified depressor substance in certain tissue extracts. *J. Physiol. (Lond)*, 72:74–87.
90. Werman, R. (1966): Criteria for identification of a central nervous system transmitter. *Comp. Biochem. Physiol.*, 18:745–766.
91. Yarbrough, G. G. (1976): TRH potentiates excitatory action of acetylcholine on cerebral cortical neurones. *Nature (Lond)*, 263:523–524.

Central Nervous System Effects of Hypothalamic Hormones and Other Peptides, edited by Collu et al. Raven Press, New York © 1979.

Effects of Purified CRF and Other Substances on the Secretion of ACTH and β-Endorphin-Like Immunoactivities by Cultured Anterior or Neurointermediate Pituitary Cells

Wylie Vale, Jean Rivier, Roger Guillemin, and Catherine Rivier

Peptide Biology Laboratory, and Laboratories for Neuroendocrinology, The Salk Institute, La Jolla, California 92037

The regulation of corticotropic cells' secretory functions is of neurobiological interest for several reasons: (a) Numerous agents including peptides, biogenic monoamines, steroids, and prostaglandins modulate secretions by corticotropic cells (50), thereby providing an excellent model for such interactions in other tissues, including the brain. (b) The secretory products of corticotropic cells such as corticotropin (ACTH), endorphins, and melanotropins (MSH) exert powerful and perhaps even physiologic effects on the central nervous system (CNS), as has been shown by the studies of many groups, including those of Kastin (24), Krivoy (26), De Wied (11), and Bloom (5). In view of the possibility that retrograde flow might occur in the hypothalamic-hypophysial portal system (3,37), such pituitary products could reach the brain in high concentrations. (c) Based on teleologic considerations and experience with other hypophysiotropic peptides, it is probable that the still-putative corticotropin releasing factor (CRF) itself possesses significant roles within the CNS.

Starting anew several years ago on a program directed toward the isolation and characterization of the putative CRF, we developed a bioassay (51,52) based on the ability of CRF to stimulate the secretion of radioimmunoassayable ACTH-like immunoactivity (ACTH-LI) by cultured anterior pituitary cells. This pituitary cell culture technique (49,51) had already been successfully applied to numerous physiologic and pharmacologic studies, including the isolation of somatostatin (48) and the development of biologically important analogs of luteinizing hormone-releasing factor (LRF) and somatostatin (51). The ACTH-LI was measured by a double-antibody radioimmunoassay employing an N-terminally directed anti-ACTH serum (38).

The sensitivity of cultured anterior pituitary cells to secretagogs was demonstrated by the cells' ACTH-LI secretory responses to a variety of substances or conditions such as cyclic AMP derivatives, phosphodiesterase inhibitors, elevated medium potassium, the calcium ionophore A23187, and the cocarcinogen phorbol myristate acetate (PMA) (50,51,55). Vasopressin (either lysine or arginine) and vasotosin have moderate stimulatory effects of ACTH-LI secretion (50,57). Although these peptides are quite potent, releasing ACTH-LI at $\geq$ 0.1 nM, the secretory V_{max} observed in response to the neurohypophysial peptides is much lower than that seen with ^{8}BrcAMP, 3-isobutylmethylxanthine, or PMA. The response to $10 \times [K^+]$ medium is intermediate between that to high concentrations of ^{8}BrcAMP and of vasopressin.

Partial purification on Sephadex G-50 of one fraction derived from an earlier program (8) purifying ovine hypothalamic LRF yields two zones of corticotropin-releasing activity (50). One zone (I) induces an ACTH-LI secretory V_{max} similar to that of ^{8}BrcAMP, and the other zone (II) gives a maximum secretory rate similar to that of vasopressin. Subsequent purification of zone II yielded a peptide with an amino acid composition identical to that of [Arg^8]vasopressin (Vale, Rivier, and Rivier, *unpublished results*).

Zone I, in our view, probably contains the physiologic CRF. This CRF-like activity was purified by SP-Sephadex carbon-exchange chromatography, filtration on Biogel P-60 in guanidine·HCl (Vale and Rivier, *in preparation*), and high-pressure liquid chromatography (42). Our most potent CRF preparations significantly stimulate ACTH-LI secretion at concentrations as low as 1 ng peptide/ml medium. The ACTH-LI releasing activity is abolished by incubation with trypsin (50). The most purified CRF preparations have an apparent molecular weight of about 2,000 daltons. It is probable that the chromatographic behavior of cruder CRF preparations reflects a noncovalent association of CRF with larger molecules.

We reported earlier that norepinephrine and other α-adrenergic agonists can stimulate ACTH-LI secretion, an effect that is inhibited by phentolamine and phenoxybenzamine. These α-adrenergic antagonists do not interfere with the activity of our purified CRF (50).

The secretion of ACTH-LI by anterior pituitary cells is also sensitive to a variety of inhibitory substances. Glucocorticoids, which are key elements in the physiologic regulation of ACTH-LI secretion, can inhibit the CRF-mediated secretion of ACTH-LI by cultured anterior pituitary cells (50, 51). This inhibition is time-dependent and is observed at lower concentrations of glucocorticoids in the cultured anterior pituitary cells than in other *in vitro* systems (15,44). Mineralocorticoids and progesterone are also effective inhibitors of CRF- or ^{8}BrcAMP-stimulated ACTH-LI secretion (50) (Fig. 1), although these steroids are considerably less potent than the glucocorticoids. Whether progesterone and the mineralocorticoids are acting by virtue of their affinities for glucocorticoid receptors has not been determined. Several prostaglandins, including PGE$_1$, PGE$_2$, and PGF$_{2\alpha}$ produce

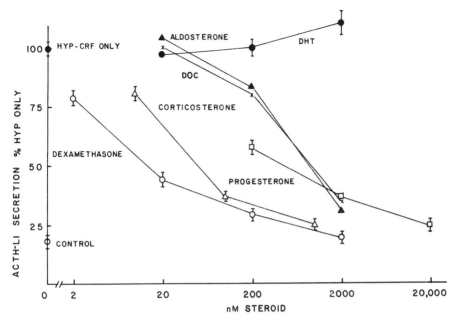

FIG. 1. Effects of steroid pretreatment (16 hr) on the secretion of ACTH mediated by purified ovine CRF (HYP-CRF) by cultured rat adenohypophysial cells.

a moderate but reproducible inhibition of the CRF-mediated release of ACTH-LI (50).

Thus a variety of substances—neuropeptides, steroids, biogenic monoamines, and prostaglandins—can act at the anterior pituitary level to modulate ACTH-LI secretion *in vitro* (Fig. 2). It is possible that each of these agents might at some time have access to the *in situ* pituitary at biologically effective concentrations and might be of physiologic significance in the regulation of ACTH secretion.

All of these substances can modulate the secretion of other products of adenohypophysial corticotropic cells, including β-lipotropin (β-LPH) and β-endorphin. β-Lipotropin (β-LPH) contains the sequences of β-melanotropin (β-LPH$_{41\text{-}58}$) and the morphinomimetic peptides β-endorphin (β-LPH$_{61\text{-}91}$) and methionine enkephalin (β-LPH$_{61\text{-}65}$) (7,21,27,28). The existence of a common precursor for ACTH and β-LPH as well as their smaller peptides is supported by several lines of evidence: immunologic determinants for ACTH and β-LPH (30) or β-endorphin (33) have been reported to occur in the same purified pituitary fraction. Furthermore, Mains et al. (35) found that the ACTH-LI secreting At-20/D-16V mouse pituitary cell line biosynthesizes 31K ACTH, which appeared to be processed to 23K, ACTH, 13K (6.7K) ACTH, ACTH (4.5K), β-LPH, and β-endorphin. Consistently, Giognoni et al. (17) reported that the parent At-20 cell line pro-

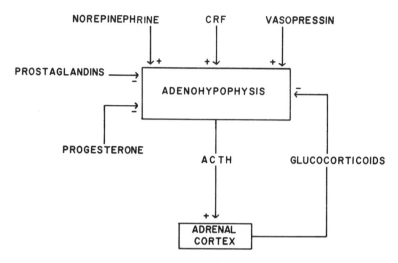

FIG. 2. Substances shown to modify the rate of ACTH secretion by cultured adenohypophysial cells.

duces opioid peptides as well as ACTH. In addition, ACTH and either β-MSH, β-LPH, or endorphins have been reported to be present in the same cells of the pituitary (4,12,35,39,40).

In view of the postulated common origin of peptides related to ACTH and β-LPH, it is reasonable to suggest that the factors regulating the secretion of these products would be similar. *In vivo* studies have shown that under numerous experimental or pathologic circumstances, the secretory rates of ACTH-LI are modified in parallel with the secretory rates of β-LPH-LI (1,16,22,45), β-MSH-LI (2,20,31), and recently, β-endorphin-like immunoactivity (β-endor-LI) (18,43).

Because of the difficulties with the separation of direct from indirect effects *in vivo,* it is critical to determine that specific substances modifying ACTH secretion *in vitro* also modify β-LPH and β-endorphin secretion *in vitro.*

The β-endorphin radioimmunoassay developed by Guillemin et al. (18) detects an internal sequence (Leu[14]-His[27]) within β-endorphin and therefore does not distinguish between β-endorphin, β-LPH, or 31K ACTH. Likewise, the N-terminally directed ACTH antiserum of Orth does not distinguish between ACTH and any of its larger forms. In selected experiments, the apparent molecular weight of the secreted and cellular β-endorphin-like immunoactivity (ACTH-LI) was determined by analytical gel filtration (34) on Biogel P-60 in denaturing solvents (4 M guanidine·HC1/0.1 N HOAc/0.02% BSA) (34,57). Chromatographs were standardized with ACTH, ovine β-LPH (10), murine 31 K ACTH, and synthetic β-endorphin (30).

The addition of general secretagogs (e.g., [8]BrcAMP or IBMX) to cultured anterior pituitary cells leads to the release of ACTH-LI and β-endor-LI, as does incubation in elevated [K⁺] medium. More specific ACTH secretagogs (e.g., norepinephrine and [Arg[8]]vasopressin) and several preparations of ovine CRF (including our most pure) that do not release growth hormone, prolactin, luteinizing hormone, or thyrotropin from these cells, stimulate the secretion of β-endor-LI (56) (Figs. 3 and 4).

Chromatographic analysis of the β-endorphin and ACTH-like immunoreactive species in culture fluids suggests that anterior pituitary cells secrete 31K ACTH, β-LPH, ACTH, and β-endorphin. Stimulation of secretion with either purified ovine CRF or ⁸BrcAMP results in larger peaks of immunoactivity resembling 31K ACTH, β-LPH, ACTH, and β-endorphin, and the appearance of a new peak corresponding to an ACTH immunoreactive molecule of approximately 6,500 molecular weight (56). This peak may represent "13K ACTH," which was recently determined by Eipper and Mains (32) to have a molecular weight of 6,700 $\pm$ 600 and to be similar to known ACTH (1–39) with one complex heterosaccharide chain attached within the carboxy terminal region of the molecule. These results are consistent with the hypothesis that CRF can stimulate the secretion of a variety of products related to 31K ACTH, including β-LPH and β-endorphin. Since another secretagog, ⁸BrcAMP, yields a similar chromatographic pattern of ACTH-LI and β-endor-LI (56), CRF does not appear to determine uniquely

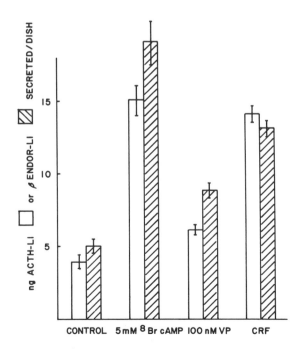

FIG. 3. Effects of ⁸BrcAMP, [Arg[8]]vasopressin (VP), and purified ovine CRF on the secretion of ACTH-LI and β-endor-LI by cultured adenohypophysial cells.

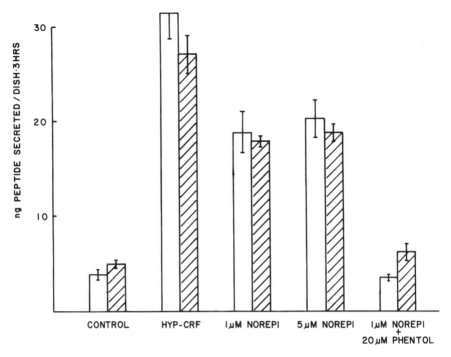

FIG. 4. Effects of purified ovine CRF (HYP-CRF), norepinephrine (NOREPI), and phentolamine (PHENTOL) on the secretion of ACTH-LI and β-endor-LI by cultured adenohypophysial cells.

the nature of the corticotropic products secreted during these acute studies.

Pretreatment of cells for 16 hr with glucocorticoids or progesterone inhibits the secretion of β-endor-LI as well as ACTH-LI. Prostaglandin (PGE_2) partially suppresses the CRF-mediated release of both β-endor-LI and ACTH-LI (57) (Fig. 5).

Thus under numerous circumstances the secretory rates of β-endorphin-LI and ACTH-LI vary in the same direction, even though the correlation between the levels of β-endor-LI and ACTH-LI appear to be better at higher rather than lower secretory rates of the two immunoactivities.

Based on these *in vitro* and the before-mentioned *in vivo* studies, it appears that CRF presumably secreted during circumstances such as "stress" affects the integrated secretion of ACTH and β-endorphin. In consideration of the actions of these peptides, as well as possible direct vascular pathways from pituitary to brain, these peptides might possibly exert endocrine, gastrointestinal, and CNS actions that could be of adaptive significance to various situations.

The intermediate lobe of the pituitary has been known for some time to consist primarily of corticotropic cells which contain and/or secrete a variety of peptides related to ACTH and β-LPH (4,12,30,35,40). It is probable

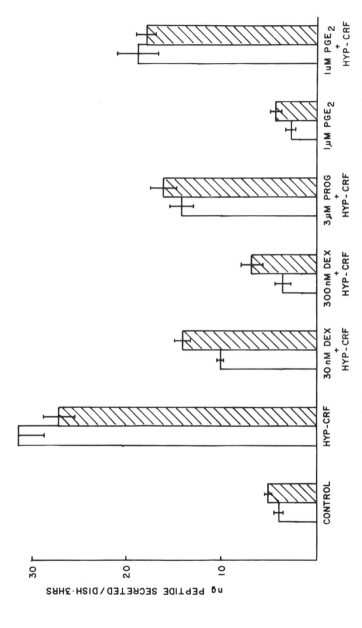

FIG. 5. Effects of dexamethasone-21-PO$_4$ (DEX) or progesterone (PROG) pretreatment (16 hr) or prostaglandin (PGE$_2$) on the purified hypothalamic ovine CRF (HYP-CRF)-mediated secretion of ACTH-LI or β-endor-LI by cultured adenohypophysial cells.

that most of the ACTH in intermediate lobe corticotropic cells is converted to α-MSH (Ac-ACTH$_{1-13}$-NH$_2$) and to CLIP (ACTH$_{17-39}$). Since the intermediate lobe secretes some α-MSH, the distinction between the two lobes is only relative. We observed that the principal β-endor-LI contained in and secreted by intermediate lobe cells co-elutes with synthetic β-endorphin, with only small amounts co-eluting with 31K ACTH and β-LPH (34,54), whereas in anterior lobe cells slightly more β-LPH than β-endorphin appears in cells or as secreted products.

Our *in vitro* studies of intermediate lobe corticotropic cells employed cultures of enzymatically dissociated neurointermediate lobe cells. These cultures were prepared essentially as per the method for the anterior lobe cells (49,51) with the exception that experiments were carried out in 4 to 10 rather than 3 to 4 days following dissociation.

As is the case with prolactin-secreting adenohypophysial cells, the spon-

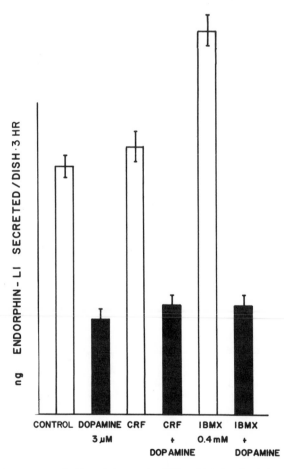

FIG. 6. Effects of dopamine, purified hypothalamic ovine CRF, and 3-isobutylmethylxanthine (IBMX), on the secretion of β-endor-LI by cultured neurointermediate lobe cells.

taneous secretion of corticotropic cells' products by neurointermediate lobe cultures increases initially and persists at a high rate for weeks (6,54). Such results are consistent with *in vivo* studies involving hypothalamic lesions (9,46) and suggest that the hypothalamus exerts a net inhibitory influence on intermediate lobe corticotropic cells.

In contrast to adenohypophysial corticotropic cells, neurointermediate lobe cell cultures do not secrete β-endor-LI in response to purified CRF preparations (53,54) (Fig. 6). These cells are responsive to some secretagogs since [8]BrcAMP and IBMX can significantly increase the β-endor-LI secretion rate. In agreement, Kraicer and Morris (25) reported that their purified CRF preparation did not stimulate ACTH release from acutely dissociated intermediate lobe cells.

Elevated medium [K^+] does not stimulate β-endor-LI by neurointermediate lobe cells (54,55). Since Hadley et al. (19) reported that neurointermediate lobe cells in culture spontaneously depolarize at a high rate, it is possible that the β-endor-LI secretory rate mediated through a depolarization-triggered mechanism is already maximal and that the elevated medium [K^+] can exert no additional effects.

Dopamine and its agonists (e.g., apomorphine) (Figs. 6 and 7) are powerful inhibitors of both spontaneous and IBMX-stimulated secretion of β-endor-LI by neurointermediate lobe cells. This inhibitory effect of dopamine

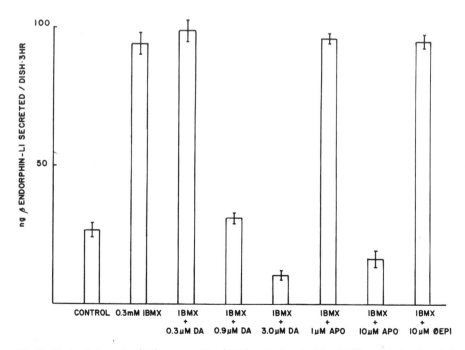

FIG. 7. Effects of dopamine (DA), apomorphine (APO), and phenylephrine (ϕEPI) on 3-isobutyl methyl xanthine (IBMX) secretion of β-endor-LI by cultured neurointermediate lobe cells.

is reversed by dopamine antagonists such as haloperidol and (+)butaclamol (Fig. 8). Hadley et al. (19) and Fischer and Moriarty (14) reported earlier that dopamine could suppress the secretion of two other intermediate lobe corticotropic cells' products (bioassayble α-MSH and ACTH). In the former study (14), dopamine was proposed to act through α-adrenergic receptors, whereas our results imply that dopamine receptors are involved in the inhibition of β-endor-LI secretion. The presence of rich dopaminergic innervation of the pars intermedia (36) of some species is consistent with there being a physiologic role of dopamine in the regulation of β-endorphin secretion by those cells.

The adenohypophysial secretion of ACTH-LI and β-endor-LI is not inhibited by dopamine agonists. Another major difference between the regulation of anterior and intermediate lobe corticotropic cells' secretions is that glucocorticoids do not inhibit the secretion of β-endor-LI by neurointermediate lobe cultures. Consistently, Fischer and Moriarty found no effects of dexamethasone on the secretion of bioassayble ACTH by neurointermediate lobes *in vitro* (14).

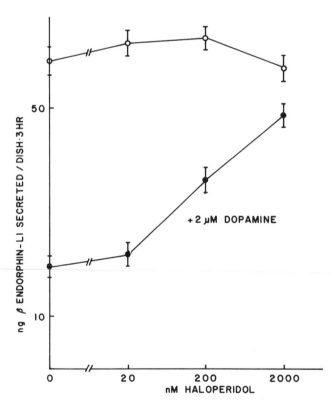

FIG. 8. Haloperidol reversal of dopamine inhibition of 3-isobutyl methyl xanthine-mediated secretion of β-endor-LI by cultured neurointermediate lobe cells.

Other peptides, including the proposed melanocyte-inhibiting factor, H-Pro-Leu-Gly-NH$_2$ (MIF-I), somatostatin, bombesin, substance P, neurotensin, vasopressin, and TRF have been found to have no effects on the basal β-endor-LI secretory rate by cultured neurointermediate lobe cells. In addition, we observed no effects of several monoamines, including serotonin, isoproterenol, phenylephrine, and carbachol by these cells.

In conclusion, intermediate and anterior lobe corticotropic cells differ from one another not only in their posttranslational processing of the putative precursor 31K ACTH but in the array of regulatory substances modulating the secretory rates of the two cell types. The differential effects of purified CRF, dopamine, and glucocorticoids might be of particular relevance. Consistently, several *in vivo* studies have shown that the secretions of α-MSH (primarily an intermediate lobe product) and of ACTH (primarily an anterior lobe product) do not always correlate (13,23,47). The physiologic and perhaps pathophysiologic roles played by peptides secreted by corticotropic cells, as well as the contributions of substances such as the putative CRF, glucocorticoids, and dopamine to such roles remain to be established.

ACKNOWLEDGMENTS

The authors appreciate the generous gift of anti-ACTH serum from Dr. David Orth. We thank Dr. Nick Ling for the synthetic β-endorphin, Dr. Michel Chrétien for the purified ovine β-lipotropin, and Drs. R. Mains and B. Eipper for the sample of murine 31K ACTH. The authors recognize the expert technical assistance of Mss. Terry Vargo, Alice Mauss, Alice Wolfe, Ermilinda Tucker, and Ginny Allen. Research in the authors' laboratories was supported by NIH grants AM18811, AM20917, NS-142631, and HD09690; The National Foundation March of Dimes NF411; The Hearst Foundation; and the Rockefeller Foundation.

REFERENCES

1. Abe, K., Nicholson, N., Liddle, G., Orth, D., and Island, D. (1969): Normal and abnormal regulation of β-MSH in man. *J. Clin. Invest.*, 48:2259–2263.
2. Bachelot, I., Wolfsen, R., and Odell, W. (1977): Pituitary and plasma lipotropins: Demonstration of the artifactual nature of β-MSH. *J. Clin. Endocrinol. Metab.*, 44:939–946.
3. Bergland, R., and Page, E. (1976): Vascular organization within the mammalian hypophysis. I. Median eminence. In: *Fifth International Congress of Endocrinology, Hamburg, FRG,* p. 503 (abstract).
4. Bloom, F., Battenberg, E., Rossier, J., Ling, N., Leppaluoto, J., Vargo, T., and Guillemin, R. (1977): Endorphins are located in the intermediate and anterior lobes of the pituitary gland, not in the neurohypophysis. *Life Sci.*, 20:43–48.
5. Bloom, F., Segal, D., Ling, N., and Guillemin, R. (1976): Endorphins: Profound behavioral effects in rats suggest new etiological factors in mental illness. *Science*, 194:630–632.
6. Bower, C., Hadley, M., and Hruby, V. (1974): Biogenic amines and control of melanophore stimulating hormone release. *Science*, 184:70–72.

7. Bradbury, A., Smyth, D., and Snell, D. (1976): Biosynthesis of β-MSH and ACTH. In: *Peptides: Chemistry, Structure, Biology*, edited by R. Walter and J. Meinhofer, pp. 609–616. Ann Arbor Science, Ann Arbor, Michigan.
8. Burgus, R., et al. (1976): Isolation and characterization of hypothalamic peptide hormones. In: *Hypothalamus and Endocrine Functions*, edited by F. Labrie, J. Meites, and G. Pelletier, pp. 355–372. Raven Press, New York.
9. Carrillo, A., Kastin, A., Dunn, J., and Schally, A. (1973): MSH activity in plasma and pituitaries of rats with large hypothalamic lesions. *Neuroendocrinology*, 12: 12–128.
10. Chrétien, M. (1979): Beta-lipotropin = pro-endorphin. *This volume.*
11. De Wied, D. (1977): Peptides and behavior. *Life Sci.*, 20:195–204.
12. Dubois, P., Vargues-Regairas, H., and Dubois, M. (1973): Human foetal anterior pituitary immunofluorescent evidence for corticotropin and melanotropin activities. *Z. Zellforsch. Mikrosc.*, 145:131–143.
13. Dunn, J., Kastin, A., Carrillo, A., and Schally, A. (1972): Additional evidence for dissociation of melanocyte-stimulating hormone and corticotropin release. *J. Endocrinol.*, 55:463–464.
14. Fischer, J., and Moriarty, C. (1977): Control of bioactive corticotropin release from the neuro-intermedia lobe of the rat. *Endocrinology*, 100:1047–1054.
15. Fleischer, N., and Vale, W. (1968): Inhibition of vasopressin-induced ACTH release from the pituitary by glucocorticoids in vitro. *Endocrinology*, 83:1232–1236.
16. Gilkes, J., Bloomfield, G., Scott, A., Lowry, P., Ratcliffe, P., Landon, J., and Rees, L. (1976): Development and validation of a radioimmunoassay for peptides related to β-melanocyte-stimulating hormone in human plasma. *J. Clin. Endocrinol. Metab.*, 40:450–457.
17. Giognoni, G., Sabol, S., and Niernberg, M. (1977): Synthesis of opiate peptides by a clonal pituitary tumor. *Proc. Natl. Acad. Sci. USA*, 74:2259–2263.
18. Guillemin, R., Vargo, T., Rossier, J., Minick, S., Ling, N., Rivier, C., Vale, W., and Bloom, F. (1977): β-Endorphin and adrenocorticotropin are secreted concomitantly by the pituitary gland. *Science*, 197:1367–1369.
19. Hadley, M., Hruby, V., and Bower, A. (1975): Cellular mechanisms controlling melanophone stimulating hormone (MSH) release. *Gen. Comp. Endocrinol.*, 26: 24–35.
20. Hirata, U., Matsukura, S., Immura, H., Nakamura, M., and Tanaka, A. (1976): Size heterogeneity of β-MSH in ectopic ACTH-producing tumors: Presence of β-LPH-like peptide. *J. Clin. Endocrinol. Metab.*, 42:33–40.
21. Hughes, J., Smith, T., Kosterlitz, H., Fothergil, L., Morgan, B., and Morris, H. (1975): Identification of two related pentapeptides from the brain with potent opiate agonist activity. *Nature (Lond)*, 258:577–579.
22. Jeffcoate, W., Gilkes, J., Rees, L., Lowry, P., and Besser, G. (1977): The use of radioimmunoassays for human β-lipotropin. *Endocrinology*, 100:318A.
23. Kastin, A., Beach, G., Hawley, W., Kendall, J., Jr., Edwards, M., and Schally, A. (1973): Dissociation of MSH and ACTH release in man. *J. Clin. Endocrinol. Metab.*, 36:770–772.
24. Kastin, A. J., Plotnikoff, N. P., Harryl, R., and Schally, A. V. (1975): Hypothalamic hormones and the central nervous system. In: *Hypothalamic Hormones: Chemistry, Physiology, Pharmacology and Clinical Uses*, edited by M. Motta, P. G. Crosignani, and L. Martini, pp. 261–268. Academic Press, New York.
25. Kraicer, J., and Morris, A. (1976): In vitro release of ACTH from dispersed rat pars intermedia cells. I. Effect of secretagogues. *Neuroendocrinology*, 20:79–96.
26. Krivoy, W., and Guillemin, R. (1961): On a possible role of α-melanocytes stimulating hormone (α-MSH) in the central nervous system of the mammalians. I. An effect of α-MSH in the spinal cord of the cat. *Endocrinology*, 69:170–175.
27. Lazarus, L., Ling, N., and Guillemin, R. (1976): β-Lipotropin as a prohormone for the morphinomimetic peptides, endorphins and enkephalins. *Proc. Soc. Acad. Sci. USA*, 73:2156–2159.
28. Li, C., and Chung, D. (1976): Isolation and structure of an untriakonotopeptide

with opiate activity from camel pituitary glands. *Proc. Natl. Acad. Sci. USA,* 73:1145–1148.

29. Ling, N. (1977): Solid phase synthesis of porcine α-endorphin and γ-endorphin, two hypothalamic pituitary peptides with opiate activity. *Biochem. Biophys. Res. Commun.,* 74:248–255.
30. Lowry, P., Hope, J., and Silman, R. (1976): *International Congress Series 402,* pp. 71–76. Excerpta Medica, Amsterdam.
31. Lowry, P., Rees, J., Tomlin, L., Gillies, S., and Landon, J. (1977): Chemical characterization of ectopic ACTH purified from a malignant thymic carcinoid tumor. *J. Clin. Endocrinol. Metab.,* 43:831–835.
32. Mains, R., and Eipper, B. (1978): *Biochemistry (in press).*
33. Mains, R., Eipper, B., and Ling, N. (1977): Common precursor to corticotropins and endorphins. *Proc. Natl. Acad. Sci. USA,* 74:3014–3018.
34. Minick, S., Vale, W., and Guillemin, R. (1978): *(Manuscript in preparation).*
35. Moriarty, G. (1973): Adenohypophysis ultrastructural cytochemistry. *J. Histochem. Cytochem.,* 21:855–894.
36. Nobin, A., Bjorklund, A., and Stenevi, U. (1972): Origin of the hypophyseal catecholamine innervation. *International Congress Series 256,* p. 50. Excerpta Medica, Amsterdam.
37. Oliver, C., Mical, R., and Porter, J. (1977): Hypothalamic-pituitary vasculature: Evidence for retrograde blood flow in the pituitary stalk. *Endocrinology,* 101:598–604.
38. Orth, D. (1974): Adrenocorticotropic hormone (ACTH). In: *Methods of Hormone Radioimmunoassay,* edited by B. Jaffe and H. Behrman, pp. 125–160. Academic Press, New York.
39. Pelletier, G., Leclerc, R., Labrie, F., Côté, J., Chrétien, M., and Lis, M. (1977): Immunohistochemical localization of β-lipotropic hormone in the pituitary gland. *Endocrinology,* 100:770–776.
40. Phifer, R., Orth, D., and Spicer, S. (1974): Specific demonstration of the human hypophyseal adrenocortico-melantropic (ACTH/MSH) cell. *J. Clin. Endocrinol. Metab.,* 39:684–692.
41. Portanova, R., and Sayers, G. (1973): An in vitro assay for corticotropin releasing factor(s) using suspensions of isolated pituitary cells. *Neuroendocrinology,* 12:236–248.
42. Rivier, J., Spiess, J., Villarreal, J., Perrin, M., Rivier, C., Brown, M., and Vale, W. (1978): Use of trialkylammonium phosphate (TAAP) or formate buffers in RP-HPLC for characterization and isolation of synthetic and naturally occurring peptide hormones and analogues. *J. Liquid Chrom.* 1:343.
43. Rossier, J., French, E., Rivier, C., Ling, N., Guillemin, R., and Bloom, F. (1977): Foot shock induced stress and the content of β-endorphin in rat brain and blood. *Nature (Lond),* 270:618–620.
44. Sayers, G., and Portanova, R. (1974): Secretion of ACTH by isolated anterior pituitary cells: Kinetics of stimulation by corticotropin-releasing factor and of inhibition by corticosterone. *Endocrinology,* 94:1723–1730.
45. Tanaka, K., Mound, C., and Orth, D. (1976): High molecular weight forms of bioactive and immunoreactive "β-MSH" in human plasma, pituitary and tumor tissue. *Endocrinology,* 98:129A.
46. Thody, A. (1974): Plasma and pituitary MSH levels in the rat after lesions of the hypothalamus. *Neuroendocrinology,* 16:323–331.
47. Usategui, R., et al. (1976): Immunoreactive α-MSH and ACTH levels in rat plasma and pituitary. *Endocrinology,* 98:189–196.
48. Vale, W., Brazeau, P., Rivier, C., Brown, M., Boss, B., Rivier, J., Burgus, R., Ling, N., and Guillemin, R. (1975): Somatostatin. *Recent Prog. Horm. Res.* 31:365–397.
49. Vale, W., Grant, G., Amoss, M., Blackwell, R., and Guillemin, R. (1972): Culture of enzymatically dispersed anterior pituitary cells: Functional validation of a method. *Endocrinology,* 91:562–572.

50. Vale, W., and Rivier, C. (1977): Substances modulating the secretion of ACTH by cultured anterior pituitary cells. *Fed. Proc.,* 36:2094–2099.
51. Vale, W., Rivier, C., Brown, M., Chan, L., Ling, N., and Rivier, J. (1976): Application of adenohypophyseal cell culture to neuroendocrinology. In: *Hypothalamus and Endocrine Functions,* edited by F. Labrie, J. Meites, and G. Pelletier, pp. 397–429. Plenum Press, New York.
52. Vale, W., Rivier, C., Brown, M., and Rivier, J. (1977): Diverse roles of hypothalamic regulatory peptides. In: *Medicinal Chemistry V,* pp. 25–62. Elsevier, Amsterdam.
53. Vale, W., Rivier, C., Minick, S., Ling, N., and Guillemin, R. (1978): Regulation of secretion of ACTH and β-endorphin-like immunoreactivities by cultured anterior or intermediate + posterior pituitary cells. *Endocrinology,* 102:A213.
54. Vale, W., Rivier, C., Minick, S., Wolfe, A., and Guillemin, R. (1978): (*Manuscript in preparation*).
55. Vale, W., Rivier, C., Rivier, J., and Brown, M. (1978): Adenohypophysial and other extracentral nervous system roles of hypothalamic regulatory peptides. In: *Psychopharmacology: A Generation of Progress,* edited by M. A. Lipton, A. Di Mascio, and K. F. Killam, pp. 403–422. Raven Press, New York.
56. Vale, W., Rivier, C., Yang, L., Minick, S., and Guillemin, R. (1978): Effects of purified hypothalamic corticotropin releasing factor and other substances on the secretion of ACTH and β-endorphin-like immunoactivities in vitro. *Endocrinology,* 103:(*in press*).
57. Yasuda, N., and Greer, M. (1976): Studies on the corticotropin-releasing activity of vasopressin, using ACTH secretion by cultured rat adenohypophyseal cells. *Endocrinology,* 98:936–942.

Central Nervous System Effects of Hypothalamic Hormones and Other Peptides, edited by Collu et al. Raven Press, New York © 1979.

Neuropeptides and Avoidance Behavior; with Special Reference to the Effects of Vasopressin, ACTH, and MSH on Memory Processes

Tj. B. van Wimersma Greidanus

Rudolf Magnus Institute for Pharmacology, Vondellaan 6, Utrecht, The Netherlands

The brain is a target organ for various peptides that originate from the neurohypophysis as well as from the intermediate and anterior lobes of the adenohypophysis. The importance of these entities was revealed by the finding that avoidance behavior was impaired after extirpation of the pituitary gland (29) and could be corrected by treatment with hypophysial factors such as adrenocorticotropic hormone (ACTH), melanocyte-stimulating hormone (MSH), vasopressin (LVP), and peptides related to these pituitary hormones (29).

This behavioral effect of ACTH and of the peptides related to it (e.g., the fragments ACTH 1–10 and ACTH 4–10) appeared to be rather short-lasting, whereas the effect of vasopressin and its analogs was longer-lasted and persisted after the injected hormone had disappeared from the body (6).

In view of these results it was postulated that the pituitary gland manufactures and releases neuropeptides related to ACTH and vasopressin, which are involved in the acquisition and maintenance of new behavior patterns.

ACTIVE AVOIDANCE BEHAVIOR OF INTACT RATS

In intact rats the effect of ACTH, MSH, and vasopressin on acquisition of avoidance behavior was not easily detected but could be demonstrated clearly when the maintenance of a previously acquired conditioned avoidance response (CAR) was the criterion. These peptides delayed extinction of the avoidance response, and again the effect of ACTH and ACTH analogs was short-lasted whereas that of vasopressin was long-lasted (30,33). A single injection of the analog ACTH 4–10 induced inhibition of extinction of a one-way pole-jumping avoidance response which lasted, depending on the dose, from 4 hr to maximally 1 day (23,31,36). In contrast, a single subcutaneous injection of LVP resulted in an inhibition of extinction of the response which lasted several weeks (34,39).

It was concluded from these results that different mechanisms and/or sites of action were involved in the effect exerted on avoidance behavior by ACTH and related peptides and by vasopressin and its analogs.

SITES OF ACTION

Studies on the sites of action of pituitary peptides revealed that midbrain limbic structures could be target tissues for the behavioral effect of these peptides. Implantation experiments with the decapeptide ACTH 1–10 demonstrated that the brain region where the mesencephalon and diencephalon shade off into each other at the posterior thalamic level was an important area for the behavioral effect of this peptide. Local application of ACTH 1–10 in the parafascicular nucleus, the lateral habenular nucleus, or the tectospinal tract effectively inhibited extinction of the pole-jumping avoidance response. In addition, injection of the peptide into the liquor of the brain ventricular system also resulted in a delay of extinction of the CAR. No effect of the peptide followed implantation in other areas of the brain, e.g., the ventral and rostral parts of the thalamus, globus pallidus, caudate nucleus (36). Microinjection of small amounts (0.1 μg) of LVP in various brain areas pointed to the same brain regions as sites of action as for ACTH 1–10 (39). The posterior thalamic region thus seems to be an essential structure for the effect of ACTH-related peptides as well as for the effect of vasopressin and its analogs on avoidance behavior.

The unilateral local application of small amounts of the peptides may not be sufficient to alter the activity of that particular region in such a way that it is reflected in a behavioral effect. Consequently the lack of effect of a local application of a behaviorally active peptide to a restricted area of the brain does not necessarily mean that this brain region is not involved in the effect of the peptide. Lesion studies were therefore performed to obtain additional information about the central sites of action of the behaviorally active pituitary peptides.

Extensive bilateral lesions in the dorsal hippocampus and the rostral septal area appeared to block the inhibitory influence of ACTH 4 – 10 and of LVP on extinction of pole-jumping avoidance behavior. In sham-operated animals doses of 1 to 3 μg induced a marked effect, but not in animals bearing lesions in the rostral septal area (35,41) or the dorsal hippocampus (37). Relatively high amounts (e.g., 9 μg) of the peptides did not inhibit extinction of the response in these animals. There is evidence for a specific uptake of a behaviorally potent ACTH analog in the septal area of the brain (27). In addition, it appeared that extensive bilateral lesions in the amygdaloid complex blocked this behavioral effect of vasopressin as well (Bouman and van Wimersma Greidanus, *in preparation*).

Different effects were observed in rats with lesions in the posterior thalamic area. ACTH 4–10 in doses up to 9 μg did not alter the rate of extinction in rats with parafascicular lesions, whereas treatment with LVP resulted in delayed extinction of the CAR, although the parafascicular-lesioned animals required higher amounts of LVP (approximately 5 μg) than did the sham-operated controls (1 μg) (40). Thus although the parafascicular region in the posterior thalamus is sensitive to the behavioral effects of ACTH 4–10 and LVP, this region is essential only for the effect of ACTH 4–10 and not for that of vasopressin on extinction of pole-jumping avoidance behavior.

In relation to these studies on the site of behavioral action of the pituitary peptides, it is interesting that the α-MPT-induced disappearance of catecholamines was enhanced in specific brain regions after central administration of arginine-8-vasopressin in comparison to saline-treated controls. The α-MPT-induced disappearance of norepinephrine was most markedly accelerated in the dorsal septal nucleus, the parafascicular nucleus, the dorsal raphe nucleus, and the nucleus tractus solitarii, whereas the disappearance of dopamine was predominantly affected in the caudate nucleus and the median eminence.

It has been suggested on the basis of these results that catecholamine neurotransmission in these regions was involved in the various behavioral effects of vasopressin (26). The intracerebroventricular administration of vasopressin antiserum, which impairs active and passive avoidance behavior, had an effect on catecholamine turnover opposite to that of vasopressin treatment (Versteeg et al., *in preparation*).

PASSIVE AVOIDANCE BEHAVIOR

The pituitary peptides ACTH, MSH, and vasopressin and their analogs affect not only active avoidance behavior but also passive avoidance behavior. In a simple one-trial passive avoidance task, rats were trained to avoid a dark compartment in which they previously experienced foot shock as aversive stimulus. Rats generally prefer darkness to light, and when placed on an illuminated platform connected to a dark box they will enter this box within a few seconds. If the animal is shocked in the dark compartment after a number of attempts to enter, its latency to reenter increases in relation to the intensity and duration of the shock (1).

A single injection of ACTH 4–10 1 hr prior to the retention trial and 23 hr after the single learning trial of shock (0.25 mA, 2 sec) markedly increased avoidance latencies. However, the effect of ACTH 4–10 disappeared the next day. In addition ACTH 4–10 did not increase avoidance latency scores when applied immediately after the learning trial (35). ACTH analogs thus again exerted a "short-term" behavioral effect. A single injection of LVP or dg-LVP immediately after the learning trial or 1 hr prior to the retention trial resulted in increased retention of the passive avoidance response as well, and this effect was still apparent at subsequent retention trials performed 48 and 120 hr after the learning trial, indicating a "long-term" effect of vasopressin in this behavioral test (2,5).

In addition, vasopressin has been shown to retard extinction of a food-reinforced black-white discrimination task (13) and to prolong extinction of a positively reinforced, sexually motivated T-maze learning (4).

ARE PITUITARY PEPTIDES PHYSIOLOGICALLY INVOLVED IN AVOIDANCE BEHAVIOR?

Passive avoidance behavior was used to explore the physiological role of endogenous ACTH, MSH, and vasopressin in the acquisition and maintenance of the avoidance response. Specific radioimmunoassays for ACTH, MSH, and vasopressin were used to determine the blood levels of these hormones during passive avoidance performance.

Animals were decapitated immediately after the learning trial or 5 min after the start of the retention trial. Plasma was kept frozen until assayed for hormone content.

No difference could be found between MSH levels in the plasma collected immediately after the learning trial or in that collected after retention, although shock levels during the learning trial varied from 0.00 mA (no shock), to 0.25 mA (low shock), to 0.75 mA (high shock) (Thody, de Rotte, and van Wimersma Greidanus, *unpublished data*). Since shock intensities were correlated with passive avoidance latency scores during retention, no correlation was found between passive avoidance performance and plasma MSH levels (Fig. 1).

In contrast, there was a good correlation between the behavioral performance and plasma ACTH levels (43). Long latencies during retention as a result of high shock intensity during the acquisition trial were associated with high plasma ACTH levels, whereas shorter latencies due to low shock intensity during the learning trial were associated with lower plasma levels of ACTH (Fig. 1). Surprisingly, plasma ACTH levels appeared to be higher during retention of the passive avoidance response than immediately after the learning trial, indicating that the "fear" or expectancy of being shocked may have been a stronger stimulus for pituitary ACTH release than electric foot shock itself (43). These data were confirmed recently by Endröczi et al. (10), who reported a significant positive correlation between retention of a passive avoidance response and the rise of the plasma ACTH level in adrenalectomized rats in a situation motivated by thirst versus fear.

Vasopressin was measured by radioimmunoassay in peripheral plasma samples obtained at 5 sec, 1 min, and 5 min after the onset of the passive avoidance retention session, or at 5 min after the acquisition trial (9). Although there were again marked differences in avoidance latencies, the plasma vasopressin levels of the experimental groups did not differ significantly from the basal values, except in the animals exposed to the highest shock intensity. The plasma vasopressin level in this group was 3.0 ± 0.5

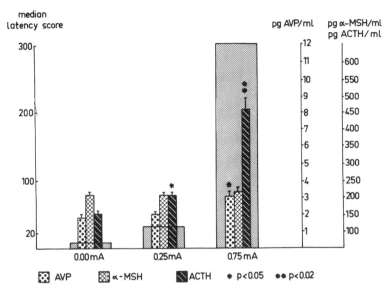

FIG. 1. Median avoidance latency scores and plasma levels of ACTH, α-MSH, and vasopressin measured 5 min after the onset of the 24-hr retention session of a passive avoidance response.

pg/ml 5 min after the retention session. This was approximately twice the level in the control groups (Fig. 1).

BEHAVIOR AND ANTISERA TO VASOPRESSIN, ACTH, OR α-MSH

In spite of the results of this last experiment it seems that the peripheral circulation is of minor importance for the behavioral effect of vasopressin. More direct support for this concept was obtained from experiments in which rats were treated with antiserum to neuropeptides in order to neutralize the endogenous hormone (42). Intravenously injected vasopressin antiserum effectively bound vasopressin in the circulation as was shown by the virtual absence of this hormone from the urine and by the marked increase in the production of urine. This antiserum treatment, performed immediately after the learning trial of a passive avoidance response, did not affect passive avoidance behavior during retention.

In contrast, vasopressin antiserum administered into one of the lateral ventricles of the brain immediately after the learning trial induced an almost complete deficit in the passive avoidance task when retention was tested 6 hr or later following acquisition of the response. Although the control group responded with maximal passive avoidance latencies (5 min) during retention, owing to a high shock level during the learning trial, the animals intraventricularly injected with vasopressin antiserum entered the dark compartment within 50 sec. This behavior was not altered when the animals were tested for retention at 2 min or at 1 or 2 hr after administration of the vasopressin antiserum. The latter observations indicate that vasopressin affects memory consolidation or long-term storage of information rather than learning processes (38,42).

From these results it may be concluded that centrally available vasopressin, rather than the vasopressin released into the peripheral circulation, plays a role in processes related to memory. In addition it was found that administration of vasopressin antiserum prior to the retention session resulted in disturbed passive avoidance behavior as well. This suggests that vasopressin is not only important for the storage of information but is also essential for the retrieval of stored information (38).

It appeared that a single subcutaneous injection of ACTH 4–10 prior to retention increased the avoidance latency scores in animals in which the retrieval process had been disturbed by treatment with vasopressin antiserum prior to retention (Fig. 2). The injection of ACTH 4–10 failed to restore the disturbed storage process or memory consolidation caused by vasopressin antiserum given immediately after the learning trial (Fig. 3). It thus seems that ACTH 4–10 can be used as a tool to differentiate between memory consolidation and retrieval processes.

Antisera to ACTH or to α-MSH do not affect passive avoidance retention when they are injected intracerebroventricularly after the learning trial. However, when the injection is made prior to the first retention session, passive

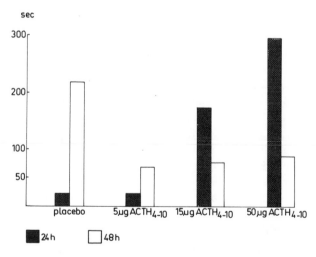

FIG. 2. Retention of passive avoidance behavior in rats following intraventricular injection of anti-AVP serum (1:10) 1 hr prior to the first retention session. Influence of graded doses of ACTH 4–10 (s.c.) 1 hr prior to the first retention session. Retention sessions at 24 and 48 hr. Shock level during learning trial (75 mA, 2 sec).

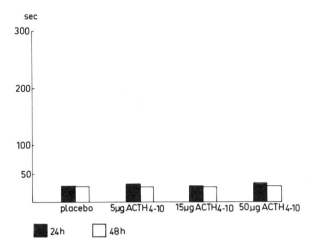

FIG. 3. Retention of passive avoidance behavior in rats following intraventricular injection of anti-AVP serum (1:10) immediately after the learning trial (75 mA, 2 sec). Influence of graded doses of ACTH 4–10 (s.c.) 1 hr prior to the first retention session. Retention sessions at 24 and 48 hr.

avoidance behavior is impaired. It is concluded that ACTH and α-MSH are involved in retrieval but not in storage processes (44).

OTHER PITUITARY PEPTIDES AND BEHAVIOR

After the behavioral effects of the pituitary peptides ACTH, MSH, and vasopressin were discovered, it appeared that the pituitary also contained other behaviorally active neuropeptides. A first indication of this was the finding that several peptides isolated from pituitary tissue extracts and probably derived from β-LPH (lipotropin) could restore the disturbed active avoidance acquisition of hypophysectomized rats (15,32). More recent information was obtained from studies on the behavioral effects of the endorphins. These peptides, designated α-endorphin (β-LPH 61–76) or β-endorphin (C-fragment; β-LPH 61–91), appeared to be as active as ACTH 4–10 in delaying the extinction of the pole-jumping avoidance response (32). It was recently shown that, under certain circumstances, oxytocin has an effect on avoidance behavior opposite to that of vasopressin (7,24). Thus it may be expected that new pituitary peptides with central nervous system (CNS) activity will be discovered in the near future.

TRANSPORT OF NEUROPEPTIDES TO THEIR SITES OF ACTION

Neurohypophysial principles may be released into the cerebrospinal fluid (CSF) in order to reach midbrain limbic structures, which probably are their sites of action. Since hypothalamic-limbic connections have been described (8,25) and suggested as an integral subsystem of a peptidergic neurosecretory system (16), neurohypophysial peptides could be transported directly through this system to their limbic sites of action as well.

Neuropeptides from anterior and intermediate lobe origin may also avoid the peripheral circulation since some evidence exists that they may enter the brain by retrograde transport along the pituitary stalk via the basilar cisterns, which seem to connect the hormone-producing cells of the pituitary gland with the liquor of the brain ventricular system, or via blood vessels connecting the pituitary and the brain (3,17,20).

Neuroanatomical studies suggest that hormones from the pars distalis may reach the brain by backflow through the neurohypophysis and portal vessels (20) or by retrograde ependymal tanycyte transport to the CSF with selective absorption by specific areas of the brain (22). The presence of neuropeptides in the CSF, relative impermeability of the brain, rapid degradation in the systemic circulation, etc. all point to direct transport from the pituitary to the brain. The synthesis of pars distalis-like hormones in the brain cannot be excluded; however, growth hormone activity (21), ACTH (14,18; van Dijk, de Kloet, and van Wimersma Greidanus, *unpublished data*), thyroid-stimulating activity (21), MSH (19), β-lipotropin (28), and endorphins (12) are reported to occur in several brain regions which belong to the limbic system.

CONCLUSION

The hypothalamo-pituitary system contains various peptides related to ACTH, MSH, β-LPH, vasopressin, and oxytocin which are designated as neuropeptides and which act on the CNS (11). At least part of these neuropeptides may well be generated from larger precursor molecules, e.g., ACTH and β-LPH. It is possible that the enzymatic cleavage of these precursor molecules into behaviorally active peptides occurs in the pituitary; it may also be that these processes take place in the brain. It is postulated that the neuropeptides are transported to their limbic sites of action directly or by means of the CSF. Through these neuropeptides the hypothalamo-pituitary axis plays an essential role in the brain processes involved in motivation, learning, and/or memory, and enables the organism to display the appropriate behavioral response for coping adequately with environmental changes.

ACKNOWLEDGMENTS

The author is deeply indebted to Gerda Croiset, Angèle Balvers, Jan Dogterom, André van Dijk, Hans Goedemans, Guus de Rotte, and Hein Verspaget for their enthusiastic participation in the experiments; to Marie-

Louise Schönbaum and Marianne van Grondelle for correcting and typing the manuscript; and to Ton van den Brink for the illustrations.

REFERENCES

1. Ader, R., and de Wied, D. (1972): Effects of lysine vasopressin on passive avoidance learning. *Psychon. Sci.,* 29:46–48.
2. Ader, R., Weijnen, J. W. A. M., and Moleman, P. (1972): Retention of a passive avoidance response as a function of the intensity and duration of electric shock. *Psychon. Sci.,* 26:125–128.
3. Allen, J. P., Kendall, J. W., McGilvra, R., and Vancura, C. (1974): Immunoreactive ACTH in cerebrospinal fluid. *J. Clin. Endocrinol. Metab.,* 38:586–593.
4. Bohus, B. (1977): Effect of desglycinamide-lysine vasopressin (DG-LVP) on sexually motivated T-maze behavior of the male rat. *Horm. Behav.,* 8:52–61.
5. Bohus, B., Ader, R., and de Wied, D. (1972): Effects of vasopressin on active and passive avoidance behavior. *Horm. Behav.,* 3:191–197.
6. Bohus, B., Gispen, W. H., and de Wied, D. (1973): Effect of lysine vasopressin and ACTH 4–10 on conditioned avoidance behavior of hypophysectomized rats. *Neuroendocrinology,* 11:137–143.
7. Bohus, B., Urban, I., van Wimersma Greidanus, Tj. B. and de Wied, D. (1978): Opposite effects of oxytocin and vasopressin on avoidance behavior and hippocampal theta rhythm in the rat. *Neuropharmacology,* 17:239–247.
8. Buys, R. M., Swaab, D. F., Dogterom, J., and van Leeuwen, F. W. (1978): Intra- and extrahypothalamic vasopressin and oxytocin pathways in the rat. *Cell Tissue Res.,* 186:423–433.
9. Dogterom, J. (1977): The release and presence of vasopressin in plasma and cerebrospinal fluid as measured by radioimmunoassay; studies on vasopressin as a mediator of memory processes in the rat. Thesis, Utrecht.
10. Endröczi, E., Hrachek, Á., Nyakas, Cs., and Szabó, G. (1977): Correlation between passive avoidance learning and plasma ACTH response in adrenalectomized rats. *Acta Physiol. Acad. Sci. Hung.,* 50:35–37.
11. Gispen, W. H., Reith, M. E. A., Schotman, P., Wiegant, V. M., Zwiers, H., and de Wied, D. (1977): CNS and ACTH-like peptides; neurochemical response and interaction with opiates. In: *Neuropeptide Influences on the Brain and Behavior,* edited by L. H. Miller, C. A. Sandman, and A. J. Kastin, pp. 61–80. Raven Press, New York.
12. Guillemin, R., Ling, N., and Burgus, R. (1976): Endorphines, peptides d'origine hypothalamique et neurophypophysaire à activité morphinomimétique; isolement et structure moléculaire d'α-endorphine. *CR Acad. Sci.* [D] (*Paris*), 282:783–785.
13. Hostetter, G., Jubb, S. L., and Kozlowski, G. P. (1977): Vasopressin affects the behavior of rats in a positively-rewarded discrimination task. *Life Sci.,* 21:1323–1328.
14. Krieger, D. T., Liotta, A., and Brownstein, M. J. (1977): Presence of corticotropin in limbic system of normal and hypophysectomized rats. *Brain Res.,* 128:575–579.
15. Lande, S., de Wied, D., and Witter, A. (1973): Unique pituitary peptides with behavioral-affecting activity. In: *Drug Effects on Neuroendocrine Regulation,* edited by E. Zimmermann, W. H. Gispen, B. H. Marks, and D. de Wied, pp. 421–427. Elsevier, Amsterdam.
16. Martin, J. B., Renaud, L. P., and Brazeau, P. (1975): Hypothalamic peptides; new evidence for peptidergic pathways in the CNS. *Lancet,* 2:393–395.
17. Mezey, E., Palkovits, M., de Kloet, E. R., Verhoef, J., and de Wied, D. (1978): Evidence for pituitary-brain transport of a behaviorally potent ACTH analog. *Life Sci.,* 22:831–838.
18. Moldow, R., and Yalow, R. S. (1978): Extrahypophysial distribution of corticotropin as a function of brain size. *Proc. Natl. Acad. Sci. USA,* 75:994–998.

19. Oliver, C., Barnea, A., Warberg, J., Eskay, R. L., and Porter, J. C. (1977): Distribution characterization and subcellular localization of MSH in the brain. In: *Frontiers of Hormone Research*, Vol. 4, edited by F. J. H. Tilders, D. F. Swaab, and Tj. B. van Wimersma Greidanus, pp. 162–166. Karger, Basel.

20. Oliver, C., Mical, R. S., and Porter, J. C. (1977): Hypothalamic-pituitary vasculature: Evidence for retrograde blood flow in the pituitary stalk. *Endocrinology*, 101:598–604.

21. Pacold, S. T., Kirsteins, L., Hojvat, S., Lawrence, A. M., and Hagen, T. C. (1978): Biologically active pituitary hormones in the rat brain amygdaloid nucleus. *Science*, 199:804–805.

22. Page, R. B., Munger, B. L., and Bergland, R. M. (1976): Scanning microscopy of pituitary vascular casts. *Am. J. Anat.*, 146:273–301.

23. Schotman, P., Reith, M. E. A., van Wimersma Greidanus, Tj. B., Gispen, W. H., and de Wied, D. (1976): Hypothalamic and pituitary peptide hormones and the central nervous system. In: *Molecular and Functional Neurobiology*, edited by W. H. Gispen, pp. 309–344. Elsevier, Amsterdam.

24. Schulz, H., Kovács, G. L., and Telegdy, G. (1974): Effects of physiological doses of vasopressin on avoidance and exploratory behaviour in rats. *Acta Physiol. Acad. Sci. Hung.*, 45:211–215.

25. Sterba, G. (1974): Ascending neurosecretory pathways of the peptidergic type. In: *Neurosecretion—The Final Neuroendocrine Pathway*, edited by F. Knowles and L. Volbrath, pp. 38–47. Springer, Berlin.

26. Tanaka, M., de Kloet, E. R., de Wied, D., and Versteeg, D. H. G. (1977): Arginine-8-vasopressin affects catecholamine metabolism in specific brain nuclei. *Life Sci.*, 20:1799–1808.

27. Verhoef, J., Palkovits, M., and Witter, A. (1977): Distribution of a behaviorally highly potent ACTH 4–9 analog in rat brain after intraventricular administration. *Brain Res.*, 126:89–104.

28. Watson, S. J., Barchas, J. D., and Li, C. H. (1977): β-Lipotropin: Localization of cells and axons in rat brain immunocytochemistry. *Proc. Natl. Acad. Sci. USA*, 74:5155–5158.

29. Wied, D. de (1969): Effects of peptide hormones on behaviour. In: *Frontiers in Neuroendocrinology*, edited by W. F. Ganong and L. Martini, pp. 97–140. Oxford University Press, New York.

30. Wied, D. de (1971): Long term effect of vasopressin on the maintenance of a conditioned avoidance response in rats. *Nature (Lond)*, 232:58–60.

31. Wied, D. de (1974): Pituitary-adrenal system hormones and behavior. In: *The Neurosciences, 3rd Study Program*, edited by F. O. Schmitt and F. G. Worden, pp. 653–666. MIT Press, Cambridge, Mass.

32. Wied, D. de (1977): ACTH effects on learning processes. In: *Endocrinology; Proceedings of the V International Congress of Endocrinology, Hamburg, Vol. 1*, edited by V. H. T. James, pp. 51–56. International Congress Series No. 402. Excerpta Medica, Amsterdam.

33. Wied, D. de, and Bohus, B. (1966): Long term and short term effect on retention of a conditioned avoidance response in rats by treatment respectively with long acting pitressin or α-MSH. *Nature (Lond)*, 212:1484–1486.

34. Wied, D. de, van Wimersma Greidanus, Tj. B., Bohus, B., Urban, I., and Gispen, W. H. (1976): Vasopressin and memory consolidation. *Prog. Brain Res.*, 45:181–194.

35. van Wimersma Greidanus, Tj. B. (1977): Effects of MSH and related peptides on avoidance behavior in rats. In: *Frontiers of Hormone Research*, Vol. 4, edited by F. J. H. Tilders, D. F. Swaab, and Tj. B. van Wimersma Greidanus, pp. 129–139. Karger, Basel.

36. Wimersma Greidanus, Tj. B. van, and de Wied, D. (1971): Effects of systemic and intracerebral administration of two opposite acting ACTH-related peptides on extinction of conditioned avoidance behavior. *Neuroendocrinology*, 7:291–301.

37. Wimersma Greidanus, Tj. B. van, and de Wied, D. (1976): Dorsal hippocampus;

a site of action of neuropeptides on avoidance behavior? *Pharmacol. Biochem. Behav. (Suppl. 1)*, 5:29–33.

38. Wimersma Greidanus, Tj. B. van, and de Wied, D. (1976): Modulation of passive avoidance behavior of rats by intracerebroventricular administration of anti-vasopressin serum. *Behav. Biol.,* 18:325–333.

39. Wimersma Greidanus, Tj. B. van, Bohus, B., and de Wied, D. (1973): Effects of peptide hormones on behaviour. In: *Progress in Endocrinology, Proceedings of the 4th International Congress of Endocrinology, Washington, D.C.,* pp. 197–201. International Congress Series No. 273. Excerpta Medica, Amsterdam.

40. Wimersma Greidanus, Tj. B. van, Bohus, B., and de Wied, D. (1974): Differential localization of the influence of lysine vasopressin and of ACTH 4–10 on avoidance behavior: A study in rats bearing lesions in the parafascicular nuclei. *Neuroendocrinology,* 14:280–288.

41. Wimersma Greidanus, Tj. B. van, Bohus, B., and de Wied, D. (1975): CNS sites of action of ACTH, MSH and vasopressin in relation to avoidance behavior. In: *Anatomical Neuroendocrinology; International Conference of Neurobiology of CNS-Hormone Interactions, Chapel Hill,* edited by W. F. Stumpf and L. D. Grant, pp. 284–289. Karger, Basel.

42. Wimersma Greidanus, Tj. B. van, Dogterom, J., and de Wied, D. (1975): Intraventricular administration of anti-vasopressin serum inhibits memory consolidation in rats. *Life Sci.,* 16:637–644.

43. Wimersma Greidanus, Tj. B. van, Rees, L. H., Scott, A. P., Lowry, P. J., and de Wied, D. (1977): ACTH release during passive avoidance behavior. *Brain Res. Bull.,* 2:101–104.

44. Wimersma Greidanus, Tj. B. van, van Dijk, A. M. A., de Rotte, A. A., Goedemans, J. H. J., Croiset, G., and Thody, A. J. (1978): Involvement of ACTH and MSH in active and passive avoidance behavior. *Brain Res. Bull.,* 3:227–230.

Central Nervous System Effects of Hypothalamic Hormones and Other Peptides, edited by Collu et al. Raven Press, New York © 1979.

Role of Monoamines in Mediating the Action of ACTH, Vasopressin, and Oxytocin

G. Telegdy and G. L. Kovács

Department of Pathophysiology, University Medical School, Szeged P.O.B. 531, Hungary

During the last few years our department has been engaged in studying the actions of different peptide hormones on brain neurotransmitter levels in correlation with certain behavioral patterns (36). In this chapter we report findings in connection with the effects of ACTH, vasopressin, and oxytocin on the catecholamine and serotonin metabolism in correlation with certain behavioral reactions.

ACTION OF ACTH ON BRAIN MONOAMINES

The actions of ACTH and ACTH fragments on certain behavioral patterns have already been well documented in different laboratories. It has been shown that ACTH delays the extinction of an active avoidance reflex, improves passive avoidance behavior by an antiamnestic action, influences approach behavior and sexually motivated behavior, increases the maintenance of reflex activity in an avoidance situation, and enhances the electrical activity of the brain (1,3,4,6,7,11,12,14,18,20,23,24,41,43,44,47).

Whether the action of ACTH or ACTH fragments is direct or through influencing other systems (e.g., neurotransmitters) is still unsolved. In the present series of experiments we demonstrated the actions of ACTH on catecholamine and serotonin levels in normal and adrenalectomized animals.

ACTH (2.0 IU/animal; Exacthin Richter), given i.p. 30 min prior to the animals being killed, significantly increased the dopamine (DA) levels in the striatum and mesencephalon (Fig. 1). In adrenalectomized animals the same amount of ACTH decreased the DA content of the hypothalamus, whereas in the striatum a further increase could be observed. The action of ACTH on the norepinephrine (NE) content was somewhat different. No effect was observed on the NE contents of the hypothalamus, striatum, and mesencephalon, but there were decreases in the septum and dorsal hippocampus (Fig. 2). Following adrenalectomy, no significant alteration was obtained in any of the brain areas studied. ACTH increased the serotonin levels in the hypothalamus and mesencephalon in normal animals but had

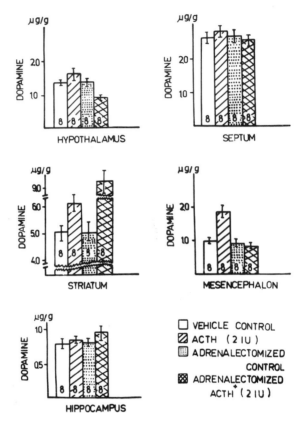

FIG. 1. Action of ACTH (2.0 IU) on the DA contents of different brain areas in normal and adrenalectomized rats.

no effect in adrenalectomized rats under otherwise identical conditions (Fig. 3).

The catecholamine levels and the serotonin content of the brain were determined according to the methods of Shellenberger and Gordon (26) and Snyder et al. (34).

Our data support the findings of other investigators (8,13,16,17,38–40) that the brain catecholaminergic system might be responsible for the central nervous action of ACTH. This is further supported by the findings of Wiegant et al. (51), who demonstrated that a dopaminergic receptor blocker injected into the substantia nigra prevented some of the behavioral action of ACTH.

It seems that the serotoninergic system does not play an important role in the behavioral action of ACTH, since adrenalectomy may eliminate the action on serotonin (37); furthermore, the behavioral action is clearer in adrenalectomized rats (4).

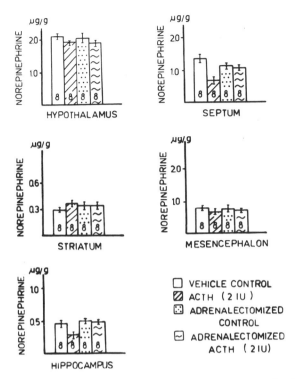

FIG. 2. Action of ACTH (2.0 IU) on the NE contents of different brain areas in normal and adrenalectomized rats.

ACTIONS OF VASOPRESSIN ON BEHAVIOR AND NEUROTRANSMITTER METABOLISM

The effect of vasopressin on behavioral reaction has already been shown (2,10,28,29,42,50). Vasopressin treatment can improve memory (1,48) and delays extinction in active avoidance behavior (45), and desglycinamide-lysine-vasopressin restores retrograde amnesia (24,25).

Hereditary diabetes insipidus rats (Brattleboro strain) display learning and memory defects that could be restored by vasopressin treatment (5,22, 46,49,50). Desglycinamide-lysine-vasopressin can avert a puromycin-caused memory blockade (14). Even in a physiological dose, it can delay extinction of an active avoidance reflex (28,29) and self-stimulation (32). These data indicate that vasopressin can play a physiological role in memory processes, and that part of its action may involve protein synthesis.

In our study the effects of vasopressin on catecholamine and serotonin metabolism were studied in relation to active and passive avoidance behaviors. The action of vasopressin on the acquisition of an active avoidance reflex was studied in the bench-jumping apparatus described in detail earlier (35). The animals were trained in an experimental box, with 10 condition-

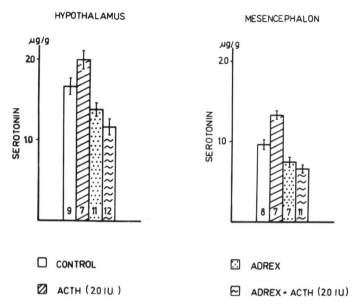

FIG. 3. Action of ACTH (2.0 IU) on the serotonin contents of different brain areas in normal and adrenalectomized rats.

ing trials per day. The conditioning signal was light associated with electric shock delivered through the feet of the animal. In order to avoid electric shock the animal could jump onto a bench on the wall of the box. The learning and the extinction were studied. During the extinction period no reinforcement was given.

Vasopressin (lysine-8-vasopressin) in a dose of 300 mU/kg i.p. given 10 min prior to the training session had no marked effect on the acquisition of the conditioned reflex (Fig. 4). Alpha-methyl-p-tyrosine (α-MT) in a dose of 80 mg/kg 4 hr prior to conditioning significantly inhibited the synthesis of catecholamine (19,27) and reduced the learning of the conditioned avoidance reflex (Fig. 4). However, vasopressin was able to counteract the effect of α-MT on learning and thus compensated the learning deficit elicited by the administration of α-MT.

Lysine-8-vasopressin delayed the extinction. This effect was described earlier (28,29,45). α-MT facilitates extinction of the active avoidance reflex. Vasopressin, however, was not able to compensate the facilitatory action of α-MT on the extinction.

The action of vasopressin on passive avoidance behavior (Fig. 5) was studied according to Fibiger et al. (9) and Kovács et al. (15). The animals were placed on the grid floor of a bench-jumping conditioning apparatus and were trained to jump onto the bench. Current (1.0 mA) was applied through the grid floor until the animal jumped onto the bench, and the total

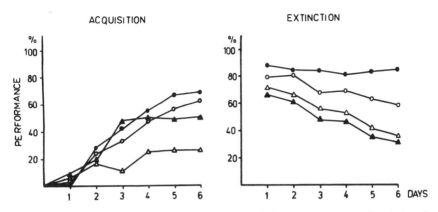

FIG. 4. Effects of vasopressin (300 mU/kg) and α-MT (80 mg/kg) on the acquisition and extinction of an active avoidance reflex. [O—O, Control; △—△, α-MT (80 mg/kg); ●—●, lysine-8-vasopressin (300 mU/kg); ▲—▲, α-MT + lysine-8-vasopressin.]

time to reach the criterion (remaining on the bench for 180 sec) was measured. This time was called the "step-on latency." Having met this criterion, the animal was removed from the apparatus and tested 24 hr later. The animal was placed on the bench and the latency to step-down ("step-down latency") was measured up to 180 sec. Prior to the behavioral session

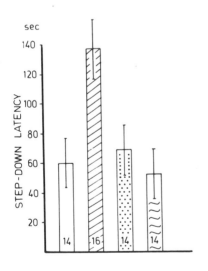

FIG. 5. Effects of vasopressin (300 mU/kg) and α-MT (80 mg/kg) on passive avoidance ("step-down latency") behavior.

☐ CONTROL

▨ VASOPRESSIN (300 mU / kg)

⸬ αMT (80 mg / kg)

∿ αMT + VASOPRESSIN

the animals were treated with α-MT (80 mg/kg) 3 hr before or with lysine-8-vasopressin (300 mU/kg) 10 min before the training session, alone or in combination with each other.

Neither vasopressin nor α-MT had any effect on the "step-on latency," but the "step-down latency" was considerably lengthened. α-MT per se had no effect on the "step-down latency," but it was able to prevent the action of vasopressin when given in combination with vasopressin.

Lysine-vasopressin administered 10 min prior to the animals being killed decreased the DA contents of the hypothalamus, septum, striatum, and mesencephalon (Fig. 6). It had no effect on the NE and serotonin contents of any of the brain areas studied.

The action of vasopressin on the catecholamine turnover (Fig. 7) was studied by the method of Nagatsu et al. (21) using α-MT (250 mg/kg). The

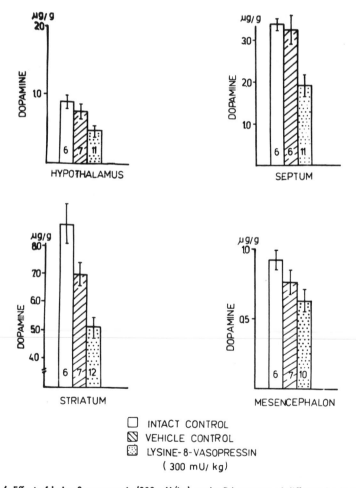

FIG. 6. Effect of lysine-8-vasopressin (300 mU/kg) on the DA contents of different brain areas.

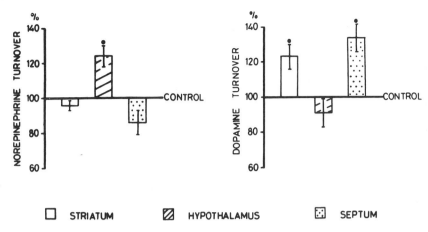

STRIATUM   HYPOTHALAMUS   SEPTUM

FIG. 7. Effect of vasopressin (300 mU/kg) on catecholamine turnover in different brain areas.

NE and DA contents were measured 4 hr later. Following vasopressin, DA turnover was increased in the striatum and septum, but that of NE only in the hypothalamus.

The animals having a genetic defect of the vasopressin system, the Brattleboro strain, in which the homozygous animal has diabetes insipidus, revealed that this strain was inferior in acquisition of the two-way active avoidance reflex and displayed a severe memory deficit that could be restored by vasopressin administration (5,46,49) (Fig. 8). In active avoidance reflex the Brattleboro homozygous rats improved less during the first 3 days in the learning procedure, which became normalized after 4 to 6 days.

α-MT (80 mg/kg) significantly reduced the learning in all three groups when given 3 hr before the trial session (Fig. 9). However, vasopressin

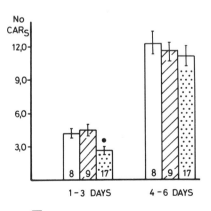

FIG. 8. Acquisition of active avoidance behavior in Brattleboro homozygous and heterozygous and CFY strain rats.

☐ CFY
▨ BRATTLEBORO HETEROZYGOUS
⬚ BRATTLEBORO HOMOZYGOUS

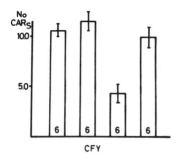

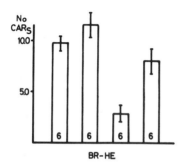

FIG. 9. Effects of α-MT and vasopressin treatment on learning in Brattleboro homozygous (BR-HO) and heterozygous (BR-HE) and CFY rats.

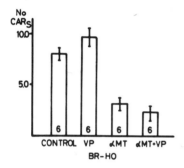

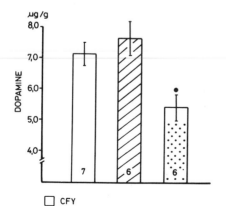

FIG. 10. DA contents of the striatum in Brattleboro homozygous and heterozygous and CFY rats.

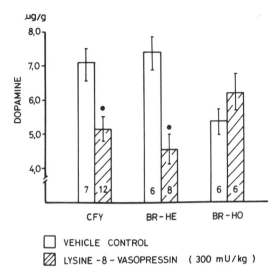

VEHICLE CONTROL

LYSINE -8 - VASOPRESSIN   (300 mU/kg)

FIG. 11. Effect of vasopressin on the dopamine levels of the striatum in Brattleboro homozygous (BR-HO) and heterozygous (BR-HE) and CFY rats.

(300 mU/kg) given i.p. 10 min before training restored the α-MT-induced learning deficit in Brattleboro heterozygous and CFY strain rats but not in Brattleboro homozygotes.

The dopamine content of the striatum is lower in the hereditary diabetes insipidus rats (Brattleboro homozygous) than in heterozygous or in normal CFY animals (Fig. 10). Lysine-8-vasopressin (300 mU/kg) decreased the dopamine level of the striatum in CFY and heterozygous rats but had no influence in the homozygous animals (Fig. 11). The NE content of the septum is higher in Brattleboro heterozygous and homozygous rats than in the normal CFY animals (Fig. 12). Following vasopressin treatment, the

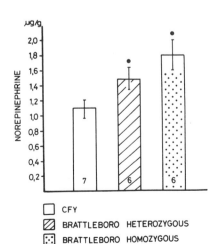

CFY

BRATTLEBORO HETEROZYGOUS

BRATTLEBORO HOMOZYGOUS

FIG. 12. NE contents of the septum in CFY and Brattleboro heterozygous and homozygous rats.

turnover rates of NE in the septum and DA in the striatum were greater in homozygous than in heterozygous Brattleboro rats (Fig. 13).

The results show that although Brattleboro rats suffer from diabetes insipidus for genetic reasons, the condition is not absolutely equal to a simple vasopressin deficiency, since these animals show other signs of their genetic defect in relation to brain transmitter metabolism. Even the hetero-

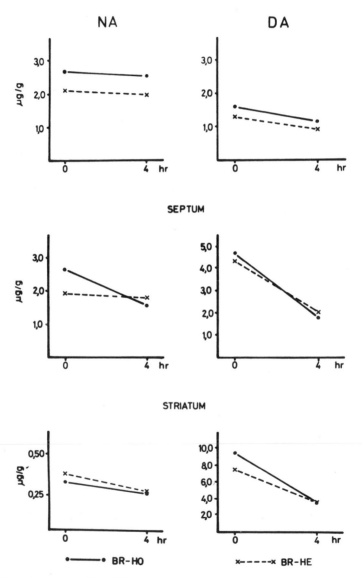

FIG. 13. Effect of vasopressin (300 mU/kg) on catecholamine turnover in Brattleboro homozygous (BR-HO) and heterozygous (BR-HE) rats. (NA) Norepinephrine. (DA) Dopamine.

zygous animals, which show no sign of diabetes insipidus, differ from other strains in relation to their transmitter level.

ACTIONS OF OXYTOCIN ON BEHAVIOR AND BRAIN MONOAMINES

The effect of oxytocin on brain function was first demonstrated by electrophysiological methods (30,31,33). Oxytocin was able to decrease the activity of hypothalamic neurons (31); the reaction time was shortened by oxytocin treatment (33). In behavior studies, oxytocin facilitated the extinction of an active avoidance reflex (28,29) and facilitated self-stimulation behavior (32). All these actions were opposite to those of vasopressin.

In a study of the action of oxytocin on the acquisition of an active avoidance reflex, oxytocin in a dose of 300 mU/kg i.p. 10 min before the training session caused no significant alteration in acquisition (Fig. 14). α-MT given 3 hr prior to the training led to a deficit in learning which could not be counteracted by oxytocin (Fig. 14); 30 mU/kg caused facilitation in the extinction of active avoidance training. The effect was opposite to that of vasopressin.

The effects of oxytocin and vasopressin on self-stimulation behavior were tested. Insulated stainless steel electrodes were implanted into the left lateral hypothalamic area. Four days after the postoperative recovery period, self-stimulation was established with the following stimulation parameters: 0.2-sec trains of rectangular stimuli with frequency of 90 to 130 cps, impulse duration of 0.15 to 0.50 msec, intensity of 3.5 to 20.0 volts. The ani-

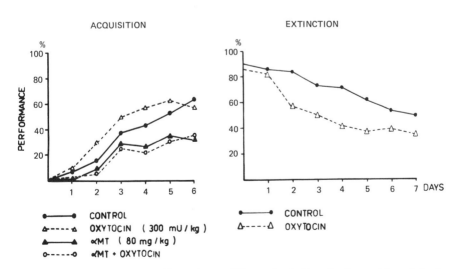

FIG. 14. Effects of oxytocin and α-MT on the acquisition and extinction of active avoidance behavior.

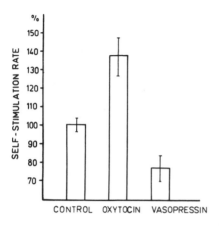

FIG. 15. Effects of intraventricular administration of oxytocin (500 μU/animal) and vasopressin (50 μU virgule animal) on self-stimulation behavior.

mals were trained until a stable level of self-stimulation behavior was reached (32).

Oxytocin (Richter, Budapest) in a dose of 500 μU/animal, and vasopressin (Sandoz Co., Basel) in a dose of 50 μU/animal, were dissolved in artificial cerebrospinal fluid and injected in 5 μl volume into the lateral ventricle. The self-stimulation was tested between 10 and 20 min after injection. Oxytocin significantly increased the self-stimulation rate, whereas vasopressin decreased it (Fig. 15). The self-stimulation rate was expressed as a percent of the control value.

The effect of oxytocin on the passive avoidance behavior (Fig. 16) was tested as described earlier (10,27). Following oxytocin (300 mU/kg) the "step-on latency" did not change, although the "step-down latency" was considerably shortened. This effect was also opposite to that of vasopressin.

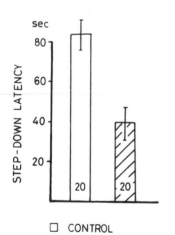

FIG. 16. Effect of oxytocin (300 mU/kg) on passive avoidance behavior ("step-down latency").

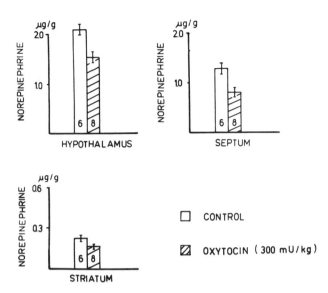

FIG. 17. Effect of oxytocin (300 mU/kg) treatment on NE content of different brain areas.

The NE contents of the hypothalamus, septum, and striatum decreased following oxytocin (300 mU/kg i.p.) given 10 min following treatment, but there was no effect on the dopamine in the same regions (Fig. 17). Following 300 mU/kg, the serotonin content decreased in the septum but was unchanged in the hypothalamus, striatum, and mesencephalon (Fig. 18). The DA turnover rate increased in the hypothalamus and decreased in the striatum; the NE turnover also decreased in the striatum (Fig. 19).

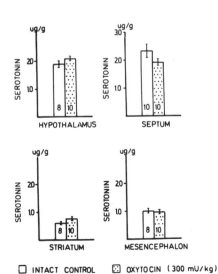

FIG. 18. Effect of oxytocin (300 mU/kg) treatment on serotonin content of different brain areas.

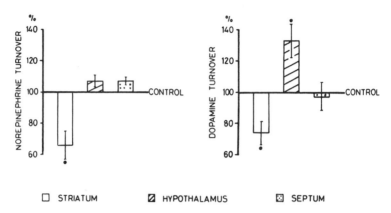

FIG. 19. Effects of oxytocin (300 mU/kg) treatment on DA and NE turnover in different brain areas.

CONCLUSIONS

The presented data show that the actions of ACTH, vasopressin, and oxytocin on different behavioral models can be modified by influencing brain monoamine levels and metabolism. The actions of these peptide hormones on the brain transmitter levels and metabolism indicate that in certain behavioral reactions action mediated via the brain monoamines also must be considered.

ACKNOWLEDGMENT

Research has been supported by the Scientific Research Council, Ministry of Health, Hungary (4–08–0302–03–0/T).

REFERENCES

1. Ader, R., and De Wied, D. (1972): Effects of lysine vasopressin on passive avoidance learning. *Psychon. Sci.,* 29:46–48.
2. Bohus, B., Gispen, W. H., and De Wied, D. (1973): Effect of lysine vasopressin and ACTH 4–10 on conditioned avoidance behavior of hypophysectomized rats. *Neuroendocrinology,* 11:137–143.
3. Bohus, B., Hendrickx, H. H. L., Van Kolfschoten, A. A., and Krediet, T. G. (1975): Effect of ACTH$^{4-10}$ on copulatory and sexually motivated approach behavior in the male rat. In: *Sexual Behavior: Pharmacology and Biochemistry,* edited by M. Sandler and G. L. Gessa, pp. 269–275. Raven Press, New York.
4. Bohus, B., Nyakas, C., and Endröczi, E. (1968): Effects of adrenocorticotrophic hormone on avoidance behaviour of intact and adrenalectomized rats. *Int. J. Neuropharmacol.,* 7:307–314.
5. Bohus, B., Van Wimersma Greidanus, Tj. B., and De Wied, D. (1975): Behavioral and endocrine responses of rats with hereditary hypothalamic diabetes insipidus (Brattleboro strain). *Physiol. Behav.,* 14:609–615.
6. Endröczi, E., and Fekete, T. (1971): Thalami-cortical synchronization, habituation and hormone action. In: *Recent Developments of Neurobiology in Hungary,* Vol. III, edited by K. Lissák, pp. 115–131. Akadémiai Kiadó, Budapest.

7. Endröczi, E., Lissák, K., Fekete, T., and De Wied, D. (1970): Effects of ACTH on EEG habituation in human subjects. *Prog. Brain Res.,* 32:254–263.
8. Endröczi, E., Hraschek, A., Nyakas, C., and Szabó G. (1976): Brain catecholamines and pituitary-adrenal function. In: *Cellular and Molecular Bases of Neuroendocrine Processes,* edited by E. Endröczi, pp. 607–618. Akadémiai Kiadó, Budapest.
9. Fibiger, H. C., Robert, D. C. S., and Price, M. T. C. (1975): The role of telencephalic noradrenaline in learning and memory. In: *Chemical Tools in Catecholamine Research,* Vol. 1, edited by G. Jonsson, T. Malmfors, and C. Sachs, pp. 349–356. Elsevier, Amsterdam.
10. Garrud, P. (1975): Effects of lysine-8-vasopressin on punishment-induced supression of a level-holding response. *Prog. Brain Res.,* 42:173–186.
11. Gray, J. A., Mayes, A. R., and Wilson, M. (1971): A barbiturate-like effect of adrenocorticotropic hormone on the partial reinforcement acquisition and extinction effects. *Neuropharmacology,* 10:223–230.
12. Guth, S., Levine, S., and Seward, J. P. (1971): Appetitive acquisition and extinction effects with exogenous ACTH. *Physiol. Behav.,* 7:195–200.
13. Hökfelt, T., and Fuxe, K. (1972): On the morphology and the neuroendocrine role of hypothalamic catecholamine neurons. In: *Brain-Endocrine Interaction. Median Eminence: Structure and Function,* edited by K. M. Knigge, D. E. Scott, and A. Weindl, pp. 181–223. Karger, Basel.
14. Kovács, G. L., and Telegdy, G. (1978): Indoleamines and behaviour: The possible role of serotoninergic mechanisms in the pituitary-adrenocortical hormone-induced behavioural action. In: *Recent Development of Neurobiology in Hungary,* edited by K. Lissák. Akadémiai Kiadó, Budapest *(in press).*
15. Kovács, G. L., Vécsei, L., Szabó, G., and Telegdy, G. (1977): The involvement of catecholaminergic mechanisms in the behavioural action of vasopressin. *Neurosci. Lett.,* 5:337–344.
16. Leonard, B. F. (1974): The effect of two synthetic ACTH analogues on the metabolism of biogenic amines in the rat brain. *Arch. Int. Pharmacodyn.,* 207:242–253.
17. Leonard, B. E., Ramaekers, F., and Rigter, H. (1975): Effects of adrenocorticotrophin-(4–10)-heptapeptide on changes in brain monoamine metabolism associated with retrograde amnesia in the rat. *Biochem. Soc. Transact.,* 3:113–115.
18. Levine, S., and Jones, L. E. (1965): Adrenocorticotrophic hormone (ACTH) and passive avoidance learning. *J. Comp. Physiol. Psychol.,* 59:357–360.
19. Levitt, M., Spector, S., Sjoerdsma, A., and Udenfriend, S. (1965): Elucidation of the rate limiting step in norepinephrine biosynthesis in the perfused guinea pig heart. *J. Pharmacol. Exp. Ther.,* 148:1–8.
20. Lissák, K., Kovács, G. L., and Telegdy, G. (1977): Involvement of serotoninergic system in mediation of corticosteroid action on avoidance behaviour (in Russian). In: *Novoe o Gormonah i Mehanisme ih Dejstvijah,* edited by M. F. Gulij, R. E. Kaveckij, P. G. Kostuk, K. P. Zak, and R. C. Filatova, pp. 180–192. Naukova Dumka, Kiev.
21. Nagatsu, J., Levitt, J., and Udenfriend, S. (1964): Tyrosine hydroxylase. *J. Biol. Chem.,* 239:2910–2917.
22. Ramaekers, F., Rigter, H., and Leonard, B. E. (1977): Parallel changes in behaviour and hippocampal serotonin metabolism in rats following treatment with desglycinamide lysine vasopressin. *Brain. Res.,* 120:485–492.
23. Rigter, H., and Van Riezen, H. (1975): Anti-amnestic effect of $ACTH_{4-10}$: Its independence of the nature of the amnestic agent and the behavioral test. *Physiol. Behav.,* 14:563–566.
24. Rigter, H., Van Riezen, H., and De Wied, D. (1974): The effects of ACTH- and vasopressin-analogues on CO_2-induced retrograde amnesia in rats. *Physiol. Behav.,* 13:381–388.
25. Rigter, H., Elbertse, R., and Van Riezen, H. (1975): Time-dependent anti-amnestic effect of ACTH 4–10 and desglycinamide-lysine vasopressin. *Prog. Brain Res.,* 42:163–171.

26. Shellenberger, M. K., and Gordon, J. H. (1971): A rapid simplified procedure for simultaneous assay of norepinephrine, dopamine, and 5-hydroxytryptamine from discrete brain areas. *Anal. Biochem.*, 39:356–372.
27. Spector, S., Sjoerdsma, A., and Udenfriend, S. (1965): Blockade of endogenous norepinephrine synthesis by alpha-methyl-tyrosine an inhibitor of tyrosine hydroxylase. *J. Pharmacol. Exp. Ther.*, 147:86–102.
28. Schulz, H., Kovács, G. L., and Telegdy, G. (1974): Effect of physiological doses of vasopressin and oxytocin on avoidance and exploratory behaviour in rats. *Acta Physiol. Acad. Sci. Hung.* 45:211–215.
29. Schulz, H., Kovács, G. L., and Telegdy, G. (1976): The effect of vasopressin and oxytocin on avoidance behaviour in rats. In: *Cellular and Molecular Bases of Neuroendocrine Processes*, edited by E. Endröczi, pp. 555–564. Akadémiai Kiadó, Budapest.
30. Schulz, H., Unger, H., and Schwarzberg, H. (1973): Einfluss von intraventrikulär applizierter Glutaminsäure und Oxytocin auf die Impulsentladungerate hypothalamischer Neuronengebiete. *Acta Biol. Med. Germ.*, 30:197–202.
31. Schulz, H., Unger, H., Schwarzberg, H., Pommrich, G., and Stolze, R. (1971): Neuronenaktivität hypothalamischer Kerngebiete von Kaninchen nach intraventrikulärer Applikation von Vasopressin und Oxytocin. *Experientia*, 27:1482.
32. Schwarzberg, H., Hartman, G., Kovács, G. L., and Telegdy, G. (1976): The effect of intraventricular administration of oxytocin and vasopressin on self-stimulation in rats. *Acta Physiol. Acad. Sci. Hung.*, 47:127–131.
33. Schwarzberg, H., and Unger, H. (1970): Anderung der Reaktionszeit von Ratten nach Applikation von Vasopressin, Oxytocin und Na-thiglykolat. *Acta Biol. Med. Germ.*, 24:507–516.
34. Snyder, S. H., Axelrod, J., and Zweig, M. (1967): Circadian rhythm in the serotonin content of the rat pineal gland. *J. Pharmacol. Exp. Ther.*, 158:206–213.
35. Telegdy, G., Hadnagy, J., and Lissák, K. (1968): The effect of gonads on conditioned avoidance behaviour of rats. *Acta Physiol. Acad. Sci. Hung.*, 33:439–446.
36. Telegdy, G., and Kovács, G. L. (1978): The role of monoamines in mediating the action of hormones on learning and memory. In: *IBRO Monograph Series*, edited by M. A. B. Brazier (*in press*).
37. Vermes, I., Telegdy, G., and Lissák, K. (1973): Correlation between hypothalamic serotonin content and adrenal function during acute stress: Effect of adrenal corticosteroids on hypothalamic serotonin content. *Acta Physiol. Acad. Sci. Hung.*, 43:33–42.
38. Versteeg, D. H. G. (1973): Effects of two ACTH-analogs on noradrenaline metabolism in rat brain. *Brain Res.*, 49:483–485.
39. Versteeg, D. H. G., Gispen, W. H., Schotman, P., Witter, A., and De Wied, D. (1972): Hypophysectomy and rat brain metabolism: Effects of synthetic ACTH analogs. *Adv. Biochem. Psychopharmacol.*, 6:219–239.
40. Versteeg, D. H. G., and Wurtman, R. J. (1975): Effect of $ACTH_{4-10}$ on the rate of synthesis of (H^3)catecholamines in the brains of intact, hypophysectomized and adrenalectomized rats. *Brain Res.*, 93:552–557.
41. Wied, D. De (1966): Inhibitory effect of ACTH and related peptides on extinction of conditioned avoidance behavior. *Proc. Soc. Exp. Biol. Med.*, 122:28–32.
42. Wied, D. De (1971): Long term effect of vasopressin on the maintenance of a conditioned avoidance response in rats. *Nature (Lond)*, 232:58–60.
43. Wied, D. De (1976): ACTH effects on learning processes. In: *International Congress Series 402*, Vol. 1, pp. 51–56. Excerpta Medica, Amsterdam.
44. Wied, D. De (1977): Peptides and behavior. *Life Sci.*, 20:195–204.
45. Wied, D. De, and Bohus, B. (1966): Long term and short term effect on retention of a conditioned avoidance response in rats by treatment with long acting pitressin or α-MSH. *Nature (Lond)*, 212:1484–1486.
46. Wied, D. De, Bohus, B., and Van Wimersma Greidanus, Tj. B. (1975): Memory deficit in rats with hereditary diabetes insipidus. *Brain Res.*, 85:152–156.
47. Wied, D. De, Bohus, B., Gispen, W. H., Urban, I., and Van Wimersma Greidanus, Tj. B. (1975): Pituitary peptides on motivational, learning and memory processes.

In: *CNS and Behavioural Pharmacology,* Vol. 3, edited by M. Airaksinen, pp. 19–30. Finnish Pharmacological Society, Helsinki.

48. Wied, D. De, Bohus, B., and Van Wimersma Greidanus, Tj. B. (1976): The significance of vasopressin for pituitary ACTH release in conditioned emotional situations. In: *Cellular and Molecular Bases of Neuroendocrine Processes,* edited by E. Endröczi, pp. 547–553. Akadémiai Kiadó, Budapest.

49. Van Wimersma Greidanus, Tj. B., Dogterom, J., and De Wied, D. (1975): Intraventricular administration of anti-vasopressin serum inhibits memory consolidation in rats. *Life Sci.,* 16:637–644.

50. Van Wimersma Greidanus, Tj. B., Bohus, B., and De Wied, D. (1975): The role of vasopressin in memory processes. *Prog. Brain Res.,* 42:135–141.

51. Wiegant, V. M., Cools, A. R., and Gispen, W. H. (1977): ACTH-induced excessive grooming involves brain dopamine. *Eur. J. Pharmacol.,* 41:343–346.

Central Nervous System Effects of Hypothalamic Hormones and Other Peptides, edited by Collu et al. Raven Press, New York © 1979.

Control of Prolactin Secretion at the Pituitary Level: A Model for Postsynaptic Dopaminergic Systems

F. Labrie, M. Beaulieu, L. Ferland, V. Raymond, T. Di Paolo, M. G. Caron, R. Veilleux, F. Denizeau, C. Euvrard, J. P. Raynaud, and J. R. Boissier

Medical Research Council Group in Molecular Endocrinology, Le Centre Hospitalier de l'Université Laval, Québec G1V 4G2, Canada; and Centre de Recherches Roussel-UCLAF, Romainville 93230, France

Secretion of prolactin from the anterior pituitary gland is controlled by stimulatory and inhibitory influences of hypothalamic origin. Morphological and physiological studies indicate that these substances are released from nerve endings in the median eminence and reach the adenohypophysial portal blood system. At least part of the stimulatory hypothalamic influence appears to be mediated by the tripeptide thyrotropin-releasing hormone (TRH), which has been shown to stimulate prolactin secretion in the human *in vivo* (8,41) and in the rat *in vivo* and *in vitro* (29,68).

The predominant influence of the hypothalamus on prolactin secretion, however, is inhibitory (58). Rapidly accumulating evidence suggests that dopamine (DA) may be the main or even the only inhibitory substance involved. In fact, destruction of the dopaminergic cell bodies and terminals resulted in a marked elevation of plasma prolactin levels (7). Moreover, the prolactin release-inhibiting activity contained in purified hypothalamic extracts could be accounted for by their catecholamine content (78), and preincubation of hypothalamic extracts with aluminum oxide or monoamine oxidase led to a complete loss of prolactin release-inhibiting activity (73). In support of this physiological role of DA in the control of prolactin secretion, DA was recently measured in portal blood (5).

It thus appeared important to study in detail the specificity of the control of prolactin secretion and the properties of the adenohypophysial dopaminergic receptor. Since estrogens are known to be potent stimulators of prolactin secretion, the interaction of estrogens with dopaminergic action was then studied at the pituitary level *in vitro* and *in vivo*.

The present data show a close correlation between specificity of binding of the ergot derivative [³H]dihydroergocryptine and the specificity of control of prolactin release measured in anterior pituitary cells in culture. Estrogens were found to act directly at the pituitary level and, more surprisingly, to have potent antidopaminergic activity on prolactin secretion. Since changes of prolactin secretion in anterior pituitary cells in culture can be measured with a high degree of precision, it provides a sensitive and specific screening test for potential antiparkinsonian and antischizophrenic drugs. Moreover, since dopamine is involved in various brain functions and in some diseases, knowledge gained about the pituitary dopamine receptor should help our understanding of dopaminergic action in various brain functions.

SPECIFICITY OF CONTROL OF PROLACTIN SECRETION

Much information about the factors controlling prolactin release could be obtained using rat hemipituitaries (6,52,57,64,73). However, since adeno-hypophysial cells in primary culture proved to be a more precise system for studying control of the secretion of many pituitary hormones (30,31,48), we used this model in the present report to investigate in detail the specificity of action of a large series of DA agonists and antagonists on prolactin release. The high degree of precision obtained with the pituitary cell system made possible study of the correlation between the biological activity (effect on prolactin release) of the various substances and their affinity for the adenohypophysial DA receptor (13,47). Moreover, compounds so far classified as DA or serotonergic antagonists were found to be mixed DA agonist-antagonists.

Specificity of the Inhibitory Effect of Catecholamines

Figure 1 shows the inhibitory effect of increasing concentrations of various catecholamines and analogs on prolactin release during a 2-hr incubation of rat anterior pituitary cells in primary culture. As measured by the concentration giving a 50% inhibition of hormone release, the following order of potency was obtained: DA (35 nM) > epinephrine (420 nM) $\geq$ norepinephrine (540 nM); the α- and β-agonists phenylephrine and isoproterenol were without effect up to 10 μM. Apomorphine, the prototype of DA agonists (2), was approximately 10 times more potent than DA as inhibitor of prolactin release at an ED_{50} value of 3 nM (Table 1).

At high concentrations, apomorphine, DA, epinephrine, and norepinephrine led to a maximal 85 to 90% inhibition of basal prolactin release. Serotonin, a neurotransmitter potentially involved in the control of prolactin secretion *in vivo* (46,77) was a very weak inhibitor of prolactin release in cells in culture (Table 1). The inhibition of prolactin release by catecholamines showed the expected stereoselectivity since ($-$)epinephrine and ($-$)norepinephrine affected prolactin release with a potency approximately eight times greater than the corresponding ($+$)enantiomers (Table 1).

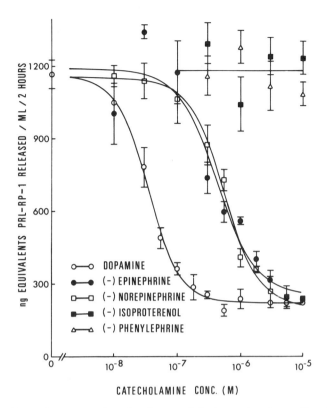

FIG. 1. Effect of increasing concentrations of various catecholamines and analogs on the release of prolactin in anterior pituitary cells in primary culture. Four days after plating, cells obtained from adult female
Sprague-Dawley rats at random stages of the estrous cycle were incubated for 2 hr in the presence of the
indicated drug concentrations. The experiment was performed as described (13).

TABLE 1. *Apparent dissociation constants of dopaminergic agents in anterior pituitary*

Agents	Prolactin release from rat anterior pituitary cells in culture		[³H]DHEC binding to bovine anterior pituitary membranes	
	K_D (nM)	Relative potency	K_D (nM)	Relative potency
Agonists				
Apomorphine	3	1,170	78	628
Dopamine	35	100	490	100
(—)Epinephrine	420	8.33	1,700	28.8
(+)Epinephrine	3,100	1.13	16,500	2.97
(—)Norepinephrine	540	6.48	3,200	15.3
(+)Norepinephrine	4,200	0.83	15,000	3.27
(—)Isoproterenol	—	—	> 100,000	< 0.5
Clonidine	—	—	> 100,000	< 0.5
Phentolamine	> 10,000	< 0.35	3,200	15.3
Propranolol	—	—	> 100,000	< 0.5
Dihydroergocryptine	0.2	17,500	4.7	10,400
Dihydroergocornine	0.4	8,750	10.8	4,530

TABLE 1. Continued

Agents	Prolactin release from rat anterior pituitary cells in culture		[³H]DHEC binding to bovine anterior pituitary membranes	
	K_D (nM)	Relative potency	K_D (nM)	Relative potency
Ergocryptine	0.2	17,500	6.5	7,540
2-Bromo-α-ergocryptine	2.9	1,210	24	2,040
Antagonists				
(+)Butaclamol	0.3	11,700	1.3	37,700
(−)Butaclamol	> 1,000	< 3.5	> 100,000	< 0.5
α-Flupenthixol	2.4	1,460	6.7	7,310
β-Flupenthixol	330	10.6	1,600	30.6
cis-Thiothixene	4.6	760	27	1,810
trans-Thiothixene	44	79.5	1,300	37.7
Haloperidol[a]	0.7	5,000	12	4,080
Pimozide[a]	0.3	11,700	33	1,480
Fluphenazine	0.6	5,830	3.4	14,400
Triflupromazine	n.t.	n.t.	9.1	5,380
Perphenazine	n.t.	n.t.	30	1,630
Chlorpromazine	28	125	44	1,110
Serotonin	n.t.	n.t.	23,000	2.13
Cyproheptadine[a]	14	250	230	213
Methysergide[a]	190	18.4	1,100	44.5

(−) indicates effect of agent was too weak to calculate a valid K_D value.

n.t. = not tested.

Several catecholamine analogs, precursors, and metabolites were tested for their ability to compete for binding. Ephedrine, L-DOPA, α-methyl-DOPA, and (±)dihydroxymandelic acid did not interact significantly with the binding sites below 100 μM. Normetanephrine inhibited binding by 50% at 100 μM. Various other agents having a presumable influence on dopaminergic systems in vivo have been screened for possible interactions with the receptor sites. None of the following drugs tested had any effect at 10 to 100 μM: morphine, β-endorphin, thyrotropin releasing hormone, triiodothyronine, α-melanocyte-stimulating hormone, 17β-estradiol, 5α-dihydrotestosterone, substance P, neurotensin, somatostatin, and γ-aminobutyric acid.

Apparent dissociation constants (K_D) of dopaminergic agonists and antagonists and other compounds for their effects on prolactin release in anterior pituitary cells in primary culture and their ability to compete for [³H]dihydroergocryptine binding to bovine anterior pituitary membranes are shown. K_D values for agonistic activity were taken directly as the concentration of an agent giving 50% (ED₅₀) of maximal inhibition of prolactin release by that agent. For antagonistic activity, compounds were tested in the presence of 3 nM DHE or 50 nM dopamine, and apparent K_D values were calculated according to the equation $K_D = IC_{50}/(1 + S/K)$, where S is the concentration of dopaminergic agonist, K is the ED₅₀ value of dopamine or DHE for inhibition of prolactin release, and IC₅₀ is the concentration of the agent giving 50% reversal of the inhibitory action of dopamine or DHE. For the effects of agonists and antagonists on [³H]DHE binding, K_D values were calculated according to the equation $K_D = IC_{50}/(1 + S/K)$. In this equation, S = the concentration of labeled ligand present in the assay mixture, K = the apparent K_D of [³H]DHEC for the binding sites as estimated by equilibrium or kinetic analysis (2.2 nM was used). IC₅₀ is the concentration of an agent giving 50% competition of specific binding. Relative potencies for agonists and antagonists were calculated in reference to dopamine: K_D of dopamine/K_D of agent × 100. Thus arbitrarily dopamine was chosen as having a relative potency of 100.

[a] When tested these antagonists were found also to have agonistic activity as judged by their ability to inhibit prolactin release. The following K_D values were obtained: haloperidol (> 10,000 nM), pimozide (27 nM), cyproheptadine (500 nM), and methysergide (> 10,000 nM). K_D values for antagonist activity of these agents were calculated from the concentrations giving 50% reversal of inhibition of prolactin release by an agent. At these concentrations pimozide, cyproheptadine, and methysergide had significant agonist activity and did not reverse the dopaminergic inhibition of prolactin completely. Note that not all antagonists were tested for agonist activity.

Effect of Ergot Alkaloids

Ergot alkaloids, which are thought to act mainly through a dopaminergic mechanism on prolactin secretion *in vivo* (17), were tested for their potency in this *in vitro* system. It can be seen in Fig. 2 that dihydroergocornine (DHE) and dihydroergocryptine (DHEC) had approximately the same potency in inhibiting prolactin release. In fact, they were about 100 times more potent than DA, the ED_{50} values of DHEC and DHE being 0.2 and 0.4 nM, respectively. Ergocryptine was highly potent at an ED_{50} value of 0.2 nM (Table 1). 2-Bromo-α-ergocryptine (CB-154), a compound used as inhibitor of prolactin secretion in hyperprolactinemia in humans (25,80), was also tested. It was somewhat less potent, with an ED_{50} value of 2.9 nM. As illustrated in Fig. 2, high concentrations of ergot alkaloids led to the same maximal inhibition of prolactin release (80 to 90%) as obtained with high concentrations of catecholamines (Fig. 1).

It is of interest to mention on Fig. 2 that [³H]DHEC, the tracer used to study characteristics of the adenohypophysial putative dopaminergic recep-

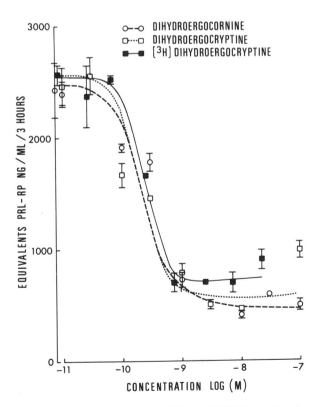

FIG. 2. Effect of increasing concentrations of DHE, DHEC, and [³H]DHEC on the release of prolactin in anterior pituitary cells in primary culture. Cells in monolayer culture were incubated for 3 hr in the presence of the indicated drug concentrations.

tor, inhibited prolactin release with a potency identical to that of the un-labeled material, thus indicating that the labeled compound used had a biological activity similar to the authentic DHEC.

Assessment of DA Antagonistic Activity

To study further the specificity of the dopaminergic control of prolactin release, we took advantage of the precision of the *in vitro* system to examine the ability of various dopaminergic antagonists and their enantiomers to reverse the inhibition of prolactin release induced by DHE (3 nM) or DA (50 nM). As previously observed (Fig. 2), 3 nM DHE decreased basal prolactin release by more than 75% (Fig. 3). This inhibitory action of 3 nM DHE could be progressively and completely reversed by the addition of increasing concentrations of the potent neuroleptic (+)butaclamol ($K_D = 0.3$ nM) whereas its clinically inactive enantiomer (−)butaclamol had only slight activity at 10 μM (Fig. 3).

In agreement with their relative dopaminergic-blocking activities in pharmacological tests, α-flupenthixol was approximately 100-fold more potent than β-flupenthixol to reverse the DHE-induced inhibition of PRL release (Fig. 3) whereas *cis*-thiothixene was more active than *trans*-thiothixene by about an order of magnitude (Fig. 3). Almost identical results were obtained when 50 nM DA was used to inhibit PRL release (data not shown).

Assessment of Mixed DA Agonistic-Antagonistic Activity

When assayed in the presence of 3 nM DHE, the classic DA antagonist haloperidol led to a complete reversal of the inhibitory effect of the ergot alkaloid at a relatively low concentration ($K_D = 0.7$ nM) (Fig. 4A). However, at concentrations above 1 μM, haloperidol caused a decrease of prolactin release characteristic of a DA agonistic activity (40% inhibition at 10 μM). This weak DA agonistic activity of haloperidol was confirmed when the neuroleptic was tested alone, a 45% inhibition of PRL release being measured at 10 μM haloperidol.

As illustrated in Fig. 4B, pimozide, so far classified as a DA antagonist, is also a fairly potent DA agonist. In fact, when pimozide was present alone, it inhibited prolactin release at a potency similar ($ED_{50} = 25$ nM) to that of DA itself (35 nM), thus suggesting that pimozide may act as a relatively potent DA agonist. At low concentrations, pimozide could, however, reverse by about 75% the inhibitory effect of 3 nM DHE, thus indicating the DA antagonistic properties of the compound. However, at concentrations above 10 nM, the agonistic properties of pimozide become predominant and a progressive decrease of prolactin release was observed.

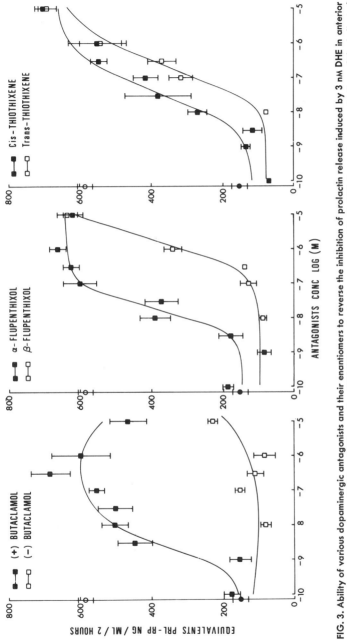

FIG. 3. Ability of various dopaminergic antagonists and their enantiomers to reverse the inhibition of prolactin release induced by 3 nM DHE in anterior pituitary cells in primary culture. (○) Basal PRL secretion. (●) PRL secretion in the presence of 3 nM DHE. Increasing concentrations of the indicated compounds were tested in the presence of 3 nM DHE during a 2-hr incubation.

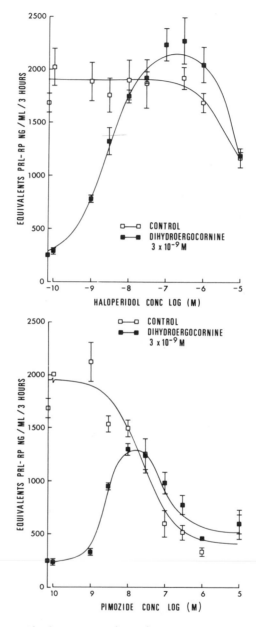

FIG. 4. Effects of haloperidol (top) and pimozide (bottom) on prolactin secretion in anterior pituitary cells in monolayer culture. The effects of increasing concentrations of haloperidol or pimozide on prolactin release were tested alone (measurement of DA agonistic activity; *open symbols*) or in the presence of 3 nM DHE (measurement of DA antagonistic activity; *closed symbols*) during a 3-hr incubation.

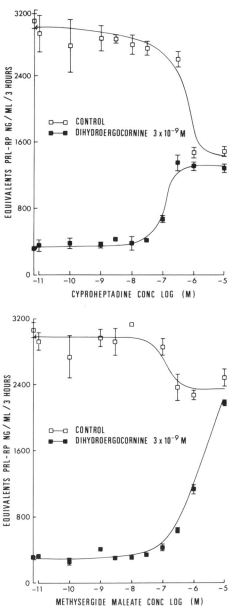

FIG. 5. Effect of the putative serotonergic agents cyproheptadine (top) and methysergide (bottom) on the release of prolactin from anterior pituitary cells in primary culture. The assay was as described in Fig. 4: effect of the agent alone as inhibitor of prolactin release (measurement of DA agonistic activity; *open symbols*) or in the presence of 3 nM DHE for its ability to reverse the inhibitory effect of the ergot alkaloid on prolactin release (measurement of DA antagonistic activity; *closed symbols*).

Effects of Serotonergic Agents

In view of the reported stimulatory action of serotonergic agents in the control of PRL secretion *in vivo* (46,47), it was of interest to study the effect of putative serotonergic agents at the pituitary level on prolactin release. As shown in Fig. 5, the putative serotonergic antagonists cyproheptadine and methysergide showed weak prolactin release-inhibiting activity. In addition, both compounds, at concentrations higher than 100 nM, partially reversed the inhibition of prolactin release induced by 3 nM DHE. These data indicate that both compounds can act as partial DA agonists and antagonists on prolactin secretion at the level of the anterior pituitary gland.

Other compounds were tested for their effects on prolactin release. Thus phenothiazines (e.g., fluphenazine and chlorpromazine) were able to reverse the inhibition of prolactin release caused by 3 nM DHE (Table 1).

Discussion

The present data demonstrate clearly that the order of potency of various inhibitors of prolactin release in anterior pituitary cells in culture (apomorphine > DA > epinephrine ≥ norepinephrine >> isoproterenol = phenylephrine) is typical of a dopaminergic process. Many previous investigations performed *in vitro* using intact pituitaries (38,45,52,56,58, 66,73) and *in vivo* (7,27,28,51,78) have clearly shown a direct inhibitory effect of DA on prolactin release at the anterior pituitary level. The present experiments performed in cells in culture extend these observations and demonstrate the specificity of the dopaminergic action.

The high degree of stereoselectivity of the prolactin response is well illustrated by the relative potencies of the neuroleptics (+)- and (−) butaclamol, α- and β-flupenthixol and *cis*- and *trans*-thiothixene (Fig. 3). The stereospecificity of dopamine action is also well demonstrated by the finding that (−)epinephrine and (−)norepinephrine are approximately eight times more potent inhibitors of prolactin release than the (+)enantiomers (Table 1). The high degree of precision of the system used permitted the somewhat unexpected findings that compounds so far classified as DA antagonists, haloperidol and pimozide (2,57), do in fact have mixed agonist-antagonist properties (Fig. 4). The inhibitory effect of high concentrations of haloperidol are, however, in agreement with previous *in vitro* findings (54,66).

The findings (Fig. 5) of a direct action of the serotonergic antagonists methysergide and cyproheptadine at the anterior pituitary level on prolactin release could offer an explanation for the *in vivo* observations of a stimulation of plasma prolactin levels after administration of these compounds (46, 47). The present data clearly demonstrate that the control of prolactin release, as assessed by the specificity of action of a large variety of compounds of known pharmacological potency, is a typically dopaminergic process.

CHARACTERISTICS OF THE PITUITARY
DOPAMINE RECEPTOR

Attempts to correlate binding to the dopaminergic receptor with a physiological or biochemical response have been less successful than with α- and β-adrenergic receptors. In the brain, where most dopaminergic binding studies have been performed (11,12,20,71), dopamine receptors appear to be coupled to adenylate cyclase (37,40,44). However, the potency of dopaminergic antagonists to inhibit dopamine-sensitive adenylate cyclase activity did not always correlate well with the ability of all classes of compounds to compete with [³H]haloperidol or [³H]dopamine binding (9,11,18, 21,39,43,60).

Since agents have been shown to modulate prolactin secretion by a direct action at the anterior pituitary level *in vivo* and *in vitro* (28,58,79), and we recently studied the specificity of action of a series of dopaminergic agonists and antagonists on prolactin secretion in adenohypophysial cells in culture, it seemed important to study properties of the putative dopamine receptor in the anterior pituitary gland.

Our original goal was to study control of prolactin secretion and binding of a specific dopaminergic ligand in the rat anterior pituitary system. In preliminary experiments, we were able to demonstrate binding of [³H]DHEC to rat anterior pituitary membranes or whole cells in culture that appears to possess features of dopaminergic specificity. However, due to the very small amount of membrane protein that can be derived from rat anterior pituitary, the relatively low concentration of receptors in these preparations, and the modest specific activity of the labeled ligand, it was felt that the bovine anterior pituitary would be a preferable tissue to carry out such detailed studies of binding to dopaminergic receptors.

Equilibrium Studies of [³H]DHEC Binding to Anterior Pituitary Membranes

As shown in Fig. 6A, specific binding of [³H]DHEC increased with increasing concentrations of free [³H]DHEC and was saturable. Nonspecific binding increased linearly from 20 to 25% of total binding at low concentrations of ligand ($\sim$5 nM) to reach $\sim$75% of total binding at the highest concentrations used. Represented in Fig. 6B are data of specific binding plotted according to Scatchard (70). Since the Scatchard plot yielded a straight line (69), these results are consistent with there being a single class of [³H]DHEC binding sites. As calculated from the slope of the line, a K_D value of 2.2 ± 0.6 nM was obtained from the pooled data of five experiments. In these experiments, a mean saturation value of 0.32 ± 0.02 pmole/mg protein was obtained.

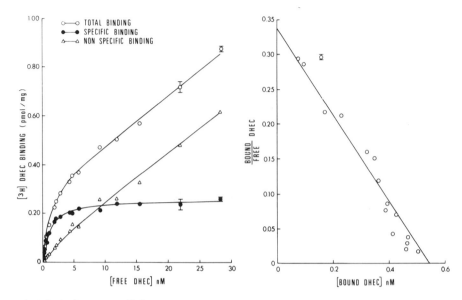

FIG. 6. (A: left): Binding of [³H]DHEC to bovine anterior pituitary membranes as a function of increasing concentrations of ligand. Membrane preparations were incubated with increasing concentrations of [³H]DHEC (0.35 to 30 nM) for 180 min. A longer incubation period was chosen to ensure that binding at low ligand concentrations had reached equilibrium. Specific binding (●) was calculated from the difference between total and nonspecific [10 μM (+)butaclamol] binding. Saturation binding was 0.32 ± 0.02 pmole/mg (N = 5 experiments). (B: right): Scatchard plot of [³H]DHEC binding. Results from the experiment shown in A are plotted here. An apparent dissociation constant (K_D) of 1.6 nM was obtained in this experiment. A mean apparent K_D value of 2.2 ± 0.6 nM was obtained from five such experiments. Results shown in A and B are means ± SEM of triplicate determinations from a representative experiment. Data where no bracket is shown indicate that the SEM was smaller than the symbol used.

Specificity and Affinity of Interaction of Dopaminergic and Other Agents With [³H]DHEC Binding Sites

Binding of [³H]DHEC to bovine anterior pituitary membranes displayed a specificity typical of a dopaminergic process. As shown in Fig. 7, agonists competed for [³H]DHEC binding with the following order of potency: apomorphine > dopamine > epinephrine ≥ norepinephrine >> isoproterenol = clonidine. This relative order of potency closely resembles the potency of these agonists in inhibiting prolactin secretion from rat anterior pituitary (Fig. 1), in stimulating the dopamine-sensitive adenylate cyclase (40,44), and in competing for [³H]haloperidol (11,71), [³H]dopamine (11,27,37,44, 71), and [³H]apomorphine binding (72) in brain tissue.

Ergot alkaloids which act as potent dopaminergic agonists on prolactin secretion (35) are also potent competitors of [³H]DHEC binding. These ergot compounds did in fact compete for binding with a potency which

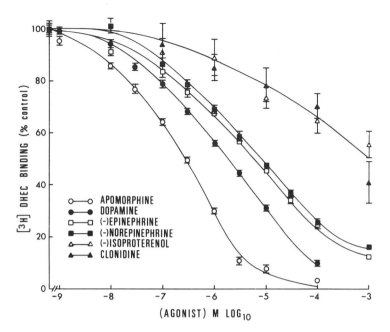

FIG. 7. Competition of various agonists for [³H]DHEC binding to bovine anterior pituitary membranes. Membranes were pretreated at 25°C for 10 min with 0.1% ascorbic acid and 10 μM pargyline. Control specific binding (100%) was 0.185 ± 0.009 pmole/mg (N = 3). Results shown are means ± SEM of three experiments determined in triplicate.

closely parallels their inhibitory effect on prolactin release in anterior pituitary cells in culture (data not shown).

[³H]DHEC binding sites in bovine anterior pituitary displayed marked stereoselectivity toward various neuroleptics and their isomers. Thus (+)butaclamol, which possesses potent pharmacological dopamine-blocking activity (44), was more than 10,000 times more effective than its inactive (−)isomer in competing for binding (Fig. 8). Accordingly, we have taken as specific binding to the dopamine receptor sites in these pituitary preparations the amount of [³H]DHEC binding displaceable by 1 to 10 μM (+)butaclamol. Also, as apparent from Fig. 4, agonists such as apomorphine, dopamine, and the various ergot alkaloids competed for binding of [³H]DHEC to the same extent as (+)butaclamol, thus suggesting that these compounds interact with the same sites.

Figure 8 also shows that [³H]DHEC binding sites exhibit marked stereoselectivity toward other thioxanthene derivatives. α-Flupenthixol inhibited binding more potently (1,000 times) than its geometrical isomer β-flupenthixol. Similarly, *cis*-thiothixene competed for binding more potently (75 to 100 times) than *trans*-thiothixene. The characteristics of interaction of these

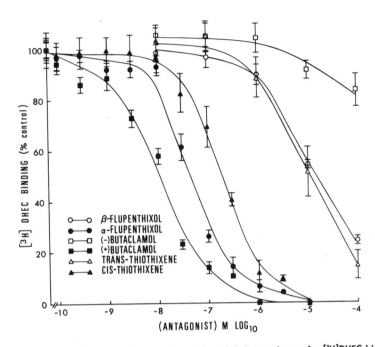

FIG. 8. Competition of various dopaminergic antagonists and their enantiomers for [³H]DHEC binding to bovine anterior pituitary membranes. [³H]DHEC (14.1 nM) binding was determined in the presence and absence of various concentrations of these agents. Control binding was 0.234 ± 0.005 pmole/mg. Results shown are means of triplicate determinations, and this experiment is representative of two.

neuroleptics with these binding sites correlate well with their ability to reverse the dopaminergic inhibition of prolactin release (Fig. 2) and their dopamine-blocking activity in pharmacological tests (61,65,82).

Various other compounds that possess dopamine antagonist activity *in vivo* were tested for their ability to compete for [³H]DHEC binding. Haloperidol reduced specific [³H]DHEC binding with high affinity to about the same extent as (+)butaclamol (Table 1). Pimozide and chlorpromazine also competed for binding with relatively high affinity, whereas clozapine inhibited binding with somewhat lower potency. The α-adrenergic antagonist phentolamine was a relatively weak competitor of [³H]DHEC binding in pituitary membranes with a half-maximal effect at about 10 μM in the presence of 12 nM labeled ligand. Propranolol, a selective β-adrenergic antagonist, did not compete for binding below 100 μM. These data further support the contention that [³H]DHEC interacts with specific dopaminergic sites in pituitary membranes.

Since putative antiserotonergic agents have been found to stimulate prolactin secretion *in vivo* (46), we examined the ability of serotonin and two serotonergic antagonists, methysergide and cyproheptadine, to compete for binding. Serotonin was a very weak competitor, whereas cyproheptadine and methysergide inhibited 50% of binding at 1 and 3 μM, respectively (Table 1). The very weak activity of serotonin is consistent with its negligible effects on prolactin secretion in rat pituitary cells in culture (Table 1). The potency of the two serotonergic antagonists [1/100 that of (+)butaclamol] was comparable to their ability to antagonize the dopaminergic inhibition of prolactin secretion and to compete for [³H]haloperidol binding sites in brain (11).

Several catecholamine analogs, precursors, and metabolites were tested for their ability to compete for binding. Ephedrine, L-DOPA, α-methyl-DOPA, and ($\pm$)dihydroxymandelic acid did not interact significantly with the binding sites below 100 μM. Normetanephrine inhibited binding by 50% at 100 μM. Various other agents having a presumable influence on dopaminergic systems *in vivo* have been screened for possible interactions with the receptor sites. None of the following drugs tested had any effect at 10 to 100 μM: morphine, β-endorphin, thyrotropin-releasing hormone, triiodothyronine, α-melanocyte-stimulating hormone, 17β-estradiol, 5α-dihydrotestosterone, substance P, neurotensin, somatostatin, and γ-aminobutyric acid.

Correlation of [³H]DHEC Binding to Bovine Anterior Pituitary Membranes and the Dopaminergic Inhibition of Prolactin Release from Rat Anterior Pituitary Cells in Culture

Table 1 lists the calculated K_D values of various compounds and their relative ability to compete for [³H]DHEC binding to bovine anterior pituitary membranes. When a comparison is made with their ability to inhibit or antagonize the dopaminergic inhibition of prolactin secretion in rat anterior pituitary cells in culture, it can be seen that a close correlation exists between the relative potencies of these agents as modulators of prolactin release (agonists or antagonists) and competitors of [³H]DHEC binding in bovine pituitary membrane preparations.

Discussion

Ergot alkaloids are known to interact with a variety of drug receptors including α-adrenergic, serotonergic, and dopaminergic receptors. [³H]DHEC has proved to be a useful ligand for studying α-adrenergic receptor binding sites in membranes derived from uterine smooth muscle (49,83), parotid acinar cells (76), and human platelets (62). In membranes from brain, binding of the ligand is more complex, appearing to label more than one type of receptor site (23). However, in membrane preparations from specific parts of the brain, under appropriate assay conditions, the α-adrenergic receptors can be exclusively labeled with [³H]DHEC (36). A recent report suggested that [³H]dihydroergotamine may label serotonergic sites in brain (19).

The present study indicates that in anterior pituitary membranes, where α-adrenergic receptors cannot be detected by present methodology, [³H]DHEC appears to label dopaminergic sites selectively and exclusively. In the anterior pituitary system, haloperidol and (+)butaclamol have been found to be, respectively, 300 and 2,500 times more potent in competing for [³H]DHEC binding than the α-adrenergic antagonist phentolamine, whereas in α-adrenergic systems the reverse situation is observed. Similarly, whereas apomorphine and dopamine are more potent than epinephrine and norepinephrine in competing for binding in this system, epinephrine and norepinephrine were the more potent agonists in α-adrenergic systems (83). As summarized in Table 1, the order of potency of a large variety of drugs to displace [³H]DHEC binding in adenohypophysial membranes closely parallels their ability to compete for [³H]dopamine (11,37,71) and [³H]apomorphine (72) binding in rat brain. Moreover, the specificity of binding is essentially identical to that of the dopaminergic response of whole pituitary cells, i.e., inhibition of prolactin secretion.

As expected of a dopaminergic receptor, the interaction of various neuroleptics with the [³H]DHEC binding sites was stereoselective. Thus (+)butaclamol, α-flupenthixol, and *cis*-thiothixene competed for binding with high potencies, whereas their corresponding pharmacologically and clinically inactive or less active enantiomers (−)butaclamol, β-flupenthixol, and *trans*-thiothixene were much less effective in competing for binding (Fig. 7; Table 1). The interaction of agonists with the sites also displayed stereoselectivity. (−)Isomers of epinephrine and norepinephrine were more potent competitors of binding than their respective (+)isomers. This stereoselective interaction of both agonists and the neuroleptic antagonists with the pituitary receptors was also reflected in their ability to modulate prolactin secretion in rat anterior pituitary cells. Similarly, ergo alkaloids and phenothiazines competed for binding in parallel to their ability to affect prolactin secretion.

Estimation of the dissociation constant (K_D) of [³H]DHEC for the sites (0.6 nM) by analysis of binding kinetics is in reasonable agreement with that observed by equilibrium binding analysis (2.2 nM). These equilibrium studies also indicate the presence of a finite number of sites in these membranes (0.32 pmole/mg). This mean saturation binding value is of the same order as those found for other dopaminergic ligands in brain tissues (2,12,48).

Somewhat surprisingly, compounds such as cyproheptadine and methysergide with presumed serotonergic specificity were found to interact with [³H]DHEC binding sites. This is probably due to a lack of specificity of these compounds, since in parallel to their interaction with the binding sites they were found to modulate prolactin secretion (29). It is thus possible that the stimulatory effect of these agents on prolactin secretion *in vivo* (28,60) is mediated by the dopaminergic receptors at the anterior pituitary level.

Dissociation constant (K_D) values for all agents calculated from their effects on prolactin release (29) were somewhat lower than those calculated for their interaction with the [³H]DHEC binding sites (2- to 20-fold). These differences could possibly be due to differences in the two species used in these studies. They might also be due to the use of high concentrations of proteins in our binding assays.

Previous studies of dopaminergic receptors in membranes derived from brain have utilized either the antagonist [³H]haloperidol (11,12,37,44,71) or the agonists [³H]dopamine (11,12,71) and [³H]apomorphine (72). As noted above, in no previous study has it been possible to observe a correlation of binding to putative dopaminergic receptors with a specific dopaminergic biological response as was done in the present investigation. Marked differences have been observed in the relative affinities of dopaminergic agonists and antagonists for [³H]haloperidol versus [³H]dopamine binding sites in brain membranes (41). Dopaminergic antagonists are relatively more potent in competing for [³H]haloperidol, whereas agonists are more potent toward [³H]dopamine binding. It has therefore been proposed that the two ligands label, respectively, "antagonist" and "agonist" states of the dopamine receptors (11).

Data presented in this study are of particular interest with regard to this model. As shown in the previous section, DHEC behaves as a full agonist, causing the same maximum inhibition of prolactin secretion as dopamine. Nonetheless, the pattern of [³H]DHEC binding in pituitary membranes has some characteristics of antagonist binding. However, the differences in affinity of agonists and antagonists are not as pronounced as those observed with [³H]haloperidol and [³H]dopamine in brain membranes (72).

Several reports have previously presented supportive evidence that specific dopamine receptors might be present in pituitary (10,14,22,53,55). However, the studies reported here represent the first direct study and characterization of these binding sites in anterior pituitary. The close correlation observed between the properties of [³H]DHEC binding sites with those of the dopaminergic inhibition of prolactin release strongly suggest that these sites correspond to the physiologically relevant dopamine receptors which regulate prolactin secretion.

The present data indicate that the anterior pituitary gland, besides its own intrinsic interest, should represent a useful model for detailed study of the mechanisms of dopaminergic action. In fact, changes of [³H]DHEC binding to the dopaminergic receptor can be correlated with an easily accessible and highly precise parameter of biological activity: prolactin release in cells in culture. Such a model of dopamine action has not been previously available and should be useful for a better understanding of the mechanisms controlling dopamine receptor-mediated actions.

POTENT ANTIDOPAMINERGIC ACTIVITY OF ESTRADIOL AT THE PITUITARY LEVEL

Effects of Estrogens in Pituitary Cells in Culture

It is well known that estrogens are potent stimulators of prolactin secretion in man (34) and rats (15,24). Moreover, the increased rate of prolactin secretion on the afternoon of proestrus in the rat is presumably under estrogenic influence (42,63). These *in vivo* effects of estrogens could, however, be exerted at the hypothalamic and/or pituitary level(s).

Since anterior pituitary cells in culture proved to be an excellent system to study the specificity of action of sex steroids at the anterior pituitary

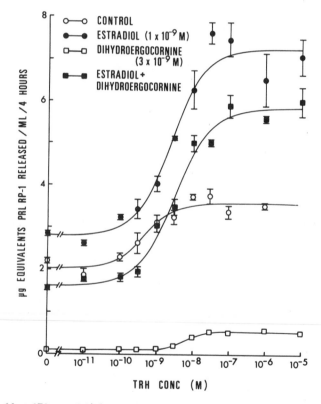

FIG. 9. Effect of 1 nM 17β-estradiol (E₂), 3 nM DHE, E₂ + DHE, or the vehicle alone (control) on the prolactin response to increasing concentrations of TRH in female rat anterior pituitary cells in primary culture. Cells were preincubated for 120 hr in the presence or absence of E₂ before a 4-hr incubation in the presence or absence of the dopamine agonist DHE and the indicated concentrations of TRH. Data are expressed as mean ± SEM of duplicate measurements of triplicate Petri dishes. Note that E₂ led to an almost complete reversal of the inhibitory effect of DHE on prolactin release.

level (29), we used this system, instead of intact pituitaries, to study the interactions of 17β-estradiol and dopamine on prolactin release. The present data show that 17β-estradiol stimulates basal as well as TRH-induced prolactin release by a direct action at the pituitary level. Moreover, somewhat unexpectedly, 17β-estradiol led to an almost complete reversal of the dopamine-induced inhibition of prolactin release.

As illustrated in Fig. 9, TRH led to a maximal 50% increase of prolactin release in anterior pituitary cells in culture at an ED_{50} value of $4.8 \pm 1.8 \times 10^{-10}$ M. It can also be seen that at a concentration of 3×10^{-9} M, the dopamine agonist dihydroergocornine (DHE) led to a 90 to 95% inhibition of basal and TRH-induced prolactin release. In fact, basal prolactin release in the presence of DHE alone was 78 ± 1 ng equivalents PRL-RP-1/ml/4 hr, and addition of E_2 to DHE increased prolactin release to $1,551 \pm 7$ ng. The maximal prolactin responses to high concentrations of TRH was 519 ± 11 and $5,855 \pm 100$ ng in the corresponding groups.

A more detailed analysis of the antagonism between E_2 and dopaminergic action on prolactin release is presented in Fig. 10. It can be seen that whereas the potent dopamine agonist RU24213 led to a 80 to 85% inhibition of spontaneous prolactin release in the absence of E_2 (Fig. 10A), the maximal

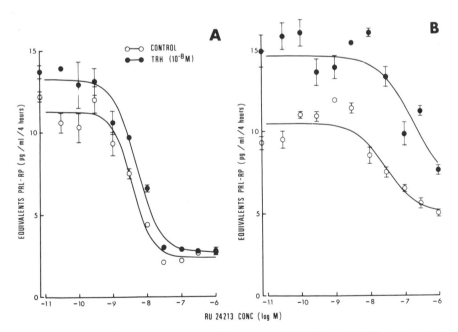

FIG. 10. Effect of TRH (10 nM), in the presence (B) or absence (A) of 17β-estradiol (E_2), on the prolactin response to increasing concentrations of the dopamine agonist RU24213 in female rat anterior pituitary cells in primary culture. Cells were preincubated for 120 hr in the presence or absence of TRH and the indicated concentrations of RU 24213. Note that the inhibitory effect of the dopamine agonist RU 24213 on prolactin release was more than 50% reversed by E_2 pretreatment.

inhibition was reduced to 40 to 45% in cells preincubated with E_2 (Fig. 10B). It can also be noted that 1×10^{-8} M TRH did not significantly affect the RU24213 ED_{50} value of inhibition of prolactin release in the presence or absence of E_2 pretreatment. Exposure to the estrogen did, however, lead to a significant increase of the RU24213 ED_{50} value ($p < 0.01$) as reflected by the higher concentrations of the dopamine agonist required to inhibit prolactin release after exposure to estrogens.

Implantation studies had already suggested an action of estrogens at the pituitary level on prolactin secretion (42). The present data clearly demonstrate a direct pituitary site of action of estradiol on prolactin secretion and extend previous information obtained with pituitary explants (63).

Antidopaminergic Effect of Estrogens at the Pituitary Level In Vivo

Following our *in vitro* data showing a potent antidopaminergic effect of estrogens on prolactin secretion, it then became of interest to investigate if such a potent activity of estrogens also occurs under *in vivo* conditions. The

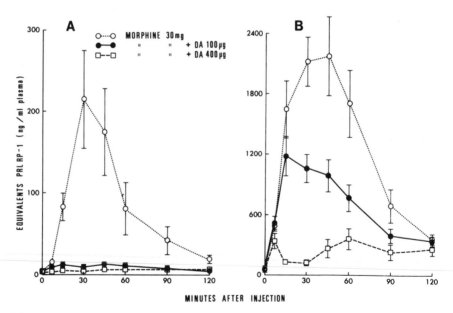

MINUTES AFTER INJECTION

FIG. 11. Effect of estrogens treatment on the inhibitory effect of dopamine on prolactin release in the female rat. Adult Sprague-Dawley female rats ovariectomized 2 weeks previously were injected with estradiol benzoate (10 μg s.c. twice a day) for 7 days or the vehicle alone (0.2 ml 1% gelatin in 0.9% NaCl) before insertion of a catheter into the right superior vena cava under anesthesia (Surital, 50 mg/kg body weight, i.p.). Two days later, undisturbed, freely moving animals were injected with morphine sulfate (30 mg s.c.) alone or in combination with dopamine (100 or 400 μg). Blood samples (0.7 ml) were then withdrawn at the indicated time intervals for measurement of plasma prolactin concentration by double-antibody radioimmunoassay as described using materials kindly provided by NIAMDD. Data are expressed as mean ± SEM of duplicate determinations of samples obtained from 8 to 10 animals per group.

present study was facilitated by our recent findings that the endogenous inhibitory dopaminergic influence on prolactin secretion can be eliminated by administration of opiates, thus making possible study of the effect of exogenous dopaminergic agents without interference by endogenous dopamine.

As illustrated in Fig. 11A, the subcutaneous administration of 100 or 400 μg dopamine completely prevented the increased plasma prolactin levels following morphine injection in rats ovariectomized 2 weeks previously. Treatment with estradiol benzoate (20 μg/day) for 7 days led to stimulation of basal plasma prolactin levels (from 14 ± 1 to 56 ± 8 ng/ml) and to a marked increase of the maximal plasma prolactin response to morphine from 215 ± 60 to $2,175 \pm 390$ ng/ml. The most interesting finding, however, is that the 100- and 400-μg doses of dopamine, which could maintain plasma prolactin levels at undetectable levels after morphine injection in control rats, led only to 40% and 85% inhibition of prolactin levels, respectively, in animals treated with estrogens (Fig. 11B).

A similar potent antidopaminergic activity of estrogens was obtained in male animals. In fact, whereas 50 and 250 μg dopamine led to, respectively, 75% and 90% inhibition of the morphine-induced rise of plasma prolactin levels in control orchidectomized animals, the same doses of dopamine led only to 25% and 65% inhibition of plasma prolactin levels in animals treated with estrogens (data not shown).

Discussion

The present findings of a potent antagonistic effect of E_2 on the action of dopamine agonists may well explain the observation of a much lower decrease of prolactin release by L-DOPA injection in normal than in stalk-sectioned female monkeys (26). Since the stalk had been cut 8 weeks previously, these animals were likely to be under low estrogenic stimulation. The antagonistic effect of E_2 on dopaminergic action may be also responsible, to an unknown extent, for the observation that apomorphine inhibited prolactin secretion to a greater degree and for a longer period (14 days) than after destruction of the medial basal hypothalamus as compared to one day (16).

The present data clearly demonstrate that estrogens, which were previously shown to have potent antidopaminergic activity on prolactin secretion in anterior pituitary cells in culture (67), can exert similar effects *in vivo,* the effect being qualitatively similar in female and male animals. As reflected by an increase of the ED_{50} value of dopamine agonists, the *in vitro* effect of estrogens was due to a decreased sensitivity to dopaminergic agents. Since the effect of estrogens occurs predominantly at low doses of dopamine, the *in vivo* antidopaminergic activity of estrogens is also apparently due to a decreased sensitivity of prolactin release to dopamine action at the anterior pituitary level. Such findings indicate that higher concentrations of dopamine in the hypothalamo-hypophysial portal blood system are likely to be required to inhibit prolactin secretion under conditions of high estrogenic influence. The almost complete reversal of the inhibitory effect of low doses of dopamine by estrogen treatment clearly indicates an important interaction between estrogens and dopamine at the adenohypophysial level (Fig. 12).

As mentioned earlier, dopamine appears to be the main factor of hypothalamic origin involved in the control of prolactin secretion (47,57). Moreover, using the dopamine agonist [³H]DHEC as tracer and measurement of prolactin release in pituitary cells in culture, we found that the characteristics of binding to the pituitary receptor and the control of prolactin secretion are typically dopaminergic (67).

The role of dopamine in various brain functions has become increasingly evident during recent years (1,4). Moreover, malfunction of dopaminergic systems can lead to neurological and psychiatric diseases (74,75). It is thus hoped that knowledge gained about the pituitary dopaminergic system, where the effects (changes of prolactin secretion) can be measured with a high degree of precision, can help our understanding of less accessible dopa-

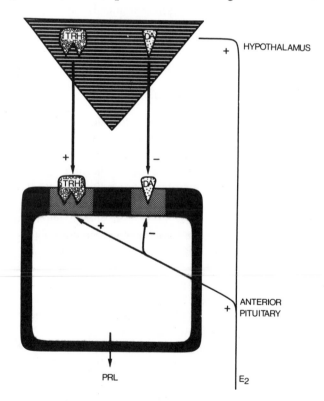

FIG. 12. Interaction between estrogens, dopamine, and TRH in the control of prolactin secretion at the anterior pituitary level. The stimulatory effect of estrogens on prolactin secretion appears to be exerted mainly through blockade of the inhibitory action of the dopaminergic receptor.

minergic systems in the central nervous system. It is of great interest that treatment with estrogens was recently found to inhibit the action of dopaminergic agents on circling behavior in rats bearing a unilateral lesion of the nigrostriatal dopaminergic pathways (3) and on striatal acetylcholine accumulation in the rat (33). Moreover, symptoms of tardive dyskinesia following chronic treatment with neuroleptics have been found to be improved by estrogen treatment in the human (81).

It should be mentioned that the present data, which clearly establish a direct antidopaminergic effect of estrogens at the pituitary level, also suggest a hypothalamic site of estrogen action. The higher stimulation of prolactin release by morphine in female than male animals and the marked increase of the prolactin response following estrogen treatment in animals of both sexes indicate an increased dopaminergic tone under the influence of estrogens. Such an interpretation is in agreement with the findings of increased dopamine turnover in the external layer of the median eminence after estrogen treatment (32,50). The potent antidopaminergic action of estrogens at the pituitary level, however, is predominant over that at the hypothalamic level and results in increased prolactin secretion under all conditions of high estrogenic influence.

SUMMARY

Since dopamine appears to be the main or even the only inhibitory substance of hypothalamic origin involved in the control of prolactin secretion, we took advantage of the pituitary cell culture system to study the specificity of control of prolactin secretion. It could be clearly demonstrated that the order of potency of various inhibitors of prolactin release in anterior pituitary cells in culture is typical of a dopaminergic process. Moreover, using a stable tracer, [^{3}H]DHEC, it was demonstrated that the pituitary receptor has binding characteristics almost superimposable to the specificity of action of a large variety of compounds on prolactin release, thus supporting the role of dopamine as physiological modulator of prolactin secretion. The high degree of precision of the pituitary system has permitted the somewhat unexpected finding that compounds so far classified as dopamine antagonists (e.g., pimozide and haloperidol) or serotonergic antagonists (e.g., methysergide and cyproheptadine) do in fact have mixed agonist-antagonist properties that could lead to a different interpretation of their reported *in vivo* actions. We next studied the possible interaction of estrogens and dopamine in the control of prolactin secretion. It was found that 17β-estradiol stimulates basal as well as TRH-induced prolactin release by a direct action at the anterior pituitary level. Moreover, somewhat unexpectedly, 17β-estradiol led to an almost complete reversal of the dopamine-induced inhibition of prolactin release. *In vivo* experiments performed in the rat confirmed the potent antidopaminergic action of estrogens at the pituitary level. In fact, the inhibitory effect of intravenously injected dopamine on prolactin secretion could be markedly inhibited by treatment with estrogens. Since dopamine receptors are not only involved with prolactin secretion but appear to play a major role in the modulation of mood and behavior and in some diseases, the control of prolactin secretion, besides its inherent interest, could well serve as a model system for studying the interaction of peripheral hormones with dopaminergic action. Moreover, the pituitary cell system appears to be the most precise screening test for potential dopaminergic and antidopaminergic drugs to be used in Parkinson's disease and schizophrenia, respectively.

REFERENCES

1. Andèn, N. E. (1972): Dopamine turnover in the corpus striatum and the limbic system after treatment with neuroleptic and anti-acetylcholine drugs. *J. Pharmacol.,* 24:905–906.
2. Andèn, N. E., Rubenson, A., Fuxe, L., and Hökfelt, T. (1967): Evidence for dopamine receptor stimulation by apomorphine. *J. Pharm. Pharmacol.,* 19:627–629.
3. Bedard, P., Dankova, J., Boucher, R., and Langelier, P. (1978): Effect of estrogens on apomorphine-induced circling behavior in the rat. *Can. J. Physiol. Pharmacol.,* 56:538–541.
4. Beiger, D., Larochelle, L., and Hormykiewicz, O. (1972): A model for the quantitative study of central dopaminergic and serotoninergic activity. *Eur. J. Pharmacol.,* 18:128–136.
5. Ben-Jonathan, N., Oliver, C., Weiner, H. J., Mical, R. S., and Porter, J. C. (1977): Dopamine in hypophyseal portal plasma of the rat during the estrous cycle and throughout pregnancy. *Endocrinology,* 100:452–458.
6. Birge, C. A., Jacobs, L. S., Hammer, C. T., and Daughaday, W. H. (1970): Catecholamine inhibition of prolactin secretion by isolated rat adenohypophysis. *Endocrinology,* 86:120–130.
7. Bishop, W., Fawcett, C. P., Krulich, L., and McCann, S. M. (1972): Acute and chronic effects of hypothalamic lesions on the release of FSH, LH and prolactin in intact and castrated cats. *Endocrinology,* 91:643–656.
8. Bowers, C. Y., Friesen, H. G., Hwang, P., Guyda, H. J., and Folkers, K. (1971): Prolactin and thyrotropin release in man by synthetic pyroglutamyl-histidyl-prolinamide. *Biochem. Biophys. Res. Commun.,* 45:1033–1041.
9. Brown, J. H., and Makman, M. H. (1973): Influence of neuroleptic drugs and apomorphine on dopamine-sensitive adenylate cyclase of retina. *J. Neurochem.,* 21:477–479.
10. Brown, G. M., Seeman, P., and Lee, T. (1976): Dopamine/neuroleptic receptors in basal hypothalamus and pituitary. *Endocrinology,* 99:1407–1410.
11. Burt, D. R., Creese, I., and Snyder, S. H. (1976): Binding interactions of lysergic acid diethylamide and related agents with dopamine receptors in the brain. *J. Mol. Pharmacol.,* 12:631–638.
12. Burt, D. R., Enna, S., Creese, I., and Snyder, S. H. (1975): Dopamine receptor binding in the corpus striatum of mammalian brain. *Proc. Natl. Acad. Sci. USA,* 72:4655–4659.
13. Caron, M. G., Beaulieu, M., Raymond, V., Gagné, B., Drouin, J., Lefkowitz, R. J., and Labrie, F. (1978): Dopamine receptors in the anterior pituitary gland: Correlation of [^{3}H]dihydroergocryptine binding with the dopaminergic control of prolactin release. *J. Biol. Chem.,* 253:2244–2253.
14. Caron, M. G., Raymond, V., Lefkowitz, R. J., and Labrie, F. (1977): Identification of dopaminergic receptors in anterior pituitary: Correlation with the dopaminergic control of prolactin release. *Fed. Proc.,* 36:278.

15. Chen, C. L., and Meites, J. (1970): Effects of estrogen and progesterone on serum and pituitary prolactin levels in ovariectomized rats. *Endocrinology,* 86:503–505.
16. Cheung, C. Y., and Weiner, R. I. (1976): Supersensitivity of anterior pituitary dopamine receptors involved in the inhibition of prolactin secretion following destruction of the medial basal hypothalamus. *Endocrinology,* 99:914–917.
17. Clemens, J. A. (1974): Neuropharmacological aspects of the neural control of prolactin secretion. In: *Hypothalamus and Endocrine Functions,* edited by F. Labrie, J. Meites, and G. Pelletier, pp. 283–301. Plenum Press, New York.
18. Clement-Cormier, Y. C., Kababian, J. W., Petzold, G. L., and Greengard, P. (1974): Dopamine-sensitive adenylate cyclase in mammalian brain: A possible site of action of antipsychotic drugs. *Proc. Natl. Acad. Sci. USA,* 71:1113–1117.
19. Closse, An., and Hauser, D. (1976): Dihydroergotamine binding to rat brain membranes. *Life Sci.,* 19:1851–1864.
20. Creese, I., Burt, D. R., and Snyder, S. H. (1975): Dopamine receptor binding: Differentiation of agonist and antagonist states with ^{3}H-dopamine and ^{3}H-haloperidol. *Life Sci.,* 17:993–1001.
21. Creese, I., Burt, D. R., and Snyder, S. H. (1976): Dopamine receptor binding predicts clinical and pharmacological potencies of antischizophrenic drugs. *Science,* 192:481–483.
22. Cronin, M., Robert, J., and Weiner, R. (1977): Dopamine receptor binding to the anterior pituitary in rat. *Fed. Proc.,* 36:46.
23. Davis, J. N., Strittmatter, W. J., Hoyler, E., and Lefkowitz, R. J. (1977): [^{3}H]Dihydroergocryptine binding in rat brain. *Brain Res.,* 132:327–336.
24. De Léan, A., Garon, M., Kelly, P. A., and Labrie, F. (1977): Changes in pituitary thyrotropin-releasing hormone receptor level and prolactin response to TRH during the rat estrous cycle. *Endocrinology,* 100:1505–1510.
25. Del Poso, E., Varga, L., Scutz, K. D., Künzig, H. J., Marbach, P., Lopez del Campo, D., and Eppenberger, U. (1975): Pituitary and ovarian response patterns to stimulation in the postpartum and in galactorrhea-amenorrhea, the role of prolactin. *Obstet. Gynecol.,* 46:539–543.
26. Diefenbach, W. M. P., Carmel, P. W., Frantz, A. G., and Ferin, M. (1976): Suppression of prolactin secretion by L-DOPA in the stalk-sectioned rhesus monkey. *J. Clin. Endocrinol. Metab.,* 43:638–642.
27. Donoso, A. O., Banzan, A. M., and Barcaglioni, J. C. (1974): Further evidence of the direct action of L-DOPA on prolactin release. *Neuroendocrinology,* 15:236–239.
28. Donoso, A. O., Bishop, W., and McCann, S. M. (1973): The effects of drugs which modify catecholamine synthesis on serum prolactin in rats with median eminence lesions. *Proc. Soc. Exp. Biol. Med.,* 143:360–363.
29. Drouin, J., De Léan, A., Rainville, D., Lachance, R., and Labrie, F. (1976): Characteristics of the interactions between TRH and somatostatin for the thyrotropin and prolactin release. *Endocrinology,* 98:514–521.
30. Drouin, J., and Labrie, F. (1976): Selective effect of androgens on LH and FSH release in anterior pituitary cells in culture. *Endocrinology,* 98:1528–1534.
31. Drouin, J., Lagacé, L., and Labrie, F. (1976): Estradiol-induced increase of the LH responsiveness to LHRH in anterior pituitary cells in culture. *Endocrinology,* 99:1477–1481.
32. Eikenburg, D. C., Ravitz, A. J., Gudelsky, G. A., and Moore, K. E. (1977): Effects of estrogen on prolactin and tuberoinfundibular dopaminergic neurons. *J. Neural. Transm.,* 40:235–244.
33. Euvrard, C., Boissier, J. R., Labrie, F., and Raynaud, J. P. Antidopaminergic activity of estrogens on cholinergic neurons in the rat striatum. In: *Proc. 7th Int. Congr. Pharmacology,* p. 442.
34. Frantz, A. G., Kleinberg, D. L., and Noel, G. L. (1972): Studies on prolactin in man. *Recent Prog. Horm. Res.,* 28:527–590.
35. Fuxe, K., Agnati, L. F., Corrodi, H., Everett, B. J., Hökfelt, T., Lofstrom, A., and Ungerstedt, U. (1975): Action of dopamine receptor agonists in forebrain and hypothalamus, rotational behavior, ovulation and dopamine turnover. *Adv. Neurol.,* 9:223–242.

36. Greenberg, D. A., and Snyder, S. H. (1977): Selective labelling of alpha-noradrenergic receptors in rat brain with [³H]dihydroergocryptine. *Life Sci.,* 20: 927–931.
37. Greengard, P. (1975): Cyclic nucleotides, protein phosphorylation and neuronal function. *Adv. Cyclic Nucleotide Res.,* 5:585–601.
38. Hill, M. K., MacLeod, R. M., and Orcutt, P. (1976): Dibutyryl cyclic AMP, adenosine and guanosine blockage of the dopamine, ergocryptine and apomorphine inhibition of prolactin release in vitro. *Endocrinology,* 99:1612–1617.
39. Iversen, L. L. (1975): Dopamine receptors in the brain. *Science,* 188:1084–1089.
40. Iversen, L. L., Horn, A. S., and Miller, R. J. (1975): In: *Pre- and Postsynaptic Receptors,* edited by E. Usdin and W. E. Bunney, pp. 207–243. Marcel Dekker, New York.
41. Jacobs, L. S., Snyder, P. J., Utiger, R. D., and Daughaday, W. H. (1973): Prolactin response to thyrotropin releasing hormone in normal subjects. *J. Clin. Endocrinol. Metab.,* 36:1069–1075.
42. Kanematsu, S., and Sawyer, C. H. (1963): Effects of intrahypothalamic and intra-hypophysial estrogen implants on pituitary prolactin and lactation in the rabbit. *Endocrinology,* 72:243–252.
43. Karobath, M., and Leitich, H. (1974): Antipsychotic drugs and dopamine stimulated adenylate cyclase prepared from corpus striatum of rat brain. *Proc. Natl. Acad. Sci. USA,* 71:2915–2918.
44. Kebabian, J. W., Petzold, G. L., and Greengard, P. (1973): Dopamine-sensitive adenylate cyclase in caudate nucleus of rat brain and its similarity to the dopamine receptor. *Proc. Natl. Acad. Sci. USA,* 69:2145–2149.
45. Koch, Y., Lu, K. H., and Meites, J. (1970): Biphasic effects of catecholamines on pituitary prolactin release in vitro. *Endocrinology,* 87:673–675.
46. Kordon, C., Blake, C. A., Terkel, J., and Sawyer, C. H. (1973/74): Participation of serotonin-containing neurons in the suckling-induced rise in plasma prolactin levels in lactating rats. *Neuroendocrinology,* 13:213–223.
47. Labrie, F., Beaulieu, M., Caron, M., and Raymond, V. (1978): The adenohypophyseal dopamine receptor: Specificity and modulation of its activity by estradiol. In: *Progress in Prolactin Physiology and Pathology,* edited by C. Robyn and M. Harter. Elsevier-North Holland, Amsterdam, pp. 121–136.
48. Labrie, F., Pelletier, G., Lemay, A., Borgeat, P., Barden, N., Dupont, A., Savary, M., Côté, J., and Boucher, R. (1973): Control of protein synthesis in anterior pituitary gland, In: *Karolinska Symposium on Research Methods in Reproductive Endocrinology,* edited by E. Diczfalusy, pp. 301–340. Geneva.
49. Lefkowitz, R. J., and Williams, L. T. (1976): Alpha-adrenergic receptor identification by [³H]dihydroergocryptine. *Science,* 192:791–793.
50. Lofstrom, A., Eneroth, P., Gustafsson, J. A., and Skett, P. (1977): Effect of estradiol benzoate on catecholamines turnover in discrete area of median eminence and limbic forebrain and on serum luteinizing hormone follicle stimulating hormone and prolactin concentration in ovariectomized female rat. *Endocrinology,* 101:1559–1569.
51. Lu, K. H., and Meites, J. (1972): Effects of L-DOPA on serum prolactin and PIF in intact and hypophysectomized pituitary-grafted rats. *Endocrinology,* 91:868–872.
52. MacLeod, R. M. (1969): Influence of norepinephrine and catecholamine-depleting agents on the synthesis and release of prolactin and growth hormone. *Endocrinology,* 85:916–923.
53. MacLeod, R. M., and Kimura, H. (1975): Dopamine receptors and the regulation of prolactin secretion. *Endocrinology,* 96:94A.
54. MacLeod, R. M. (1976): Regulation of prolactin secretion. In: *Frontiers in Neuroendocrinology,* Vol. 4, edited by L. Martini and W. F. Ganong, pp. 169–194. Raven Press, New York.
55. MacLeod, R. M. (1977): Interaction of the dopaminergic and serotoninergic systems in regulating prolactin secretion. *Fed Proc.,* 36:45.
56. MacLeod, R. M., Fontham, E. H., and Lehmeyer, J. E. (1970): Prolactin and

growth hormone production as influenced by catecholamines and agents that affect brain catecholamines. *Neuroendocrinology,* 6:283–284.

57. MacLeod, R. M., and Lehmeyer, J. E. (1974): Restoration of prolactin synthesis and release by the administration of monoaminergic blocking agents to pituitary tumor-bearing rats. *Cancer Res.,* 34:345–350.

58. MacLeod, R. M., and Lehmeyer, J. E. (1974): Studies on the mechanism of the dopamine-mediated inhibition of prolactin secretion. *Endocrinology,* 94:1077–1085.

59. Meites, J., Nicoll, C. S., and Talwalker, P. K. (1963): The central nervous system and the secretion and release of prolactin. In: *Advances in Neuroendocrinology,* edited by A. V. Nalbandov, pp. 238–288. University of Illinois Press, Urbana, Ill.

60. Miller, R. J., Horn, A. S., and Iversen, L. L. (1974): The action of neuroleptic drugs on dopamine-stimulated adenosine cyclic 3',5'-monophosphate production in rat neostriatum and limbic forebrain. *Mol. Pharmacol.,* 10:759–762.

61. Møller Nielsen, I., Pedersen, V., Nymark, M., Franck, K. F., Boeck, V., Fjalland, B., and Christensen, A. V. (1973): The comparative pharmacology of flupenthixol and some reference: Neuroleptics. *Acta Pharmacol. Toxicol. (Kbh),* 33:353–362.

62. Newman, K. D., Williams, L. T., and Bishopric, N. H. (1978): Identification of alpha-adrenergic receptors in human platelets by [³H]dihydroergocryptine binding. *J. Clin. Invest.,* 61:395–402.

63. Nicoll, C. S., and Meites, J. (1964): Prolactin secretion "in vitro": Effects of gonadal and adrenal cortical steroids. *Proc. Soc. Exp. Biol. Med.,* 117:579–583.

64. Pelletier, G., Lemay, A., Beraud, G., and Labrie, F. (1972): Ultrastructural changes accompanying the stimulatory effect of N⁶-monobutyryl adenosine 3',5'-monophosphate on the release of growth hormone, prolactin, and adrenocorticotropic hormone in rat anterior pituitary gland in vitro. *Endocrinology,* 91:1355–1371.

65. Petersen, P. V., Møller Nielsen, I. M., Petersen, V., Jorgensen, A., and Lanssen, N. (1977): In: *Psychotherapeutic Drugs, Part II: Thioxanthines,* edited by E. Usdin and I. S. Forest, pp. 827–867. Marcel Dekker, New York.

66. Quijada, M., Illner, P., Krulich, L., and McCann, S. M. (1973/74): The effects of catecholamines on hormone release from anterior pituitaries and ventral hypothalamic incubated in vitro. *Neuroendocrinology,* 13:151–163.

67. Raymond, V., Beaulieu, M., Labrie, F., and Boissier, J. R. (1978): Potent antidopaminergic activity of estradiol at the pituitary level on prolactin release. *Science,* 200:1173–1175.

68. Rivier, C., and Vale, W. (1974): In vivo stimulation of prolactin secretion in the rat by thyrotropin-releasing factor, related peptides and hypothalamic extracts. *Endocrinology,* 95:978–983.

69. Rodbard, D. (1973): Mathematics of hormone-receptor interaction. I. Basic principles. *Adv. Exp. Med. Biol.,* 36:289–326.

70. Scatchard, G. (1949): The attractions of proteins for small molecules and ions. *Ann. NY Acad. Sci.,* 51:660–672.

71. Seeman, P., Chau-Wong, M., Tedesco, J., and Wong, K. (1975): Brain receptors for antipsychotic drugs and dopamine: Direct binding assays. *Proc. Natl. Acad. Sci. USA,* 72:4376–4380.

72. Seeman, P., Lee, T., Chau-Wong, M., Tedesco, J., and Wong, K. (1976): Dopamine receptors in human and calf brains, using [³H]apomorphine and antipsychotic drug. *Proc. Natl. Acad. Sci. USA,* 73:4354–4358.

73. Shaar, C. J., and Clemens, J. A. (1974): The role of catecholamines in the release of anterior pituitary prolactin in vitro. *Endocrinology,* 95:1202–1212.

74. Snyder, S. H., Banerjee, S. P., Yamamura, H. I., and Greenberg, D. (1974): Drugs, neurotransmitters and schizophrenia. *Science,* 184:1243.

75. Stevens, J. R. (1973): An anatomy of schizophrenia? *Arch. Gen. Psychiatry,* 29:177–189.

76. Strittmatter, W. J., Davis, J. N., and Lefkowitz, R. J. (1977): Alpha-adrenergic receptor in rat carotid cells. I. A correlation of [³H] dihydroergocryptine binding and catecholamine stimulated potassium efflux. *J. Biol. Chem.,* 252:5472–5477.

77. Subramanian, M. G., and Gala, R. R. (1976): The influence of cholinergic,

adrenergic, and serotonergic drugs on the afternoon surge of plasma prolactin in ovariectomized, estrogen-treated rats. *Endocrinology,* 98:842–848.

78. Takahara, J., Arimura, A., and Schally, A. V. (1974): Suppression of prolactin release by a purified porcine PIF preparation and catecholamines infused into a rat hypophysial portal vessel. *Endocrinology,* 96:462–465.

79. Takahara, J., Arimura, A., and Schally, A. V. (1974): Effect of catecholamines on the TRH-stimulated release of prolactin and growth hormone from sheep pituitaries in vitro. *Endocrinology,* 95:1490–1494.

80. Thorner, M. O., McNeilly, A. S., Hagan, C., and Besser, G. M. (1974): Long-term treatment of galactorrhea and hypogonadism with bromocryptine. *Br. Med. J.,* 2:419–422.

81. Villeneuve, A., Langelier, P., and Bédard, P. (1977): Estrogens, dopamine and dyskinesias. *Can. Psychiatr. Assoc. J.,* 23:68–70.

82. Weissman, A. (1974): Chemical, pharmacological, and metabolic considerations of thiothixene. In: *The Phenothiazines and Structurally Related Drugs,* edited by I. S. Forrest, C. J. Carr, and E. Usdin, pp. 471–480. Raven Press, New York.

83. Williams, L. T., Mullikin, D., and Lefkowitz, R. J. (1976): Identification of alpha-adrenergic receptors in uterine smooth muscle membranes by [^{3}H]dihydroergocryptine binding. *J. Biol. Chem.,* 251:6915–6923.

Endorphins

Central Nervous System Effects of Hypothalamic Hormones and Other Peptides, edited by Collu et al. Raven Press, New York © 1979.

Beta-Lipotropin = Pro-Endorphin

M. Chrétien, P. Crine, M. Lis, S. Benjannet, and N. G. Seidah

Protein and Pituitary Hormone Laboratory, Clinical Research Institute of Montreal, Montreal, Canada

Although preliminary indications that the pituitary gland contains lipolytic substances were found in 1931 by Anselmino and Hoffman (1), the complete characterization of two of these factors was first done in ovine pituitaries by Li et al. (28) and by Chrétien and Li (11). These molecules were called beta- and gamma-lipotropin. The former consists of 91 amino acids, of which residues 1–58 comprise the sequence of gamma-lipotropin (11,28). Both molecules comprise within their sequence the full polypeptide segment beta-MSH in positions 41–58 (11). Later on, homologous lipotropins were isolated and characterized in bovine (31,33), porcine (19–21,23,24), and human pituitaries (10,15,16,29,40). From all these studies a common structural feature of lipotropins has become apparent: their structure includes the species-specific beta-MSH sequence. This was first recognized by Chrétien and Li (11), and these authors proposed the theory that beta-MSH could be derived from beta-LPH by enzymatic cleavage with the initial production of gamma-LPH as an intermediary. The structural resemblance of the cleavage sites with pro-insulin (7,42) and pro-parathyroid hormone (26) seem to support such a view.

To strengthen such a hypothesis, Chrétien et al. (2,8,12) started a series of *in vitro* labeling experiments in whole bovine pituitary slices aiming to show the conversion of beta-LPH into beta-MSH through the initial formation of gamma-LPH. Although they were able to show the biosynthesis of beta- and gamma-LPH, they were unable to isolate newly synthesized beta-melanotropin. It was therefore proposed that the conversion of gamma-LPH to beta-MSH was a slow process in bovine pituitaries (12).

Unexpectedly, at the end of 1975, Hughes et al. (27) published the sequence of two morphine-like pentapeptides from porcine brain. One of them, named methionine-enkephalin, is structurally identical to the 61–65 sequence of the pituitary peptide beta-lipotropin. The other, named leucine-enkephalin, shares only the 61–64 sequence with beta-LPH, and leucine is at the carboxy-terminal (27). The discovery of these pentapeptides raised the possibility that beta-LPH is not only the precursor of beta-MSH but could also be the precursor of met-enkephalin. Indeed, Li and Chung (30) soon after isolated a peptide from camel pituitaries corresponding to the sequence 61–91 of beta-LPH. Bradbury et al. (5) also had earlier found a similar peptide in extracts of porcine pituitary. This 31-amino acid peptide was named beta-endorphin. Chrétien et al. (9) simultaneously reported on the isolation and purification of human and sheep beta-endorphin. Guillemin et al. (25) also reported on the isolation of two fragments of beta-endorphin from old fractions of porcine neurohypophysis and hypothalamic tissue extracts, namely, segments 61–76 and 61–77 of beta-LPH, named alpha- and gamma-endorphins.

This chapter reviews our recent studies on the purification and chemical characterization of human and sheep beta-endorphin, and on biosynthesis of beta-endorphin in both whole and intermediate lobe of bovine and rat pituitaries.

The results obtained during the last 2 years in our laboratory have answered basic questions:

1. Human pituitaries as well as sheep pituitaries contain beta-endorphin, and their primary structure (amino acid sequence) has been completely characterized.

2. The pituitary gland and most particularly the intermediate lobe biosynthesizes, *de novo,* beta-endorphin from its precursor beta-lipotropin, thus beta-lipotropin is a pro-endorphin.

COMPLETE CHARACTERIZATION OF TWO MORPHINE-LIKE PEPTIDES FROM HUMAN AND SHEEP PITUITARIES

Isolation and Purification of Human and Sheep Beta-Endorphin (9)

When human or sheep pituitaries were extracted in acetone/HCl followed by a stepwise NaCl precipitation, we obtained a fraction called fraction D (28), which, when passed on a carboxymethyl cellulose (CMC) column gave peaks that contained beta-LPH, gamma-LPH, beta-MSH, and beta-endorphin. We were the first to isolate human and sheep beta-endorphin (9).

These two peptides were then analyzed for their amino acid composition as shown in Table 1. It is seen that their composition fits very well with that expected for the portion 61–91 of their respective lipotropins (28,29). The exclusive presence of tyrosine at their amino terminal further confirms their purity and identity. The morphine-like activity on the vas deferens of these peptides and their respective lipotropins is presented in Fig. 1.

Amino Acid Sequence of Human and Sheep Pituitaries (17,41)

Once we had isolated and purified these peptides, it remained to prove unequivocably that these were indeed beta-endorphins, i.e., that their sequence was identical to the carboxy-terminal portion 61–91 of their

TABLE 1. *Amino acid analysis of human and sheep 61–91 peptides*

| | Hydrolysis time | | | | | | | |
| | Human[a] | | | | Sheep[a] | | | |
Amino acid	24 hr	48 hr	72 hr	Nearest integer	24 hr	48 hr	72 hr	Nearest integer
Lys	4.53	5.28	4.80	5	4.96	4.34	5.00	5
His					0.91	0.91	0.90	1
Asp	2.08	2.22	2.06	2	2.28	1.93	2.09	2
Thr	2.71	2.61	2.28	3	2.98	2.49	2.59	3
Ser	1.84	1.58	1.32	2	1.94	1.53	1.51	2
Glu	2.99	2.76	3.21	3	3.01	2.67	2.78	3
Pro	1.20	1.09	1.21	1	1.32	1.23	1.11	1
Gly	3.27	3.24	3.01	3	3.00	2.66	2.75	3
Ala	2.20	2.06	1.98	2	2.32	2.08	2.06	2
Val	1.08	0.86	1.06	1	1.18	1.00	1.04	1
Met	0.67	0.40	0.79	1	0.91	0.83	0.73	1
Ile	1.28	1.34	1.73	2	1.32	1.69	1.82	2
Leu	2.03	1.80	2.11	2	2.25	2.13	2.15	2
Tyr	1.86	1.94	1.65	2	0.94	0.87	0.94	1
Phe	1.87	1.84	1.85	2	2.16	1.93	1.96	2

[a] Dansylation revealed that the N-terminal residue of both peptides is exclusively Tyr.

respective beta-lipotropins. Only then could we discuss the possibility of beta-LPH as being the precursor of these peptides.

Due to the extreme rarity of human pituitaries and the limited amount of human beta-endorphin purified, we opted to sequence the sheep analogue

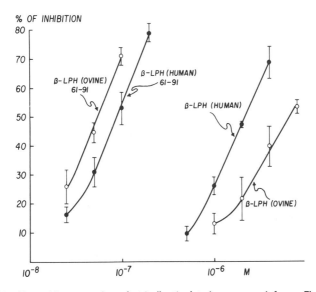

FIG. 1. Morphine-like activity assayed on electrically stimulated mouse vas deferens. The activity is expressed as percent inhibition of vas deferens concentrations. All the points are the means of 4 measurements ±SE.

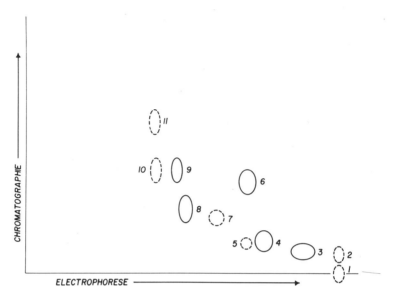

FIG. 2. Peptide map of tryptic digest of human beta-endorphin. Broken lines represent faint spots.

first, in order to establish the conditions for maximum sequence information. It soon became apparent that the automatic sequence on the intact peptide could not proceed further than 17 residues, due to peptide extractive losses during the sequenator cycles (41). It was thus decided to increase the

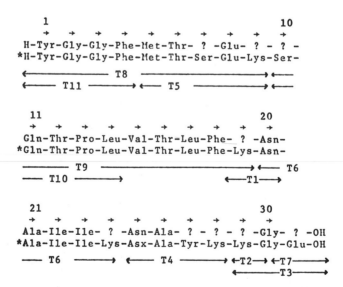

FIG. 3. Results of automatic sequencing of Braunitzer III derivatized beta-endorphin (*top lines*). Proposed sequence of beta-endorphin (*bottom lines*). The numbers refer to the positions of the tryptic peptides isolated (T1 — T11). (→) Automatic sequencing; (*) proposed sequence.

hydrophilicity of the peptide by reaction with a sufonyl naphthalene derivative, Braunitzer III (6), prior to automatic sequencing. Such a reagent reacts with all free amino groups. Upon sequencing we would thus expect blanks at the amino terminal and at all lysine residues, since the phenylthiohydantoins of so derivatized lysines are not easily detected. However, by sequencing the derivatized peptides, we identified 24 out of 31 residues with a repetitive yield of 95%. The remaining blanks at residues 10, 19, 24, 28, 29, 30, and 31 were positioned by peptide mapping on a tryptic digest of the native peptide. The eluates from each spot were submitted to amino acid and dansyl analysis. The results obtained permitted the unequivocal positioning of the tryptic peptides. It was clearly demonstrated that the sheep opiate-like peptide purified was identical to the portion 61–91 of sheep beta-lipotropin (28). In Figs. 2 and 3 we present a similar approach to the human peptide. This permitted the complete characterization of this peptide and its unequivocal identification as the segment 61–91 of human beta-lipotropin (15,29).

BIOSYNTHESIS OF BETA-ENDORPHIN IN WHOLE PITUITARY GLAND (13,14)

Although the biosynthesis of beta-LPH and gamma-LPH in whole pituitary was demonstrated 3 years ago in this laboratory (2,12), it remained to identify newly biosynthesized beta-endorphin.

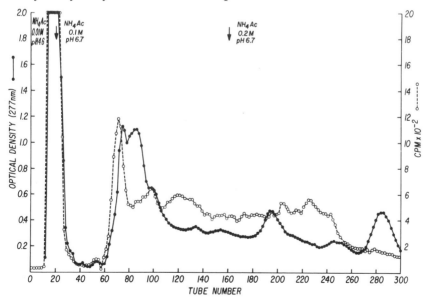

FIG. 4. CMC elution profile on the material obtained after extraction of pituitary slices incubated for 4 hr with ^{35}S-methionine. The column (1 × 40) was eluted with the gradient system of Li et al. (28). The arrows indicate the positions of gradient change.

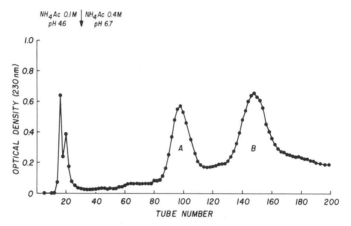

FIG. 5. CMC chromatography (1 × 25 cm) of material in fractions 236–265. The material was eluted with a concave gradient of NH₄OAc from pH 4.6 and 0.1 M to pH 6.7 and 0.4 M. Fractions of 1 ml were collected.

Incubation of whole bovine pituitary slices with ^{35}S-methionine for 4 hr, followed by acetone/HCl extraction and stepwise NaCl precipitation with an excess carrier of sheep pituitary homogenate to prevent degradation, gave the fraction D, which when passed on a CMC column showed the chromatogram illustrated in Fig. 4. Since we knew the elution position of beta-endorphin on this column (9), the fraction 236–265 was pooled and rechromatographed on another CM-Sephadex column with a faster gradient, and this material was further resolved into two components (Fig. 5). Fraction 80–114 (peak A) containing a total of 20,000 cpm was shown to contain a radioactive material migrating as a single band on acid polyacrylamide gel co-migrating with cold ovine beta-endorphin. Finally, the

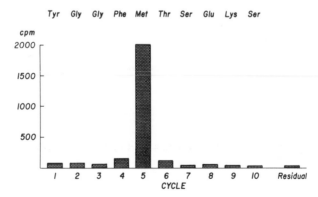

FIG. 6. Radioisotope sequence analysis of a purified bovine beta-endorphin labeled with ^{35}S-methionine. About 4,000 cpm was used as starting material. The sequence given at the top is that known for beta-endorphin.

conclusive proof that this newly labeled material was indeed bovine beta-endorphin was obtained upon microsequencing of this radioactive material as shown in Fig. 6. From the appearance of methionine at the fifth cycle, as expected from the sequence of bovine beta-endorphin (31,33), the purity and identity of this biosynthetic peptide were established.

BIOSYNTHESIS OF BETA-LPH, GAMMA-LPH, AND BETA-ENDORPHIN IN BOVINE AND RAT NEUROINTERMEDIATE PITUITARY LOBE

The pars nervosa and pars intermedia were carefully dissected from the anterior lobe of 25 fresh beef pituitary glands. By gentle mechanical treatment, the cells of the pars intermedia were then obtained and suspended in 10 ml of Krebs-Ringer bicarbonate (KRBG) containing 0.2% bovine serum albumin. After an initial preincubation period of 1 hr, the cells were incubated for 3 hr in a KRBG-containing solution with 1 mCi of ^{35}S-methionine and 4.8 mCi of ^{3}H-lysine. The cells were then homogenized and extracted in 5 ml of 10^{-3} M EDTA (pH 10.35) solution containing 5 mg/ml sheep

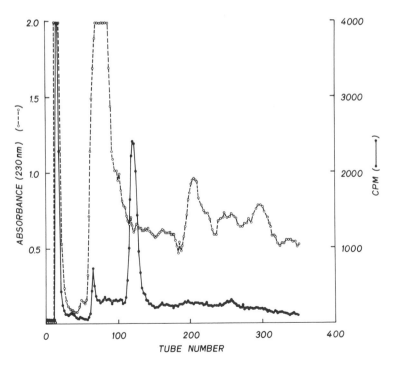

FIG. 7. CMC chromatography of the labeled proteins extracted from the isolated cells of beef pituitaries pars intermedia incubated *in vitro* for 3 hr with 1 mCi ^{35}S-methionine and 4.8 mCi ^{3}H-lysine. The column was eluted with the same gradient used in Fig. 4.

pituitary fraction D (28). After it was desalted, the extract was chromatographed on a CMC column as shown in Fig. 7.

Analysis of Fraction 59–77, Gamma-LPH

Upon polyacrylamide gel electrophoresis of the material obtained from fraction 59–77 at both pH 4.5 and pH 8.3 (Fig. 8), we obtained a single radioactive band. At both pHs the migration position was identical to that of standard sheep gamma-LPH.

Again a chemical proof of identity was judged necessary. It can be seen from Fig. 9 that within the sequence 1–58 of beta-LPH, i.e., gamma-LPH, methionine occupies position 47 and is preceded by a lysine residue at position 46. Also, lysine is present at 39 and 40. Thus if we treat gamma-LPH (1–58) with trypsin and we sequence directly the digest mixture, we expect a methionine at N-terminal and position 7 depending on whether the digestion was complete or not. A digestion of 10 min shows a methionine in positions 1 and 7, whereas an exhaustive digestion for 24 hr shows methionine

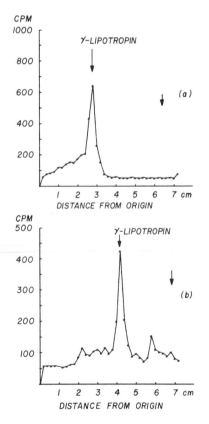

FIG. 8. Polyacrylamide gel electrophoresis at pH 4.5 (a) and pH 8.3 (b) of the radioactive material recovered in fractions 59–77 of CMC (Fig. 7).

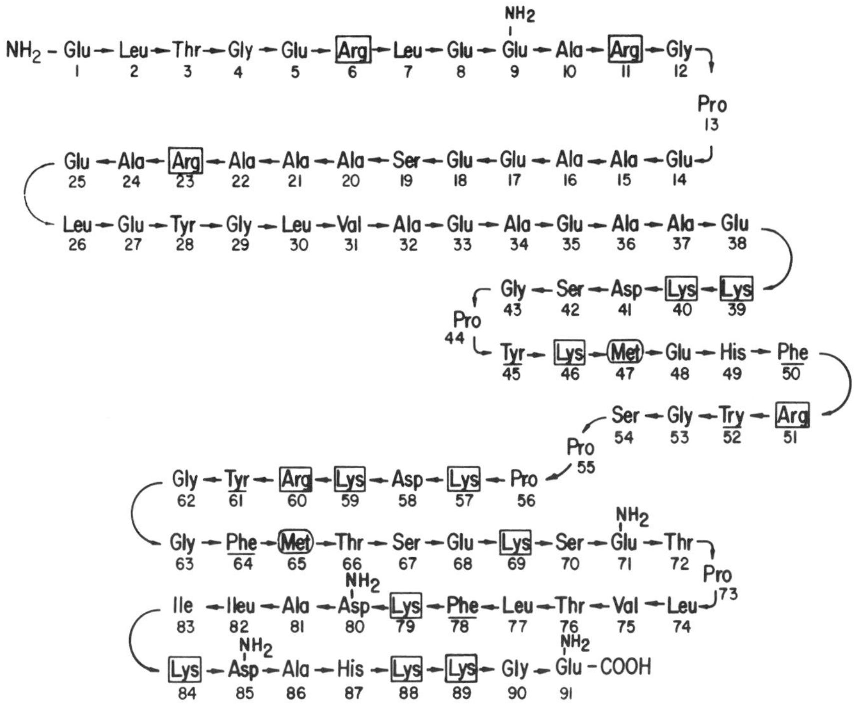

NH₂ - Glu → Leu → Thr → Gly → Glu → [Arg] → Leu → Glu → Glu → Ala → [Arg] → Gly
1　　2　　3　　4　　5　　6　　7　　8　　9(NH₂)　10　　11　　12

Pro 13

Glu → Ala → [Arg] → Ala → Ala → Ala → Ser → Glu → Glu → Ala → Ala → Glu
25　　24　　23　　22　　21　　20　　19　　18　　17　　16　　15　　14

Leu → Glu → Tyr → Gly → Leu → Val → Ala → Glu → Ala → Glu → Ala → Ala → Glu
26　　27　　28　　29　　30　　31　　32　　33　　34　　35　　36　　37　　38

Gly → Ser → Asp → [Lys] → [Lys]
43　　42　　41　　40　　39

Pro 44

Tyr → [Lys] → (Met) → Glu → His → Phe
45　　46　　47　　48　　49　　50

Ser → Gly → Try → [Arg]
54　　53　　52　　51

Pro 55

Gly → Tyr → [Arg] → [Lys] → Asp → [Lys] → Pro
62　　61　　60　　59　　58　　57　　56

Gly → Phe → (Met) → Thr → Ser → Glu → [Lys] → Ser → Glu → Thr
63　　64　　65　　66(NH₂)　67　　68　　69　　70　　71　　72

Pro 73

Ile → Ileu → Ala → Asp → [Lys] → Phe → Leu → Thr → Val → Leu
83　　82　　81(NH₂)　80　　79　　78　　77　　76(NH₂)　75　　74

[Lys] → Asp → Ala → His → [Lys] → [Lys] → Gly → Glu - COOH
84(NH₂)　85　　86　　87　　88　　89　　90　　91

FIG. 9. Amino acid sequence of sheep beta-LPH.

only at position 1. Thus we have unequivocably identified the biosynthetic product to be gamma-lipotropin from intermediary lobe pituitary.

Analysis of Fraction 236–270, Beta-Endorphin

The polyacrylamide electrophoresis at pH 4.5 of material from fraction 236–270 gave a single band which co-migrated with standard sheep beta-endorphin, after repurification on another CMC column identical to that used in Fig. 1. Upon sequencing such material (Fig. 10), we obtained as expected ^{35}S-methionine at position 5 and ^{3}H-lysine at position 9. Clearly this identifies this biosynthetic material as pure beta-endorphin.

Analysis of Fraction 195–235, Beta-Lipotropin

Purification of this fraction on Sephadex G-75 and carboxymethyl Sephadex yielded a fraction which when passed on polyacrylamide gel electrophoresis at pH 4.5 showed the presence of a band co-migrating with standard sheep beta-lipotropin (Fig. 11). However, due to the limited availability of such material, no further chemical characterization was possible.

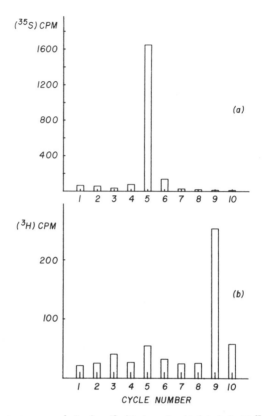

FIG. 10. Radioisotope sequence analysis of purified beta-endorphin labeled with ³⁵S-methionine and ³H-lysine. Radioactivity recovered was measured on ³⁵S-chanel (a) and ³H chanel (b) after correction for the ³⁵S spilling over. ³⁵S-Methionine and ³H-lysine were recovered at cycles 5 and 9, respectively, as expected from the primary structure of beta-endorphin.

In rat pars intermedia, similar studies have been carried out with pulse-chase experiments. As shown in Fig. 12, one can observe that a biosynthetic product of about 29,000 dalton is progressively transformed into beta-LPH and beta-endorphin. This unequivocably proves that beta-LPH is a pro-beta-endorphin, whereas the 29,000-dalton molecule which also contains ACTH is a pre-pro-beta-endorphin.

DISCUSSION

Major progress in the field of pituitary lipolytic hormones has been made due to the recent unexpected discovery of endogenous morphine-like peptides structurally related to beta-LPH. Hence this polypeptide appears unique in comprising within its sequence the structures of two biologically active peptides, beta-MSH (beta-LPH 41–58) and beta-endophin (beta-LPH 61–91).

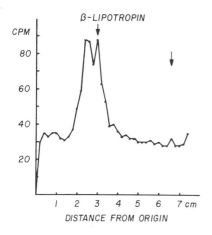

FIG. 11. Gel electrophoresis of labeled beta-LPH (fraction 195–235 in Fig. 7 purified on Sephadex G-75 and CM-Sephadex). A band comigrating with standard beta-lipotropin is seen.

Beta-lipotropin, gamma-lipotropin, and beta-endorphin have been purified from whole pituitary glands of different species including human. Immunocytofluorescence data show the presence of beta-lipotropin and beta-endorphin in anterior and intermediary lobes of rat (4). Similarly, it was shown that the major portion of opiate-like activity was found in the cells of the pars intermedia (36,39). None of these techniques unequivocably localizes the biosynthetic origin of these peptides.

Although far from being exhaustive, the biosynthetic labeling experiments have shown that beta-LPH, gamma-LPH, and beta-endorphin are actively biosynthesized in whole and intermediate lobe pituitaries. In bovine, it seems that beta-MSH is not biosynthesized in the pituitary in relatively large amounts, whereas in fish and frogs where its role is more understood (32,37) this is no longer the case. Definite proof that beta-lipotropin is also the biosynthetic precursor of beta-endorphin has been demonstrated by more extensive studies with pulse-chase labeling techniques. In rat pars intermedia, a high molecular weight protein (28 to 30 K) is transformed into beta-endorphin. Such newly biosynthesized beta-endorphin has been clearly and definitively identified in the pituitary; and because there is a striking analogy between the sequence of beta-lipotropin and that of pro-insulin at the cleavage site (43) we are tempted to propose that both beta-MSH and beta-endorphin arise from beta-lipotropin through an enzymatic process similar to the one proposed by Steiner et al. (43). That this is the case is further supported by the fact that beta-LPH has a much lower MSH and lipolytic activity than beta-MSH (28) and a much lower morphine-like activity than beta-endorphin (9), which is a situation analogous to the pro-insulin model (43).

In recent years considerable progress has been made in elucidating the mechanisms of protein biosynthesis. It now appears common that most secreted polypeptide hormones and proteins are initially synthesized from larger precursor molecules which are then converted to their respective active

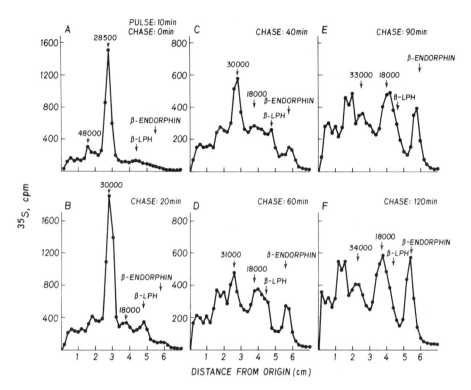

FIG. 12. SDS gel electrophoresis of desalted extracts of intermediate lobe cells obtained during a pulse-chase labeling experiment. The positions of standard labeled rat beta-LPH and beta-endorphin are marked on each figure, as well as the molecular weight corresponding to the position of the peaks.

forms by post-translational cleavage (3). Recently, Mains et al. (34) reported on the biosynthesis in a mouse pituitary tumor cell line At T-20/D-16 V of a large molecule of about 31,000 molecular weight which could be the precursor of both ACTH and beta-LPH. That this is the case was suspected long ago from immunochemical studies which showed that beta-LPH, endorphins, and ACTH occur in the same pituitary cells (18,35,36,38). The amino acid sequence of such a precursor molecule is not yet known, and its complete characterization will constitute a major step in the understanding of the enzymatic processes of maturation.

SUMMARY

The molecule beta-lipotropin, composed of 91 amino acids (beta-LPH 1–91), has gained considerable importance in recent years. Its double role as the precursor of beta-MSH (beta-LPH 41–58) and beta-endorphin (beta-LPH 61–91) makes this peptide unique. Results are presented on the role of this molecule and on the complete characterization of two morphine-like peptides from human and sheep pituitaries. One of the important synthesis sites of beta-endorphin is unequivocably in the pituitary neuro-intermediate lobe.

REFERENCES

1. Anselmino, K. J., and Hoffman, F. (1931): Nachweis der antidiuretischen komponente des hypophysenhinterlappenhormons und einer blutdrucksteigernden substanz im blute bei nephropathie und eklampsie der schwangeren. *Klin. Wochenschr.*, 10:1438–1441.
2. Bertagna, X., Lis, M., Gilardeau, C., and Chrétien, M. (1974): Biosynthèse in vitro de la béta-LPH de boeuf. *Can. J. Biochem.*, 52:349–358.
3. Blobel, G., and Dobberstein, B. (1975): Transfer of proteins across membranes. I. Presence of proteolytically processed and unprocessed nascent immunoglobulin light chains on membrane-bound ribosomes of murine myeloma. *J. Cell Biol.*, 67: 835–851.
4. Bloom, F., Battenberg, E., Rossier, J., Ling, N., Leppaluoto, J., Vargo, T. M., and Guillemin, R. (1977): Endorphins are located in the intermediate and anterior lobe of the pituitary gland, not in the neurohypophysis. *Life Sci.*, 20:43–48.
5. Bradbury, A. F., Smyth, D. G., and Snell, C. R. (1976): Lipotropin: Precursor of two biologically active peptides. *Biochem. Biophys. Res. Commun.*, 69:950–956.
6. Braunitzer, G., Chen, R., Schrank, B., et al. (1973): Die sequenzanalise des beta lactoglobulins. *Hoppe-Seylers Z. Physiol. Chem.*, 354:867–878.
7. Chance, E. R., Ellis, R. M., and Bromer, W. W. (1968): Porcine proinsulin: Characterization and amino acid sequence. *Science*, 160:165–167.
8. Chrétien, M., Benjannet, S., Bertagna, X., Lis, M., and Chrétien, M. (1974): In vitro biosynthesis of gamma-lipotropic hormone. *Clin. Res.*, 22, 730 (abstr.).
9. Chrétien, M., Benjannet, S., Dragon, N., Seidah, N. G., and Lis, M. (1976): Isolation of peptides with opiate activity from sheep and human pituitaries: Relationship to beta-lipotropin. *Biochem. Biophys. Res. Commun.*, 72:472–478.
10. Chrétien, M., Gilardeau, C., Seidah, N. G., and Lis, M. (1976): Purification and partial chemical characterization of human pituitary lipolytic hormone. *Can. J. Biochem.*, 54:778–782.
11. Chrétien, M., and Li, C. H. (1967): Isolation, purification and characterization of gamma-lipotropic hormone from sheep pituitary glands. *Can. J. Biochem.*, 45: 1163–1174.
12. Chrétien, M., Lis, M., Gilardeau, C., and Benjannet, S. (1976): In vitro biosynthesis of gamma-lipotropic hormone. *Can. J. Biochem.*, 54:566–570.
13. Chrétien, M., Seidah, N. G., Benjannet, S., Dragon, N., Routhier, R., Motomatsu, T., Crine, P., and Lis, M. (1977): A beta-LPH precursor model: Recent developments concerning morphine-like substances. *Ann. N.Y. Acad. Sci.*, 297:84–107.
14. Crine, P., Benjannet, S., Seidah, N. G., Lis, M., and Chrétien, M. (1977): In vitro biosynthesis of beta-endorphin in pituitary gland. *Proc. Natl. Acad. Sci. U.S.A.*, 74:1403–1406.
15. Cseh, G., Barat, E., Patthy, A., and Graf, L. (1972): Studies on the primary structure of human beta-lipotropic hormone. *FEBS Lett.*, 21:344–346.
16. Cseh, G., Graf, L., and Goth, E. (1968): Lipotropic hormone obtained from human pituitary glands. *FEBS Lett.*, 2:42–44.
17. Dragon, N., Seidah, N. G., Routhier, R., Lis, M., and Chrétien, M. (1977): Primary structure and morphine-like activity of human beta-endorphin. *Can. J. Biochem.*, 55:666–670.
18. Dubois, P., Vargues-Regaivaz, H., and Dubois, M. P. (1973): Human foetal anterior pituitary immunofluorescent evidence for corticotropin and melanotropin activities. *Z. Zellforsch.*, 145:131–143.
19. Gilardeau, C., and Chrétien, M. (1970): Isolation and characterization of beta-LPH from porcine pituitary glands. *Can. J. Biochem.*, 48:1017–1021.

20. Gilardeau, C., and Chrétien, M. (1972): Complete amino acid sequence of porcine beta-lipotropic hormone (beta-LPH). In: *Chemistry and Biology of Peptides, Proceedings of the 3rd Peptide Symposium,* edited by J. Meinhofer, pp. 609–611. Ann Arbor Science Publishers, Ann Arbor, Mich.
21. Graf, L., Barat, E., Cseh, G., and Sajgo, M. (1970): Amino acid sequence of porcine gamma-lipotropic hormone. *Acta Biochim. Biophys. Acad. Sci. Hung.,* 5:305–307.
22. Graf, L., Barat, E., Cseh, G., and Sajgo, M. (1971): Amino acid sequence of porcine beta-lipotropic hormone. *Biochim. Biophys. Acta,* 229:276–278.
23. Graf, L., and Cseh, G. (1968): Isolation of porcine beta-lipotropic hormone. *Acta Biochim. Biophys. Acad. Sci. Hung.,* 3:175–177.
24. Graf, L., Cseh, G., and Medzihradszky-Schweiger, H. (1969): Isolation of gamma-lipotropic hormone from porcine pituitary glands. *Biochim. Biophys. Acta,* 175: 444–447.
25. Guillemin, R., Ling, N., and Burgus, R. (1976): Endorphins, hypothalamic and neurohypophyseal peptides with morphinomimetic activity. Isolation and primary structure of alpha-endorphin. *C. R. Acad. Sci. [D] (Paris),* 282:783–785.
26. Habener, J. F., Kemper, B., Potts, J. T., Jr., and Rich, A. (1973): Bovine preparathyroid hormone: Structural analysis of radioactive peptides formed by limited cleavage. *Endocrinology,* 92:219–226.
27. Hughes, J., Smith, T. W., Kosterlitz, H. W., Fothergill, L. A., Morgan, B. A., and Morriss, H. R. (1975): Identification of two related pentapeptides from the brain with potent opiate agonist activity. *Nature,* 258:577–579.
28. Li, C. H., Barnafi, L., Chrétien, M., and Chung, D. (1965): Isolation and structure of beta-LPH from sheep pituitary glands. *Excerpta Medica Int. Congr.,* 112:349–364.
29. Li, C. H., and Chung, D. (1976): Primary structure of human beta-lipotropin. *Nature,* 260:622–624.
30. Li, C. H., and Chung, D. (1976): Isolation and structure of an untriakontapeptide with opiate activity from camel pituitary glands. *Proc. Natl. Acad. Sci. U.S.A.,* 73:1145–1148.
31. Li, C. H., Tan, L., and Chung, D. (1977): Isolation and primary structure of beta-endorphin and beta-lipotropin from bovine pituitary gland. *Biochem. Biophys. Res. Commun.,* 77:1088–1093.
32. Loh, Y. P., and Gainer, H. (1977): Biosynthesis, processing and control of release of melanotropic peptides in the neurointermediate lobe of *Xenopus laevis. J. Gen. Physiol.,* 70:37–58.
33. Lohmar, P., and Li, C. H. (1967): Isolation of ovine beta-lipotropic hormone. *Biochim. Biophys. Acta,* 147:381–383.
34. Mains, R. E., Eipper, B. A., and Ling, N. (1977): Common precursor to corticotropins and endorphins. *Proc. Natl. Acad. Sci. USA,* 74:3014–3018.
35. Moriarty, G. C. (1973): Immunocytochemistry of the pituitary glycoprotein hormones. *J. Histochem. Cytochem.,* 21:846–863.
36. Pelletier, G., Leclerc, R., Labrie, F., Côté, J., Chrétien, M., and Lis, M. (1977): Immunohistochemical localization of beta-lipotropic hormone in the pituitary gland. *Endocrinology,* 100:770–776.
37. Pezalla, P. D., Clarke, W. C., Lis, M., Seidah, N. G., and Chrétien, M. (1978): Immunological characterization of beta-lipotropin fragments (endorphin, beta-MSH and N-fragment) from fish pituitaries. *Gen. Comp. Endocrinol.,* 34:163–168.
38. Phifer, R. F., Orth, D. N., and Spicer, S. S. (1974): Specific demonstration of the human hypophyseal adrenocortico-melanotropic (ACTH-/MSH) cell. *J. Clin. Endocrinol. Metab.,* 39:684–692.
39. Queen, G., Pinsky, C., and LaBella, F. (1976): Subcellular localization of endorphin activity in bovine pituitary and brain. *Biochem. Biophys. Res. Commun.,* 72:1021–1027.
40. Scott, A. P., and Lowry, P. J. (1974): Adrenocorticotrophic and melanocyte-stimulating peptides in the human pituitary. *Biochem. J.,* 139:593–602.
41. Seidah, N. G., Dragon, N., Benjannet, S., Routhier, R., and Chrétien, M. (1977):

The complete sequence of sheep beta-endorphin. *Biochem. Biophys. Res. Commun.,* 74:1528–1535.

42. Steiner, D. F., Hallund, O., Rubenstein, A., Cho, S., and Bayliss, C. (1968): Isolation and properties of proinsulin, intermediate forms, and other minor components from crystalline bovine insulin. *Diabetes,* 17:725–736.

43. Steiner, D. F., Kemmler, W., Tager, H. S., and Peterson, J. D. (1974): Proteolytic processing in the biosynthesis of insulin and other proteins. *Fed. Proc.,* 33:2105–2115.

Central Nervous System Effects of Hypothalamic Hormones and Other Peptides, edited by Collu et al. Raven Press, New York © 1979.

Enkephalin Synthesis in Brain: Effect of Cycloheximide and Identification of Enkephalin Precursor

Steven R. Childers and Solomon H. Snyder

Departments of Pharmacology and Experimental Therapeutics and Psychiatry and Behavioral Sciences, Johns Hopkins University School of Medicine, Baltimore, Maryland 21205

The discovery by Hughes et al. (8) of the opioid peptides, methionine-enkephalin (met-enkephalin) and leucine-enkephalin (leu-enkephalin), led to the observation that the amino acid sequence of met-enkephalin was contained within the 91-amino acid pituitary hormone β-lipotropin (β-LPH). Further, the C-terminal fragment of β-LPH, β-endorphin (β-LPH$_{61\text{-}91}$), is a potent opioid peptide which also contains met-enkephalin (β-LPH$_{61\text{-}65}$) (4,6,9). These findings suggested that β-endorphin is a precursor of enkephalin, and that β-LPH is a precursor of β-endorphin. The latter hypothesis has been supported by recent studies in pituitary (10,11) which have shown that β-endorphin can be formed from β-LPH, and that both β-LPH and ACTH have a common precursor, a 31,000 molecular weight protein ("Big ACTH") that reacts with both β-endorphin and ACTH antisera. Less progress has been made in the understanding of enkephalin synthesis in brain. Smyth and his colleagues (1) have detected extracellular breakdown of β-endorphin into enkephalin in brain slices. However, the physiological significance of this conversion is not clear, since it occurs at pH 5 and since the regional distribution of β-endorphin in brain is very different from that of enkephalin (3,14). Enkephalin synthesis from labeled amino acids has been detected in brain (15), but the exact precursor relationships of enkephalin remain unclear.

One method to estimate the rate of enkephalin synthesis and utilization *in vivo* is to determine the rate of enkephalin turnover by injection of protein synthesis inhibitors. In the present study we report the inhibition of enkephalin synthesis *in vivo* by administration of cycloheximide. In addition, we report attempts to identify a precursor of enkephalin in rat brain by reacting high molecular weight proteins with specific enkephalin antisera.

MATERIALS AND METHODS

Cycloheximide Studies

Male Swiss albino mice (20 to 25 g) were anesthetized with intraperitoneal injections of Equi-Thesin (Jensen-Salisbury Labs). Cycloheximide (Sigma

Chemical Co.) was dissolved in saline at a concentration of 10 mg/ml, and 7.5 μl were injected intracerebrally at a depth of 2 mm in each of four sites: bilateral temporal and ventricular locations (7). Control mice received injections of 7.5 μl saline in identical locations. Further studies indicated that a single series of injections was not sufficient to lower brain enkephalin levels, so a second series of injections was performed 3 hr later in the same locations. In this procedure, the average mortality was 25 to 35%.

Cerebral protein synthesis was determined by a modification of the method of Barondes and Cohen (2). Mice were injected subcutaneously with 5 μCi of ^{3}H-leucine (5 Ci/mmole; New England Nuclear Corporation) and were sacrificed 40 min later. Brains were homogenized in 5 ml of 0.1 N NaOH with the Polytron; 0.5-ml aliquots of each homogenate were added to 1.5 ml of cold 12% TCA. The samples were centrifuged at 4°C for 10 min at 49,000 $\times$ g, supernatants were discarded, and pellets were washed with 1 ml of cold 10% TCA. TCA was extracted from the pellets by three 1-ml washes with ether, the pellets were dissolved in 0.5 ml of 0.1 N NaOH, and radioactivity was determined in 10 ml of aqueous scintillation fluor. Protein synthesis was calculated by determining the ratio of TCA-precipitable radioactivity to total amount of radioactivity in the homogenate.

Radioimmunoassay of Met- and Leu-Enkephalin

Antisera to met-enkephalin and leu-enkephalin were produced in rabbits as previously described (5,12). These antisera were relatively specific: over 200-fold molar excess of one enkephalin was required to cross-react in the radioimmunoassay of the other enkephalin. β-Endorphin did not cross-react with either serum at a concentration of 20 μM.

Enkephalin was extracted from cycloheximide-treated mice by homogenizing whole brain in 5 ml of 0.1 N HCl using a Brinkmann Polytron. The homogenates were then centrifuged at 4°C for 10 min at 49,000 $\times$ g, and supernatants were lyophilized, neutralized, and centrifuged at 4°C for 10 min. The supernatants were lyophilized again and samples were suspended in 0.8 ml of 50 mM sodium veronal buffer, pH 8.6. Radioimmunoassays were conducted as previously described (5) using 60,000 cpm of either ^{3}H-met-enkephalin (17.4 Ci/mmole) or ^{3}H-leu-enkephalin (21 Ci/mmole; New England Nuclear Corporation) along with antiserum and enkephalin standards or samples in a total volume of 0.25 ml.

Identification of Enkephalin Precursor

Two brains from male Sprague-Dawley rats were homogenized in 40 ml of 50 mM Tris-HCl, pH 7.7, using a Brinkmann Polytron. After centrifugation at 49,000 $\times$ g for 10 min, the supernatant was concentrated to 2 ml in an Amicon Dia-Flo apparatus with PM-10 ultrafiltration membranes.

The sample was applied to a (1.5 × 90 cm) column of Sephacryl S-200 (Pharmacia) and eluted with 50 mM Tris-HCl, pH 7.7. Fractions of 2 ml were collected and protein concentration was monitored by absorbance at 280 nm. Aliquots of 100 μl from each column fraction were assayed in triplicate in the met-enkephalin radioimmunoassay as described. In order to test for immunoglobulin binding, we incubated 300-μl aliquots of each fraction 1 hr at 25°C with 10 μl of normal rabbit serum (diluted 1:3), followed by incubation for 2 hr at 25°C with goat anti-rabbit IgG (Calbiochem). These relative concentrations of serum and anti-IgG provided maximum precipitation of immunoglobulins as determined by quantitative immunoprecipitation studies. The resulting precipitates were centrifuged at 28,000 × g for 5 min, and 100-μl aliquots of the supernatants were assayed by met-enkephalin radioimmunoassay.

In trypsin studies, brain-soluble fractions were prepared and concentrated as described above. Samples were incubated in 50 mM Tris-HCl, pH 7.7, with 1 mM $CaCl_2$, in the presence and absence of 2 mg trypsin (Worthington), at 25°C for 40 min. Samples were applied to (1 × 20 cm) columns of Bio-gel P-10 (Bio-Rad) and eluted with 50 mM Tris-HCl, pH 7.7. Fractions of 1 ml were collected and 100-μl aliquots assayed as described above.

RESULTS

Inhibition of Protein Synthesis with Cycloheximide

Cycloheximide, a potent inhibitor of protein synthesis, was injected intracerebrally in mice in an effort to halt production of met- and leu-enkephalin and thereby measure their turnover in brain. This treatment resulted in a significant loss of enkephalin 24 hr after injection, with approximately 40% loss of met-enkephalin and 30% loss of leu-enkephalin (data not shown). Analysis of cerebral protein synthesis following the two injections (Fig. 1) showed 90% loss at 4 hr, 80% loss at 10 hr, and approximately normal synthesis at 24 hr.

The effect of cycloheximide on enkephalin levels was dose dependent. Mice were given two series of injections, with each injection site receiving 25, 50, or 100 μg cycloheximide per injection. Enkephalin levels 24 hr later were only slightly decreased with 25 μg cycloheximide; however, 50 μg provided a maximal response since no further decrease was seen with 100 μg cycloheximide (data not shown).

The time course of enkephalin decrease after cycloheximide indicates a slow turnover (Fig. 2). No significant effect was seen on either met- or leu-enkephalin levels at 5 hr, and leu-enkephalin remained unchanged at 12 hr whereas met-enkephalin decreased by approximately 30%. Both peptides revealed significant decreases at 24 hr and further losses at 48 hr.

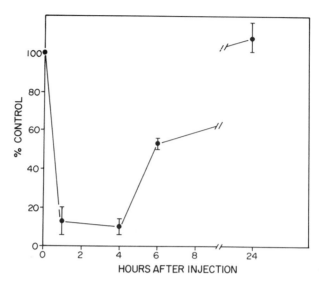

FIG. 1. Inhibition of cerebral protein synthesis by cycloheximide. Mice were injected with two series of cycloheximide (75 μg/7.5 μl) at four cerebral sites. At various times mice were injected subcutaneously with 5 μCi of ³H-leucine, and protein synthesis was determined as described in the Methods section. Results are expressed as percent of synthesis in brains of saline-injected mice.

Identification of Enkephalin Precursor

Since ACTH and β-lipotropin are produced in pituitary from high molecular weight precursors by trypsin or trypsin-like enzymes (10,11), attempts were made to produce enkephalin from tryptic digests of high molecular weight components in the brain. When the soluble fractions of rat brains were subjected to ultrafiltration on Amicon PM-10 membranes to eliminate endogenous enkephalin and eluted on a Bio-gel P-10 gel filtration column, one peak of material reacting in the met-enkephalin radioimmunoassay was detected in the void volume with an apparent molecular weight of greater than 18,000 (Fig. 3). Treatment of an identical rat brain supernatant with trypsin significantly reduced the void volume immunoreactivity and resulted in the appearance of a second peak of met-enkephalin immunoreactivity which co-migrated with authentic ³H-met-enkephalin on the same column (Fig. 3).

Further characterization of the high molecular weight precursor was accomplished by gel filtration of the soluble fraction of rat brain on Sephacryl S-200 columns (Fig. 4). Results showed the presence of two peaks of met-enkephalin immunoreactivity, with apparent molecular weights of greater than 150,000 and 50,000 to 70,000. Since these peaks may represent material which nonspecifically adsorbs ³H-met-enkephalin instead of genuine enkephalin precursors, the same column fractions were analyzed by radio-receptor assay, using ³H-met-enkephalin as a ligand (Fig. 4). No receptor

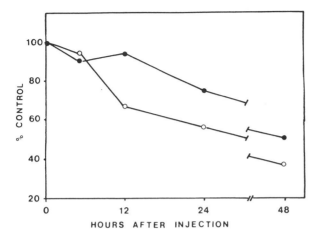

FIG. 2. Time course of cycloheximide-induced decrease of met- and leu-enkephalin. Mice were injected with two series of cycloheximide (75 µg/7.5 µl) at four cerebral sites. After sacrifice at indicated times, brains were homogenized in 5 ml of 0.1 N HCl, and met- and leu-enkephalin levels were determined by radioimmunoassay. Data represent percent of enkephalin levels in saline-injected mice. (●), leu-enkephalin; (○), met-enkephalin.

activity was detected, indicating the absence of high molecular weight components that interact with opiate receptors or nonspecifically bind ³H-enkephalin. To eliminate the possibility that the immunoreactive peaks represented endogenous enkephalin bound to macromolecules, we incubated the rat brain fraction with ³H-met-enkephalin at 0°C and eluted it on Sephacryl S-200. These results (not shown) demonstrated that essentially all en-

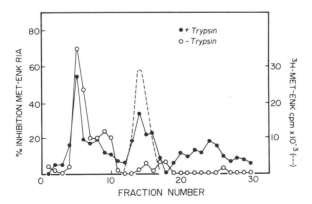

FIG. 3. Effect of trypsin treatment on enkephalin-like immunoreactivity. Soluble fractions of two rat brains were incubated in 50 mM Tris-HCl, pH 7.7, with 1 mM CaCl₂, in the presence and absence of 2 mg trypsin, for 45 min at 25°C. Sample was eluted on a (1 × 20 cm) column of Bio-gel P-10. Fractions of 1 ml were collected, and 100-µl aliquots were assayed in triplicate in the met-enkephalin radioimmunoassay. Data represent percent inhibition of ³H-met-enkephalin binding in the radioimmunoassay in the absence of unlabeled enkephalin.

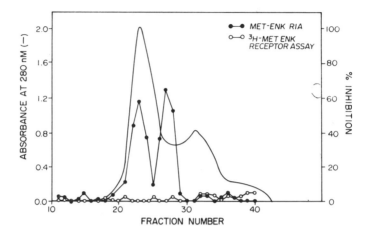

FIG. 4. Gel filtration of enkephalin-like immunoreactivity on Sephacryl S-200. Soluble fractions of two rat brains were combined and eluted on a (1.5 × 90 cm) column of Sephacryl S-200 in 50 mM Tris-HCl, pH 7.7. Fractions of 2 ml were collected and 100-μl aliquots were assayed in triplicate in the met-enkephalin radioimmunoassay, and in the opiate receptor assay with ³H-met-enkephalin as ligand (13). Data represent percent inhibition of ³H-met-enkephalin binding in either assay. (——), absorbance at 280 nm.

kephalin eluted as low molecular weight material and no detectable enkephalin bound to the macromolecular fraction.

Another possibility for artifacts is that the immunoreactive peaks may bind to immunoglobulins in the antiserum, thus displacing ³H-met-enkephalin

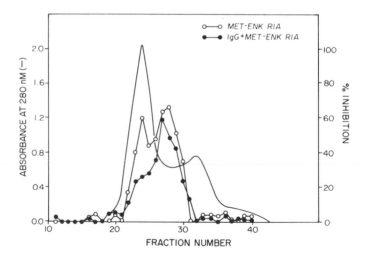

FIG. 5. Preadsorption of enkephalin-like immunoreactivity with control serum. Rat brain supernatant was fractionated on Sephacryl S-200 and assayed by radioimmunoassay as described in Fig. 4. Aliquots from each fraction (300 μl) were incubated for 1 hr at 25°C with 10 μl control rabbit serum (1:3), then incubated for 2 hr at 25°C with 50 μl of goat anti-rabbit IgG. After centrifugation, supernatants (100 μl) were assayed by radioimmunoassay as described. Data represent percent of ³H-met-enkephalin binding in the radioimmunoassay. (——), absorbance at 280 nm; (○), radioimmunoassay only; (●), preadsorbed with serum and anti-IgG.

nonspecifically in the radioimmunoassay. Therefore, each column fraction was incubated with normal rabbit serum (at the same dilution as the antiserum in the radioimmunoassay), and immunoglobulins were precipitated by goat anti-rabbit IgG. When the remaining nonprecipitated material was assayed by met-enkephalin radioimmunoassay (Fig. 5), the activity in the first peak (MW > 150,000) was eliminated, suggesting that this material bound to immunoglobulins in the control serum and was precipitated by anti-IgG. However, the 50,000 to 70,000 MW peak was only slightly decreased by anti-IgG precipitation, suggesting that this peak represents a true enkephalin precursor. Further experiments will help to reveal how this macromolecule is broken down into enkephalin in brain.

DISCUSSION

Injection of cycloheximide reduces brain enkephalin levels in a dose- and time-dependent manner. These experiments suggest, but do not confirm, that enkephalin is synthesized ribosomally, although an alternate possibility, i.e., that cycloheximide halts production of an enkephalin-synthetic enzyme, cannot be eliminated. The slow onset of the cycloheximide effect suggests that enkephalin could be released at a slow rate. Alternatively, it is consistent with the idea that much of the enkephalin in the cells is stored as a precursor that must be converted into enkephalin and released before any effect of protein synthesis inhibition can be seen.

The finding that trypsin breaks down a high molecular weight enkephalin-immunoreactive peak into a peak with the same apparent molecular weight as enkephalin indicates that enkephalin is produced in brain by proteolytic breakdown of a high molecular weight precursor. This precursor is not β-endorphin, since all molecules with molecular weight less than 10,000 were eliminated by ultrafiltration on PM-10 membranes before addition of trypsin. Further characterization on Sephacryl S-200 columns revealed that the precursor in brain is not identical to the 31,000 molecular weight precursor of β-endorphin and ACTH in the pituitary since it has an apparent molecular weight of 50,000 to 70,000. The possibility remains that the β-endorphin precursor could be formed as an intermediate product from the larger enkephalin precursor, but the major differences in regional brain distribution between enkephalin and β-endorphin/β-LPH (3) make this possibility unlikely. Further characterization of the precursor in brain will help to explain the relationships between met-enkephalin, leu-enkephalin, and β-endorphin.

ACKNOWLEDGMENTS

We thank Adele Snowman and Marla Bowman for excellent technical assistance. Supported by USPHS grant DA-1645 and USPHS post-doctoral grant MH-7329 to S.R.C.

REFERENCES

1. Austen, B. M., Smyth, D. G., and Snell, C. R. (1977): γ-Endorphin, α-endorphin and met-enkephalin are formed extracellularly from lipotropin C-fragment. *Nature,* 269:619–621.
2. Barondes, S. H., and Cohen, H. D. (1967): Delayed and sustained effect of acetoxycycloheximide on memory in mice. *Proc. Natl. Acad. Sci. U.S.A.,* 58:157–164.
3. Bloom, F. E., Rossier, J., Battenberg, E. L. F., Bayon, A., French, E., Henriksen, S. J., Siggins, G. R., Segal, D., Browne, R., Ling, N., and Guillemin, R. (1978): β-Endorphin: Cellular localization, electrophysiological and behavioral effects. In: *The Endorphins: Advances in Biochemical Psychopharmacology, Vol. 18,* edited by E. Costa and M. Trabucchi, pp. 89–110. Raven Press, New York.
4. Bradbury, A. F., Smyth, D. G., and Snell, C. R. (1976): Lipotropin: Precursor to two biologically active peptides. *Biochem. Biophys. Res. Commun.,* 69:950–956.
5. Childers, S. R., Simantov, R., and Snyder, S. H. (1977): Enkephalin: Radioimmunoassay and radioreceptor assay in morphine dependent rats. *Eur. J. Pharmacol.,* 46:289–293.
6. Cox, B. M., Goldstein, A., and Li, C. H. (1976): Opioid activity of a peptide, β-lipotropin-(61–91), derived from β-lipotropin. *Proc. Natl. Acad. Sci. U.S.A.,* 73:1821–1823.
7. Flexner, J. B., Flexner, L. B., and Stellar, E. (1963): Memory in mice as affected by intracerebral puromycin. *Science,* 141:57–59.
8. Hughes, J., Smith, T. W., Kosterlitz, H. W., Fothergill, L., Morgan, B. A., and Morris, H. R. (1975): Identification of two related pentapeptides from the brain with potent opiate agonist activity. *Nature,* 258:577–579.
9. Li, C. H., and Chung, D. (1976): Isolation and structure of an untriakontapeptide with opiate activity from camel pituitary glands. *Proc. Natl. Acad. Sci. USA,* 73:1145–1148.
10. Mains, R. E., Eipper, B. A., and Ling, N. (1977): Common precursor to corticotropins and endorphins. *Proc. Natl. Acad. Sci. USA,* 74:3014–3018.
11. Roberts, J. L., and Herbert, E. (1977): Characterization of a common precursor to corticotropin and β-lipotropin: Identification of β-lipotropin peptides and their arrangement relative to corticotropin in the precursor synthesized in a cell-free system. *Proc. Natl. Acad. Sci. USA,* 74:5300–5304.
12. Simantov, R., Childers, S. R., and Snyder, S. H. (1977): Opioid peptides: Differentiation by radioimmunoassay and radioreceptor assay. *Brain Res.,* 135:358–367.
13. Simantov, R., Childers, S. R., and Snyder, S. H. (1978): The opiate receptor binding interactions of [3H]-methionine enkephalin, an opioid peptide. *Eur. J. Pharmacol.,* 47:319–331.
14. Watson, S. J., Barchas, J. D., and Li, C. H. (1977): β-Lipotropin: Localization of cells and axons in rat brain by immunocytochemistry. *Proc. Natl. Acad. Sci. USA,* 74:5155–5158.
15. Yang, H.-Y. T., Hong, J. S., Fratta, W., and Costa, E. (1978): Rat brain enkephalins: Distribution and biosynthesis. In: *The Endorphins: Advances in Biochemical Psychopharmacology, Vol. 18,* edited by E. Costa and M. Trabucchi, pp. 149–160. Raven Press, New York.

*Central Nervous System Effects of Hypothalamic
Hormones and Other Peptides,* edited by Collu et al.
Raven Press, New York © 1979.

Effects of Endogenous Opiate Peptides on Release of Anterior Pituitary Hormones

Joseph Meites, John F. Bruni, and Dean A. Van Vugt

*Department of Physiology, Neuroendocrine Research Laboratory,
Michigan State University, East Lansing, Michigan 48824*

The recent discovery that the brain and pituitary produce opioid peptides has aroused great interest in their physiological functions. There is some evidence that they may serve as neurotransmitters in the brain and influence pain perception and behavior (6). They also may alter secretion of anterior pituitary (AP) hormones. Thus several laboratories have reported that endogenous opiate peptides (EOPs) can elevate serum concentrations of prolactin (PRL) and growth hormone (GH) in the rat (2,4,12). In addition, we have found that methionine-enkephalin and morphine can depress serum levels of LH and TSH in the male rat (2). Earlier work with morphine had shown that it similarly stimulates PRL and GH release, while inhibiting release of gonadotropins and TSH-thyroid function (3). Since high concentrations of EOPs have been found in the hypothalamus (14), these may participate in controlling AP function.

In the present chapter, we review some of the evidence that EOPs and morphine can influence AP hormone secretion, show that they may have a physiological role in regulating AP hormone release, and consider some possible hypothalamic mechanisms by which they may act to alter AP function.

EFFECTS OF MORPHINE, METHIONINE-ENKEPHALIN, AND NALOXONE ON RELEASE OF PRL, GH, LH, FSH, AND TSH

Male Sprague-Dawley rats, weighing approximately 200 to 225 g each, were injected i.p. with morphine sulfate (Mallinkrodt Labs., St. Louis, Mo.), methionine-enkephalin (Bachem, Marina Del Ray, Ca.), naloxone (Endo Labs., Garden City, N.Y.), or combinations of these drugs, in 0.1 ml 0.87% NaCl/100 g body weight at doses indicated in Table 1. The rats (10 per treatment) were decapitated 20 min after injection, and trunk blood was collected and serum separated and kept frozen at $-4°C$ until assayed.

Serum PRL, GH, LH, FSH, and TSH were assayed by standard radio-

TABLE 1. Effects of morphine, methionine-enkephalin, and naloxone on serum PRL, GH, LH, FSH, and TSH

Group (N = 10)	PRL	GH	LH	FSH	TSH
Controls, (0.87% NaCl)	14.8 ± 1.4^a	148 ± 17	22 ± 2	382 ± 19	243 ± 19
Morphine (MOR), (10.0 mg/kg)	47.0 ± 6.0^b	$1,622 \pm 129^b$	10 ± 2^b	384 ± 24	60 ± 10^b
MET-ENK, (5.0 mg/kg)	20.0 ± 4.2	258 ± 62	6 ± 2^b	306 ± 59	84 ± 17^b
Naloxone (NAL), (0.2 mg/kg)	9.0 ± 0.6^b	74 ± 24^b	57 ± 5^b	356 ± 19	207 ± 24
NAL and MOR, (0.2 + 10.0 mg/kg)	27.5 ± 3.8^b	$1,155 \pm 56^b$	16 ± 3	433 ± 48	100 ± 30^b
NAL and MET-ENK, (0.2 + 5.0 mg/kg)	13.9 ± 1.3	149 ± 16	44 ± 5^b	381 ± 35	159 ± 23

From ref. 2.

[a] $\bar{x} \pm$ SEM; all data are expressed in ng/ml serum.

[b] $p < 0.05$ compared with controls.

immunoassay procedures with NIAMDD kits provided by Dr. A. F. Parlow, Harbor General Hospital, Torrance, California. The results are expressed in terms of the standard reference preparations. Analysis of variance and Student-Newman Keuls test for multiple comparisons were used to analyze the data. The data were considered to be significant when $p < 0.05$.

It can be seen (Table 1) that morphine significantly elevated serum PRL and GH, but significantly reduced serum LH and TSH when compared with control values. Morphine had no effect on serum FSH. Methionine (met)-enkephalin produced similar, although mainly smaller, effects on serum hormone levels. Most notable was that naloxone given alone elicited a decrease in serum PRL and GH, an increase in serum LH, and had no effect on serum FSH and TSH. When naloxone was given together with morphine or met-enkephalin, the response to the latter two drugs was partially or completely counteracted.

In a second experiment (Table 2), the same drugs were given, but morphine and naloxone were injected at three dose levels each, as indicated. Essentially similar effects were observed as in the first experiment (Table 1): morphine and met-enkephalin elevated serum PRL and GH but decreased serum LH and TSH; naloxone reduced serum PRL and GH, but elevated serum LH, and in this experiment, also FSH; the combination treatments attenuated the response to any drug given alone.

It is apparent that met-enkephalin, like morphine, acts to stimulate release of PRL and GH, but to inhibit release of LH and TSH. No effect of morphine was observed on serum FSH, in agreement with earlier observations on the action of morphine on FSH secretion (3). These results therefore confirm previous reports on the effects of morphine on AP hormone

TABLE 2. *Dose-response effects of morphine, met-enkephalin, and naloxone on serum PRL, GH, LH, FSH, and TSH*

Group (N = 10)	PRL	GH	LH	FSH	TSH
Controls, (0.87% NaCl)	9.0 ± 0.4^a	131 ± 23	19 ± 1	341 ± 12	232 ± 33
Morphine (MOR), (2.0 mg/kg)	10.1 ± 0.8	839 ± 172^b	8 ± 1^b	340 ± 12	122 ± 13
Morphine, (10.0 mg/kg)	20.2 ± 2.3^b	1211 ± 185^b	9 ± 2^b	387 ± 23	77 ± 7^b
Morphine, (15.0 mg/kg)	18.5 ± 1.2^b	1775 ± 172^b	13 ± 2	333 ± 13	71 ± 9^b
MET-ENK, (5.0 mg/kg)	11.5 ± 0.6	215 ± 27^b	11 ± 2^b	314 ± 20	96 ± 17^b
Naloxone (NAL), (0.2 mg/kg)	4.6 ± 0.4^b	77 ± 10^b	44 ± 5^b	361 ± 15	272 ± 40
Naloxone, (2.0 mg/kg)	4.2 ± 0.3^b	103 ± 40	52 ± 8^b	490 ± 36^b	157 ± 22
Naloxone, (5.0 mg/kg)	4.0 ± 0.3^b	48 ± 6^b	45 ± 8^b	446 ± 29^b	191 ± 25
NAL and MOR, (0.2 + 2.0 mg/kg)	3.6 ± 0.4^b	383 ± 71^b	17 ± 3	384 ± 9	210 ± 13
NAL and MOR, (0.2 + 10.0 mg/kg)	9.0 ± 1.1	902 ± 168^b	14 ± 4	369 ± 16	134 ± 17^b
NAL and MET-ENK, (0.2 + 5.0 mg/kg)	5.4 ± 0.8^b	138 ± 37	17 ± 3	350 ± 18	191 ± 18

From ref. 2.

[a] $\bar{x} \pm$ SEM; all data are expressed in ng/ml serum.

[b] $p < 0.05$ compared with controls.

secretion, and of met-enkephalin and other EOPs on release of PRL and GH. We also show here that met-enkephalin and naloxone can influence release of gonadotropins and TSH.

What is probably most remarkable about these observations are the effects of naloxone, a specific inhibitor of EOPs, on basal levels of several AP hormones. Naloxone inhibited release of PRL and GH, in agreement with similar observations by Shaar et al. (12), but increased release of LH and FSH. This is believed to represent indirect evidence that the EOPs may have a physiological role in maintaining basal AP hormone secretion. The EOPs may chronically stimulate secretion of PRL and GH, and chronically depress secretion of LH and FSH. Further studies will be necessary to determine whether naloxone has similar effects in other species.

INHIBITION BY NALOXONE OF STRESS-INDUCED INCREASE IN PROLACTIN SECRETION

Increased release of PRL in response to many kinds of stress has been reported in man and animals, including rats (9,11). In this study, three types

TABLE 3. *Effects of naloxone (NAL) on basal serum prolactin concentrations[a]*

	Serum PRL (ng/ml)	
Method of bleeding	0.87% NaCl	NAL
Decapitation	16.3 ± 4^b	3.7 ± 0.6^c
Orbital sinus (ether anesthesia)	35.1 ± 4.3	23.9 ± 3.2^c

From ref. 13.
[a] $N = 10$.
[b] $\bar{x} \pm$ SEM.
[c] $p < 0.05$ as compared to controls.

of stresses were administered to male rats, with or without prior injection of naloxone. Male Sprague-Dawley rats, weighing 250 to 300 g each, were injected with naloxone 0.2 mg/kg body weight in 0.2 ml 0.87% NaCl per 100 g body weight or with saline solution alone just prior to stress. The stresses used were: (a) collection of blood by orbital sinus puncture under ether anesthesia as compared to collection of blood from the trunk after rapid decapitation, (b) body restraint achieved by immobilizing the rats, and (c) heat (40°C) stress. Restraint and heat stress were maintained for 30 min.

Table 3 shows that when blood was collected by orbital sinus puncture under ether anesthesia, serum PRL was significantly higher than when collected from trunk blood after decapitation. Prior administration of naloxone reduced serum PRL in the decapitated rats and partially prevented the rise in the rats subjected to orbital sinus puncture and ether. Table 4 shows that restraint or heat stress for 30 min significantly elevated serum PRL as compared to pretreatment values. Naloxone pretreatment completely prevented the rise in serum PRL by restraint stress and partially inhibited the increase in serum PRL by heat stress.

Stress induced by each of the three methods used resulted in a significant increase in serum PRL in male rats, in agreement with previous reports (9,11). Pretreatment with naloxone partially or completely prevented these increases in serum PRL. Independently, Grandison and Guidotti (7) ob-

TABLE 4. *Effects of naloxone (NAL) on stress-induced prolactin release[a]*

	Serum PRL (ng/ml)		
Treatment	Pretreatment	Post-stress	Stress + NAL
Restraint stress	9.8 ± 1.6^b	55.0 ± 14^c	11.6 ± 2.4
Heat stress	18.8 ± 2.1	91.0 ± 8.8^c	38.6 ± 14^c

From ref. 13.
[a] $N = 10$.
[b] $\bar{x} \pm$ SEM.
[c] $p < 0.05$ as compared to controls.

served that naltrexone, another EOP and morphine antagonist, inhibited PRL release induced by intermittent foot shock and ether stress. The present results therefore suggest that the EOPs may have a physiological role in regulating PRL release during stress. It has been demonstrated that an increase in EOP activity occurs in the brain during stress (1), and also that stress results in increased release of β-endorphin as well as ACTH from the pituitary into the blood (8). Since immobilization stress can increase hypothalamic serotonin activity in the rat (11), it may act to stimulate PRL release by increasing EOP activity in the hypothalamus.

EFFECTS OF MORPHINE AND NALOXONE ON
CASTRATION-INDUCED LH RELEASE IN MALE RATS

Castration is known to result in a rapid and sustained elevation of serum gonadotropins in male and female rats. In the present experiment 30 male rats, weighing 225 to 250 g each, were castrated. An additional group of 10 intact rats served as controls. Beginning 2 hr after castration and every 6 hr thereafter, 10 rats were injected i.p. with 0.87% NaCl, 10 with morphine sulfate 10 mg/kg body weight, and 10 with naloxone (0.2 mg/kg body weight). The intact control group was injected i.p. with 0.87% NaCl during the same time periods as the castrated rats. Blood samples were collected for radioimmunoassay of LH by orbital sinus puncture under light ether anesthesia 8, 14, 26, 50, 122, and 170 hr after castration. All blood samples were collected 6 hr after drug or saline administration.

Figure 1 shows that serum LH in the castrated, saline-injected controls

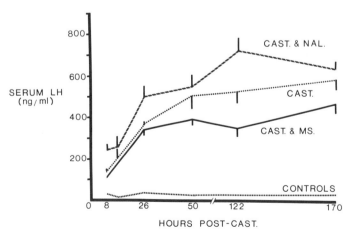

FIG. 1. Effects of castration alone (CAST), castration and naloxone (CAST & NAL), and castration and morphine sulfate (CAST & MS) on serum LH in male rats. Bottom line shows serum LH in intact male rats (CONTROLS). SEM is shown below each line. See text for other details. (From D. A. Van Vugt, J. F. Bruni, and J. Meites, *unpublished.*)

rose rapidly up to 50 hr and remained the same thereafter. Injections of morphine sulfate significantly reduced the rise in serum LH which did not increase after the first 26 hr. Naloxone treatment resulted in a greater increase in serum LH than produced by castration alone. In the intact controls there was no change in serum LH throughout this experiment. These results are believed to provide additional evidence that the EOP may normally exert a chronic inhibition on LH release and prevent a maximum rise in serum LH after castration.

INTERACTIONS OF HYPOTHALAMIC BIOGENIC AMINES WITH EOPs IN MODULATING RELEASE OF AP HORMONES

Hypothalamic biogenic amines have been demonstrated to exert an important influence on secretion of AP hormones, and may act primarily by altering release from nerve terminals in the median eminence of hypothalamic releasing or release-inhibiting factors into the pituitary portal vessels (10). An increase in hypothalamic dopamine (DA) turnover has been shown to be associated with a fall in PRL release, whereas a reduction in hypothalamic DA turnover results in an increase in PRL release (9). Serotonin (5-hydroxytryptamine, 5-HT), in contrast to DA, has been shown to produce an increase in PRL release (9). DA, norepinephrine, and 5-HT in the hypothalamus also have been observed to influence release of other AP hormones (10).

In the present study, the possible interactions of morphine and EOPs with DA and 5-HT on release of PRL were studied in male rats. The following drugs were injected once s.c. into male rats, weighing 225 to 250 g each, in doses shown in Table 5: L-DOPA, the precursor of DA; haloperidol, a dopamine receptor blocker; and morphine sulfate. The control rats were injected with 0.87% NaCl. Blood was collected by orbital sinus puncture under light ether anesthesia before, and 1 and 2 hr after administration of the drugs.

It can be seen (Table 5) that an injection of saline had no effect on serum PRL concentration in the control rats. L-DOPA significantly decreased PRL release for the 2-hr post-injection period, whereas haloperidol significantly increased serum PRL for this period. Morphine sulfate elevated serum PRL by 1 hr after injection, but this effect disappeared by 2 hr. When L-DOPA and morphine were injected simultaneously, the effect of L-DOPA predominated and morphine was unable to stimulate increased PRL release. When haloperidol and morphine were injected together, the rise in serum PRL at the end of the first hour was the same as when either drug was injected alone, and by the second hour the same as when haloperidol was given alone.

The inability of morphine to induce a rise in PRL release in the presence

TABLE 5. Relation of dopamine to morphine-induced increase in serum prolactin

Group	0 hr	1 hr	2 hr
Controls, (0.87% NaCl)	11 ± 1^a	17 ± 3	13 ± 3
L-DOPA, (50 mg/kg)	15 ± 4	3 ± 1^b	6 ± 2^b
Haloperidol (HALO) (1 mg/kg)	15 ± 3	37 ± 3^b	33 ± 3^b
Morphine sulfate, (10 mg/kg)	18 ± 3	36 ± 5^b	17 ± 7
L-DOPA + MOR	13 ± 3	6 ± 2^b	7 ± 2^b
HALO + MOR	15 ± 2	36 ± 2^b	34 ± 2^b

From D. A. Van Vugt, J. F. Bruni, and J. Meites, (unpublished observations).
[a] $\bar{x} \pm$ SEM; all data are expressed in ng/ml serum.
[b] $p < 0.05$ as compared to controls.

of an increase in DA produced by injection of L-DOPA is believed to indicate that morphine and the EOPs stimulate PRL release, at least partly, by decreasing hypothalamic DA turnover. There is recent evidence that met-enkephalin can decrease DA turnover in the median eminence of rats (5). In the presence of both haloperidol and morphine, the effect of haloperidol on PRL release predominated. Presumably because of the dose given, it maximally inhibited DA receptor activity, and any reduction in DA release from nerve terminals in the median eminence by morphine could not further decrease DA activity.

In an additional experiment, haloperidol and morphine were each injected i.p. alone in small doses that produced no significant rise in serum PRL when the rats were killed 1 hr later, but when these same doses of the two drugs were given together, a significant rise in serum PRL was seen (Fig. 2). The combined effect of a reduction in DA evoked by morphine and inhibition of DA receptor activity by haloperidol resulted in stimulation of PRL release. This observation is believed to provide further evidence that morphine and the EOPs elevate PRL release by reducing DA activity in the hypothalamus.

In the next two experiments evidence is provided that the EOPs may act via 5-HT to increase PRL release, and that 5-HT may act via EOPs. When mature male Sprague-Dawley rats were injected i.p. with quipazine, a 5-HT agonist, at doses of 5, 10, or 20 mg/kg body weight and blood was collected 60 min later from the trunk after decapitation, each of the three doses of quipazine significantly elevated serum PRL levels (Fig. 3). Quipazine at doses of 5 or 10 mg/kg given together with 5 mg morphine sulfate, a dose which does not increase prolactin release, produced no greater increase in serum PRL than quipazine alone. However, when naloxone (0.2 mg/kg body

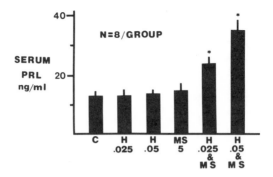

FIG. 2. Effects of haloperidol (H) and morphine sulfate (MS), each alone, and in combination on serum PRL. SEM is shown above each bar, and significant difference from controls (C) is indicated by asterisk. (From J. F. Bruni, D. A. Van Vugt, and J. Meites, *unpublished.*)

weight) was given 30 min before decapitation to rats injected with quipazine (10 or 20 mg/kg), there was a significant reduction in the ability of quipazine to increase PRL release. This may indicate that quipazine acts via the EOPs to increase PRL release, or that naloxone reduced turnover of 5-HT.

The rats were then injected i.p. with fluoxetine (Eli Lilly), a 5-HT re-uptake inhibitor, at a dose of 10 mg/kg; 5-hydroxytryptophan (5-HTP), the precursor of 5-HT, at a dose of 30 mg/kg; or morphine sulfate at a dose of 5 mg/kg. Each drug alone had no effect on serum PRL concentration (Fig. 4). Fluoxetine and 5-HTP, as well as morphine, can each increase PRL release when given at higher doses. When fluoxetine was given together with

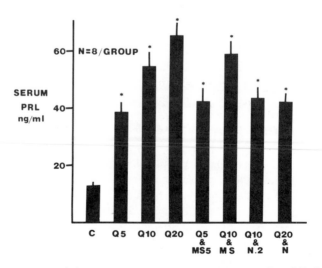

FIG. 3. Effects of quipazine (Q) alone and in combination with morphine sulfate (MS, 5 mg/kg body weight) or naloxone (N, 0.2 mg/kg body weight) on serum PRL. SEM and significant difference from controls are shown above bars. (From J. F. Bruni, D. A. Van Vugt, and J. Meites, *unpublished.*)

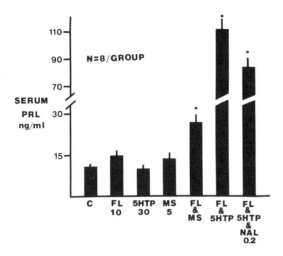

FIG. 4. Effects of fluoxetine (FL), 5-hydroxytryptophan (5HTP), morphine sulfate (MS), and naloxone (NAL) on serum PRL. See text for details. (From J. F. Bruni, D. A. Van Vugt, and J. Meites, *unpublished*.)

morphine or 5-HTP at the same doses as when given alone, a significant rise in serum PRL occurred. When fluoxetine, 5-HTP, and naloxone were given together, naloxone partially inhibited the rise in serum PRL produced by fluoxetine and 5-HTP.

The preceding experiment is believed to provide evidence that the EOPs act to increase PRL release by stimulating 5-HT activity in the hypothalamus. Thus morphine, by increasing 5-HT availability, enhanced the ability of fluoxetine to elevate PRL release. When fluoxetine and 5-HTP were given together with naloxone, the latter reduced the ability of the former two drugs to increase PRL release, presumably by reducing turnover and availability of 5-HT. It can tentatively be concluded that the EOPs promote PRL release either by increasing 5-HT activity in the hypothalamus, by decreasing DA activity, or via both mechanisms.

SUMMARY AND CONCLUSIONS

A single injection of morphine sulfate or met-enkephalin into mature male rats significantly elevated blood serum levels of PRL and GH, but significantly decreased serum levels of LH and TSH. Opposite effects were produced by injection of naloxone, a specific receptor antagonist of morphine and EOPs, which reduced serum levels of PRL and GH, but increased serum LH and FSH. This suggests a role for the EOPs in maintaining basal secretion of these hormones. When morphine or met-enkephalin was injected with naloxone, the effects of the two former drugs on AP hormone release were inhibited. Stress-induced PRL release was completely or partially prevented by prior administration of naloxone, suggesting a role for EOPs on

PRL release during stress. The castration-induced rise in LH release in male rats was partially blocked by morphine administration, and increased above control values by naloxone, suggesting that the EOPs chronically depress LH release and prevent a maximum rise in LH in response to castration.

The above observations are believed to provide strong presumptive evidence that the EOPs are involved in control of AP hormone secretion during different physiological states. This view is strengthened by the finding that the EOPs are present in high concentrations in the hypothalamus (14), the area of the brain directly controlling pituitary function. Further studies are necessary to determine whether changes in physiological states that result in altered pituitary hormone release also produce changes in EOP activity in the hypothalamus.

Through the use of CNS active drugs, evidence was provided that the EOPs may interact with hypothalamic biogenic amines in regulating AP hormone release. Thus the ability of morphine to stimulate PRL release was shown to be inhibited by an increase in hypothalamic DA produced by administering L-DOPA, and to be promoted by inhibition of DA receptor activity by haloperidol. This suggests that morphine and EOPs stimulate PRL release, at least in part, by reducing hypothalamic DA activity. Evidence also was provided that the EOPs may stimulate PRL release by increasing 5-HT activity. Thus morphine enhanced the ability of fluoxetine to increase PRL release, and quipazine, or fluoxetine and 5-HTP given together, showed reduced ability to increase serum PRL levels when naloxone was administered. The stress-induced release of PRL, shown to be associated with an increase in hypothalamic EOP (1) and 5-HT (11) activities, was blocked by prior administration of naloxone (13) or naltrexone (7). The EOPs may act similarly on 5-HT to stimulate GH and inhibit LH and TSH release.

ACKNOWLEDGMENTS

The work reported from our laboratory was supported by NIH Research Grants AM04784 from the National Institute of Arthritis, Metabolism and Digestive Diseases; CA10771 from the National Cancer Institute; AG00416 from the National Institute on Aging; and by the Michigan Agricultural Experiment Station.

REFERENCES

1. Akil, H., Madden, J., Patrick, R. L., and Barchas, J. D. (1976): Stress-induced increase in endogenous opiate peptides: Concurrent analgesia and its partial reversal by naloxone. In: *Opiates and Endogenous Opioid Peptides,* edited by H. W. Kosterlitz, pp. 63–70. North-Holland Publishing Co., Amsterdam.
2. Bruni, J. F., Van Vugt, D., Marshall, S., and Meites, J. (1977): Effects of naloxone, morphine and methionine enkephalin on serum prolactin, luteinizing hormone,

follicle stimulating hormone, thyroid stimulating hormone and growth hormone. *Life Sci.,* 21:461–466.

3. de Wied, D., van Ree, J. M., and de Jong, W. (1974): Narcotic analgesics and the neuroendocrine control of anterior pituitary function. In: *Narcotics and the Hypothalamus,* edited by E. Zimmermann and R. George, pp. 251–264. Raven Press, New York.

4. Dupont, A., Cusan, L., Labrie, F., Coy, D. H., and Li, C. H. (1977): Stimulation of prolactin release in the rat by intraventricular injection of β-endorphin and methionine-enkephalin. *Biochem. Biophys. Res. Commun.,* 75:76–82.

5. Ferland, L., Fuxe, K., Eneroth, P., Gustafsson, J. A., and Skett, P. (1977): Effects of methionine-enkephalin on prolactin release and catecholamine levels and turnover in the median eminence. *Eur. J. Pharmacol.,* 43:89–90.

6. Fredrickson, R. C. A. (1977): Enkephalin pentapeptides—A review of current evidence for a physiological role in vertebrate neurotransmission. *Life Sci.,* 21:23–42.

7. Grandison, L., and Guidotti, A. (1977): Regulation of prolactin release by endogenous opiates. *Nature,* 270:357–359.

8. Guillemin, R., Vargo, T., Rossier, J., Minick, S., Ling, N., Rivier, C., Vale, W., and Bloom, F. (1977): β-Endorphin and adrenocorticotropin are secreted concomitantly by the pituitary gland. *Science,* 197:1367–1369.

9. Meites, J., Lu, K. H., Wuttke, W., Welsch, C. W., Nagasawa, H., and Quadri, S. K. (1972): Recent studies on functions and control of prolactin secretion in rats. *Recent Prog. Horm. Res.,* 28:471–516.

10. Meites, J., Simpkins, J., Bruni, J., and Advis, J. (1977): Role of biogenic amines in control of anterior pituitary hormones. *IRCS J. Med. Sci.,* 5:1–7.

11. Mueller, G. P., Twohy, C. P., Chen, H. T., Advis, J. P., and Meites, J. (1976): Effects of l-tryptophan and restraint stress on hypothalamic and brain serotonin turnover, and pituitary TSH and prolactin release in rats. *Life Sci.,* 18:715–724.

12. Shaar, C. J., Fredrickson, R. C. A., Dininger, N. B., and Jackson, L. (1977): Enkephalin analogues and naloxone modulate the release of growth hormone and prolactin—Evidence for regulation by an endogenous opioid peptide in brain. *Life Sci.,* 21:853–860.

13. Van Vugt, D. A., Bruni, J. F., and Meites, J. (1978): Naloxone inhibition of stress-induced increase in prolactin secretion. *Life Sci.,* 22:85–90.

14. Yang, H. Y., Hong, J. S., and Costa, E. (1977): Regional distribution of leu and met-enkephalin in rat brain. *Neuropharmacology,* 16:303–307.

Central Nervous System Effects of Hypothalamic Hormones and Other Peptides, edited by Collu et al. Raven Press, New York © 1979.

Behavioral Effects of the Brain Opiates Enkephalin and Endorphin

[1]Abba J. Kastin, [2]David H. Coy, [3]Richard D. Olson, [4]Jaak Panksepp, [2]Andrew V. Schally, and [5]Curt A. Sandman

[1]*Endocrinology Section of the Medical Service, and* [2]*Endocrine and Polypeptide Laboratories, Veterans Administration Hospital and Department of Medicine, Tulane University School of Medicine, New Orleans, Louisiana 70146;* [3]*Department of Psychology, University of New Orleans, New Orleans, Louisiana 70122;* [4]*Department of Psychology, Bowling Green State University, Bowling Green, Ohio 43403; and* [5]*Department of Psychology, Ohio State University, Columbus, Ohio 43210*

The isolation of methionine- and leucine-enkephalins (met-EK, leu-EK) from brain tissue and most of the early studies with these natural opiates were performed by investigators in the field of narcotics whose interest and investigations focused on analgesia. Since early attempts at peripheral administration of met-EK failed to produce analgesia, most of the work became confined to central administration where analgesic effects were prominent.

Surprisingly little attention has been given to the fact that met-EK and leu-EK are similar in size to other small peptides known to exist in brain tissue and to exert CNS actions after peripheral administration. The behavioral effects of these other hypothalamic-pituitary peptides have been known for many years. Even though they, like EK, have short half-lives and are rapidly degraded by blood and brain enzymes, they exert central effects that last far longer than these properties would suggest.

The first test used to demonstrate the CNS effects of hypothalamic peptides was the DOPA-potentiation test. Every naturally occurring brain peptide tested in the DOPA-potentiation test has shown activity (20,38). Since other neuropharmacological tests have shown much greater specificity, it might seem that the DOPA-potentiation test is of limited value. However, the dose at which these natural peptides exert their maximum effect in the DOPA-potentiation test is substantially less than the dose at which all psychotropic agents and many analogs of the peptides tested in this assay exert the same effect (38).

Met-EK is one of two compounds shown to be at least 100 times more active in the DOPA-potentiation test than the psychotropic agents for which the test was initially devised by Everett (39). This is particularly remarkable when it is considered that met-EK was administered intraperitoneally (i.p.)

and that the observational period did not start until an hour after the injection, whereas the half-time disappearance is only a few minutes (19). In this assay, a monoamine oxidase inhibitor (pargyline) and D,L-DOPA were used at doses that resulted in minimal increases in behavioral activity. Additional increases in activity produced by the injected peptides were then rated by two methods which gave essentially the same results. The first utilized electronic activity monitors while the second used a rating scale based on observation of the motor activity, jumping, squeaking, and irritability of the mice. The potentiation of these effects by met-EK at doses $\leqslant 0.1$ mg/kg was marked (39).

No effect of met-EK was found in the serotonin-potentiation test, a test similar in design to the DOPA-potentiation except that D,L-5-hydroxytryptophan, a precursor of serotonin, is used in place of the DOPA and additional observational criteria are employed (39). A moderate reduction in foot shock-induced fighting among specially trained mice was seen after administration of low but not high doses of met-EK. This biphasic-type of response has been observed by us previously with other peptides (21) as well as with EK in the DOPA-potentiation test (39).

Some scientists might feel that the neuropharmacological tests described above do not represent "natural" behavior unconfounded by administration of other compounds. Therefore, the second behavioral test of met-EK was performed with food-restricted animals. Fifteen minutes after the i.p. injection of 80 μg/kg met-EK, hungry rats were placed in a complex Warden maze composed of 12 choice points leading either toward a single goal box containing food or into a blind alley. Animals receiving the EK pentapeptide or an analog negotiated the maze significantly faster and made reliably fewer errors than animals receiving the diluent vehicle (22). Preliminary tests tended to exclude an effect of EK on appetite, thirst, olfaction, or general activity sufficient to explain the results. An EK analog with negligible opiate activity in the mouse vas deferens bioassay and little binding affinity for opiate receptors in the brain (8) was also tested in the Warden maze. That rats injected with this analog also tended to run the maze much faster and with fewer errors than controls supported our impression that the behavioral and opiate effects of EK need not parallel each other but could be dissociated (22). This was reinforced by the opposite effects found in this study of a single dose of morphine, although it is likely that a dose of this plant opiate could be found which might give results similar to those of the natural peptide. Perhaps the strongest argument for the dissociation is the absence of analgesic effects of EK injected peripherally (6,11,25,37,43). That the actual percent of peptide crossing the blood-brain barrier might be small (19) is essentially irrelevant to this point since only a minute amount might be effective (18).

The results of these first two studies involving the DOPA-potentiation test and 12-choice maze were published in 1976. Unfortunately, they were the only ones appearing before 1978 which described behavioral actions of any natural brain opiates after peripheral administration. More recently EK has been administered to rats by the peripheral route in some other systems.

The DOPA-potentiation assay mentioned previously in this chapter has been considered an animal model of mental depression because of the activity of known antidepressant compounds in the tests. A new animal model sensitive to antidepressant treatments was described in 1977 (40). The report suggests that a rat forced to swim in an inescapable situation will eventually cease vigorous activity and make only the minimal motions required to keep its head above water. Administration of the tricyclic antidepressant imipramine reverses this "helpless" behavior. We recently found that at the dose of 1 mg/kg i.p., EK was among the most potent peptides used in an attempt to duplicate this action of imipramine (23). The observed effect was of reduced immobility which resulted from maintenance of the initial swimming activity.

Increased immobility and decreased swimming was found in goldfish tested in a paradigm of habituation with the D-Ala^2 analog of β-endorphin (β-END). This diminished activity was observed after administration of the peptide peripherally as well as into the brain cavity (31). The intracranially (i.c.) administered END acted faster than the peripherally administered material making it unlikely that the immobility originated in the periphery. The greater immobility after i.c. than i.p. injections of the β-END analog suggested the possibility of some difficulty with penetration of the blood-brain barrier by this larger peptide at the dose used (8 μg/kg). The latencies after i.c. and i.p. injections of the smaller EK analog were similar by these two routes, but since the effects were not significantly different from those obtained after injection of the diluent, penetration into the brain may not have occurred. In this regard, it has been reported that the blood-brain barrier of the goldfish is similar to that of laboratory mammals (4,30), as are the opiate receptor binding sites (36). In addition, the goldfish offers the major convenience of easy cranial injection through the cartilagenous covering of the brain.

Several opiate peptides and other compounds were injected, therefore, both i.p. and i.c., and motor activity was measured (32). In general, the effects of the materials injected into the brain cavity were manifested after 3 min, but the effects of the same dose of material injected i.p. took about twice as long. In addition, large i.c. doses of D-Ala^2-β-END have been observed in a preliminary study to reduce the electrical discharge rate of a species of electric fish, *Eigenmannia virescens* (R. D. Olson, A. J. Kastin, G. F. Michell, and D. H. Coy, *unpublished observations*).

Behavioral effects had been incidentally observed in rats injected centrally with β-endorphin. However, as with enkephalin, there was not much interest in performing studies in which the endorphins were administered i.p. This was due to the belief that the i.p. route was ineffective since it had failed to produce substantial analgesia, and to the fact that the importance of the behavioral effects was not yet widely accepted. Only a few studies have been performed in which the ENDs were injected peripherally in higher vertebrates.

In one of these studies, α-, β-, and γ-END as well as the D-Ala^2 analogs of these three ENDs were injected i.p. at the fixed dose of 100 μg/rat. Observations were made of sexual arousal, running time from the center of the field to a wall (as an index of withdrawal from a novel setting), general motor activity, hindleg rearing, grooming, and defecations (as a conventional measure of emotionality). Either the parent compound or an analog of each END seemed to affect some measure of open field behavior, although the number of rats tested was relatively small and a replication might show less specificity. One of the β-ENDs significantly increased grooming behavior, one of the α-ENDs increased sexual arousal, and the γ-ENDs increased time-to-wall or defecations (47). The D-Ala^2 analogs of the three ENDs produced dose-dependent analgesia i.c.v. which was more prolonged than that of the parent compounds; course tremors have also been observed with these peptides (50). Incubation of each of these ENDs for short periods with brain extracts revealed that substitution of D-Ala^2 significantly retarded the action of brain aminopeptidases but did not prevent cleavages by endopeptidases (13).

In another study involving peripheral injection of β-END and D-Ala^2-Met-EK-NH$_2$, the distress vocalizations accompanying social isolation of chicks were significantly reduced (35). The effect of the EK analog in this sensitive model was greater than that of an equimolar (400 nM/kg) amount of β-END when injected subcutaneously (s.c.) but not when administered i.c.v. Plant opiates are also able to diminish distress vocalizations, so that the effect would seem to be mediated by opiate receptors (15,34). It is reasonable to expect that the smaller EK could enter the brain faster after i.p. injection than the larger β-END, but analgesic effects in other species injected peripherally are easier to detect after β-END than after EK. This might be explained by a nonopiate component to the system, a species difference in degradation or sensitivity, or incomplete development of the blood-brain barrier in young chicks.

All the behavioral studies mentioned so far have involved injection of EK or END by the more convenient peripheral route. Despite the known short half-life of EK and END, and our own observations of the rapid degradation and half-time disappearance of brain opiates (13,19), we had come to feel that such considerations were not pertinent for an evaluation of behavioral effects after peripheral administration. This was based on our previous experience with other brain peptides which are rapidly degraded by rat blood yet exert CNS actions that last much longer than the intact compound in the bloodstream. Although susceptibility of EK and END to degradation helped guide the synthesis of analogs with enhanced opiate activity

(5,8,13), it did not obscure our belief that the brain opiates resemble other brain peptides which are likely to have CNS effects apart from the activity for which they were first described, and that these effects can be observed after peripheral injection.

Valuable information on the behavioral effects of EK and more particularly END has been acquired from studies involving i.c.v. administration. Some of these effects are clearly opiate related, such as emesis and hyperthermia (7), drive reduction by self-administration (2), and increased multiple-unit electrical activity in the periaqueductal gray matter (46). Other behavioral actions after i.c.v. injections are also being found by several investigators. These include effects in monkeys (Olson, Olson, Wolf, Coy, and Kastin, *unpublished observations*).

Two papers using centrally injected β-END which attracted considerable attention appeared in the same issue of *Science* (3,17). General observations of rats injected centrally with this larger brain opiate of 31 amino acids resulted in marked immobility which both groups of investigators described as resembling catatonia. However, one of these groups has recently criticized the other for speaking of a "cataleptic-like" state (42). This may seem like quibbling over semantics, but it has implications as to whether one predicts that ENDs are involved as agonists or antagonists in schizophrenia and whether naloxone would be effective therapy. That is, Jacquet and Marks (17) apparently expect a deficiency of β-END in certain forms of psychopathology, whereas the groups at the Salk Institute expect excessive endorphin to be involved (3,42).

Guillemin has spoken at many meetings of the tranquilizing effect of α-END, the violent effects of γ-END, and the catatonic effect of β-END.[13a] These speculations have been extended to an inconclusive point by a recent clinical study (24). In this report, beneficial effects of peripherally administered β-END were found in schizophrenic and depressed patients. Although the study did not involve the use of a placebo, one cannot help but recall that the DOPA-potentiation test, as well as another assay mentioned above, is considered by some investigators as animal models of mental depression. If β-END is effective in mental depression, met-EK should also be tested in this condition. Increased levels of END-like materials have been reported in the spinal fluid of chronic schizophrenics (45), but the effectiveness in schizophrenia (14) of opiate antagonists has not been confirmed (9,29). The causative material may be β-leu^5-END which appears to have been isolated from dialysates of schizophrenic patients (33), although there is some controversy about the benefits of dialysis in schizophrenia (10,26, 48,51) and other aspects of the problem.

Other behavioral effects of β-END have been observed in laboratory animals after central administration. One of the earliest was increased grooming (12), a morphine-like effect (1), and this was extended to include increased sexual behavior (28), as we had observed with centrally administered EKs (49) and β-END (50) as well as peripherally administered ENDs (47). The decreased general motor activity after central administration of β-END has been observed by many additional investigators (16,44) and extended to operant behavior; a dose-dependent suppression of lever pressing for food by hungry rats was found after β-END administered i.c.v. (27) as well as peripherally (Sandman et al., *unpublished observations*). Distress vocalizations accompanying social isolation of chicks were significantly reduced by i.c.v. injection of all the opiate peptides tested; these included met-EK, D-Ala^2-met-EK-NH$_2$, β-END, D-Ala^2-β-END, D-Ala^2-α-END, and D-Ala^2-γ-END (35). All but the met-EK were reliably active in doses as low as 100 pmoles, and the effect was reversed by naloxone.

Foot shock is a frequently employed behavioral tool known to increase the blood levels of many hormones, including α-MSH and ACTH. Recently, shock was also found to increase β-END levels in blood, but not brain (41). It is to be expected that more behavioral studies will be performed with EK, END, and their analogs as their similarity to other brain peptides is better appreciated.

CONCLUSIONS

The brain opiates EK and END have been studied extensively for their analgesic effects. Many of the behavioral actions, some of which have been observed incidentally, can be related to their opiate actions. Other effects, which may be dissociated from analgesia, were sought because of recognition that these natural opiates could be expected to share behavioral actions with other brain peptides. In spite of rapid degradation and brief duration as intact molecules in the circulation, peripheral administration of EK or EN was found to increase markedly the activity of mice in the DOPA-potentiation test and of rats in another model of depression, facilitate the running of a complex maze by hungry rats, immobilize goldfish in a habituation paradigm, affect open-field behavior, increase grooming and sexual arousal, and reduce distress vocalizations of chicks accompanying social isolation. The immobility observed after central administration of β-END has been related to similar states observed in schizophrenia, and apparently favorable clinical effects have been reported in a preliminary, unblinded study; mental depression may also have been improved, as might be anticipated from animal studies. It is expected that the actions of EK, END, and their analogs will resemble those of other brain peptides known to have CNS effects that may be involved in behavioral systems.

REFERENCES

1. Ayhan, I. H., and Randrup, A. (1973): Behavioral and pharmacological studies on morphine-induced excitation of rats. Possible relation to brain catecholamines. *Psychopharmacologia,* 29:317–328.

2. Belluzzi, J. D., and Stein, L. (1977): Enkephalin may mediate euphoria and drive-reduction reward. *Nature,* 266:556–558.

3. Bloom, F., Segal, D., Ling, N., and Guillemin, R. (1976): Endorphins: Profound behavioral effects in rats suggest new etiological factors in mental illness. *Science,* 194:630–632.

4. Brightman, M. W., Reese, T. S., Olsson, Y., and Klatzo, I. (1971): Morphologic aspects of the blood-brain barrier to peroxidase in elasmobranchs. In: *Progress in Neuropathology, Vol. 1,* edited by H. M. Zimmerman, pp. 146–161. Grune & Stratton, New York.

5. Britton, D. R., Fertel, R., Coy, D. H., and Kastin, A. J. (1978): The effect of enkephalin and endorphin analogs on receptors in the mouse vas deferens. *Biochem. Pharmacol. (in press).*

6. Chang, J. K., Fong, B. T. W., Pert, A., and Pert, C. B. (1976): Opiate receptor affinities and behavioral effects of enkephalin: Structure-activity relationship of ten synthetic peptide analogues. *Life Sci.,* 18:1473–1482.

7. Clark, W. G. (1977): Emetic and hyperthermic effects of centrally injected methionine-enkephalin in cats. *Proc. Soc. Exp. Biol. Med.,* 154:540–542.

8. Coy, D. H., Kastin, A. J., Schally, A. V., Morin, O., Caron, N. G., Labrie, F., Walker, J. M., Fertel, R., Berntson, G. G., and Sandman, C. A. (1976): Synthesis and opioid activities of stereoisomers and other D-amino acid analogs of methionine-enkephalin. *Biochem. Biophys. Res. Commun.,* 73:632–638.

9. Davis, G. C., Bunney, W. E., Jr., DeFraites, E. G., Kleinman, J. E., van Kammen, D. P., Post, R. M., and Wyatt, R. J. (1977): Intravenous naloxone administration in schizophrenia and affective illness. *Science,* 197:74–76.

10. Ferris, G. N. (1977): Letter to the editor. *Am. J. Psychiatry,* 134:1310.

11. Frederickson, R. C. A. (1977): Enkephalin pentapeptides—A review of current evidence for a physiological role in vertebrate neurotransmission. *Life Sci.,* 21: 23–42.

12. Gispen, W. H., Wiegant, V. M., Bradbury, A. F., Hulme, E. C., Smyth, D. G., Snell, C. R., and de Wied, D. (1976): Induction of excessive grooming in the rat by fragments of lipotropin. *Nature,* 264:794–795.

13. Grynbaum, A., Kastin, A. J., Coy, D. H., and Marks, N. (1977): Breakdown of enkephalin and endorphin analogs by brain extracts. *Brain Res. Bull.,* 2:479–484.

13a. Guillemin, R. *Chemical and Engineering News,* August 16, 1976. p. 18.

14. Gunne, L. M., Lindstrom, L., and Terenius, L. (1977): Naloxone-induced reversal of schizophrenic hallucinations. *J. Neural Transm.,* 40:13–19.

15. Herman, B. H., and Panksepp, J. (1978): Effects of morphine and naloxone on separation distress and approach attachment: Evidence for opiate mediation of social affect. *Pharmacol. Biochem. Behav. (in press).*

16. Izumi, K., Motomatsu, T., Chrétien, M., Butterworth, R. F., Lis, M., Seidah, N., and Barbeau, A. (1977): β-Endorphin induced akinesia in rats: Effect of apomorphine and α-methyl-p-tyrosine and related modifications of dopamine turnover in the basal ganglia. *Life Sci.,* 20:1149–1156.

17. Jacquet, Y. F., and Marks, N. (1976): The C-fragment of β-lipotropin: An endogenous neuroleptic or antipsychotogen? *Science,* 194:632–635.

18. Kastin, A. J., Coy, D. H., Schally, A. V., and Miller, L. H. (1978): Peripheral administration of hypothalamic peptides results in CNS changes. *Pharmacol. Res. Commun* 10:293–312.

19. Kastin, A. J., Nissen, C., Schally, A. V., and Coy, D. H. (1976): Blood-brain barrier, half-time disappearance, and brain distribution for labelled enkephalin and a potent analog. *Brain Res. Bull.,* 1:583–589.

20. Kastin, A. J., Plotnikoff, N. P., Schally, A. V., and Sandman, C. A. (1976): Endocrine and CNS effects of hypothalamic peptides and MSH. In: *Reviews of Neuroscience,* edited by S. Ehrenpreis and I. J. Kopin, pp. 111–148. Raven Press, New York.

21. Kastin, A. J., Sandman, C. A., Schally, A. V., and Ehrensing, R. H. (1978): Clinical effects of hypothalamic-pituitary peptides upon the central nervous system.

In: *Clinical Neuropharmacology, Vol. 3,* edited by H. L. Klawans, pp. 133–152. Raven Press, New York.

22. Kastin, A. J., Scollan, E. L., King, M. G., Schally, A. V., and Coy, D. H. (1976): Enkephalin and a potent analog facilitate maze performance after intraperitoneal administration in rats. *Pharmacol. Biochem. Behav.,* 5:691–695.

23. Kastin, A. J., Scollan, E., Ehrensing, R. H., Schally, A. V., and Coy, D. H. (1978): Enkephalin and other peptides reduce "passiveness." *Biochem. Behav. (in press).*

24. Kline, N. S., Li, C. H., Lehmann, H. E., Lajtha, A., Laski, E., and Cooper, T. (1977): β-Endorphin-induced changes in schizophrenic and depressed patients. *Arch. Gen. Psychiatry,* 34:1111–1113.

25. Kosterlitz, H. W., and Hughes, J. (1977): Peptides with morphine-like action in the brain. *Br. J. Psychiatry,* 130:298–304.

26. Levy, N. B. (1977): Letter to the editor. *Am. J. Psychiatry,* 134:1311.

27. Lichtblau, L., Fossom, L. H., and Sparber, S. B. (1977): β-Endorphin: Dose-dependent suppression of fixed-ratio operant behavior. *Life Sci.,* 21:927–932.

28. Meyerson, B. J., and Terenius, L. (1977): β-Endorphin and male sexual behavior. *Eur. J. Pharmacol.,* 42:191–192.

29. Mielke, D. H., and Gallant, D. M. (1977): An oral opiate antagonist in chronic schizophrenia: A pilot study. *Am. J. Psychiatry,* 134:1430–1431.

30. Murray, M., Jones, H., Cserr, H. F., and Rall, D. P. (1975): The blood-brain barrier and ventricular system of *Myxine glutinosa. Brain Res.,* 99:17–33.

31. Olson, R. D., Kastin, A. J., Michell, G. F., Olson, G. A., Coy, D. H., and Montalbano, D. M. (1978): Effects of endorphin and enkephalin analogs in fear habituation in goldfish. *Pharmacol. Biochem. Behav. (in press).*

32. Olson, R. D., Kastin, A. J., Montalbano, D. M., Olson, G. A., Coy, D. H., and Michell, G. F. (1978): Neuropeptides and the blood-brain barrier in goldfish. *Pharmacol. Biochem. Behav. (in press).*

33. Palmour, R. M., Ervin, F. R., Wagemaker, H., and Cade, R. (1977): Characterization of a peptide derived from the serum of psychiatric patients. *Soc. Neurosci.,* 3:320 (abst.).

34. Panksepp, J., Herman, B., Conner, R., Bishop, P., and Scott, J. P. (1978): The biology of social attachments: Opiates alleviate separation distress. *Biol. Psychiatry (in press).*

35. Panksepp, J., Vilberg, T., Bean, N. J., Coy, D. H. and Kastin, A. J. (1978): Reduction of distress vocalization in chicks by opiate-like peptides. *Brain Res. Bull. (in press).*

36. Pert, D., Aposhian, D., and Snyder, S. (1974): Phylogenetic distribution of opiate receptor bindings. *Brain Res.,* 75:356–361.

37. Pert, C. B., Pert, A., Chang, J. K., and Fong, B. T. W. (1976): (D-Ala²)-Met-enkephalin-amide: A potent, long-lasting synthetic pentapeptide analgesic. *Science,* 194:330–332.

38. Plotnikoff, N. P., and Kastin, A. J. (1977): Neuropharmacological review of hypothalamic releasing factors. In: *Neuropeptide Influences on Brain and Behavior Mechanisms,* edited by L. H. Miller, C. A. Sandman, and A. J. Kastin, pp. 81–107. Raven Press, New York.

39. Plotnikoff, N. P., Kastin, A. J., Coy, D. H., Christensen, C. W., Schally, A. V., and Spirtes, M. A. (1976): Neuropharmacological actions of enkephalin after systemic administration. *Life Sci.,* 19:1283–1288.

40. Porsolt, R. D., LePichon, M., and Jalfre, M. (1977): Depression: A new animal model sensitive to antidepressant treatments. *Nature,* 266:730–732.

41. Rossier, J., French, E. D., Rivier, C., Ling, N., Guillemin, R., and Bloom, F. (1977): Foot-shock induced stress increases β-endorphin levels in blood but not brain. *Nature,* 270:618–620.

42. Segal, D. S., Browne, R. G., Bloom, F., Ling, N., and Guillemin, R. (1977): β-Endorphin: Endogenous opiate or neuroleptic? *Science,* 198:411–413.

43. Snyder, S. G. (1977): Public Lecture: The Brain's Own Morphine and Its Receptor. Presented at Seventh Annual Meeting of Society for Neuroscience, Nov. 7–9, Anaheim, California.

44. Tache, Y., Lis, M., and Collu, R. (1977): Effects of thyrotropin-releasing hormone on behavioral and hormonal changes induced by β-endorphin. *Life Sci.,* 21:841–846.
45. Terenius, L., Wahlstrom, A., Lindstrom, L., and Widerlov, E. (1976): Increased CSF levels of endorphines in chronic psychosis. *Neurosci. Lett.,* 3:157–162.
46. Urca, G., Frenk, H., Liebeskind, J. C., and Taylor, A. N. (1977): Morphine and enkephalin: Analgesic and epileptic properties. *Science,* 197:83–86.
47. Veith, J. L., Sandman, C. A., Walker, J. M., Coy, D. H., and Kastin, A. J. (1978): Systemic administration of the endorphins selectively alters open field behavior of rats. *Physiol. Behav.* 20:539–542.
48. Wagemaker, H., Jr., and Cade, R. (1977): The use of hemodialysis in chronic schizophrenia. *Am. J. Psychiatry,* 134:684–685.
49. Walker, J. M., Berntson, G. G., Sandman, C. A., Coy, D. H., Schally, A. V., and Kastin, A. J. (1977): An analogue of enkephalin having a prolonged opiate-like effect in vivo. *Science,* 196:85–87.
50. Walker, J. M., Sandman, C. A., Berntson, G. G., McGivern, R., Coy, D. H., and Kastin, A. J. (1977): Endorphin analogs with potent and long-lasting analgesic effects. *Pharmacol. Biochem. Behav.,* 7:543–548.
51. Weddington, W. W. (1977): Letter to the editor. *Am. J. Psychiatry,* 134:1310.

Central Nervous System Effects of Hypothalamic Hormones and Other Peptides, edited by Collu et al. Raven Press, New York © 1979.

Evidence for a Role of Endorphins in the Control of Prolactin Secretion

André Dupont, Lionel Cusan, Louise Ferland, André Lemay, and Fernand Labrie

Laboratory of Molecular Endocrinology, Le Centre Hospitalier de l'Université Laval; and Department of Obstetrics and Gynecology, Hôpital St-François d'Assise, Quebec, Canada

The opiates morphine and methadone are well known to be potent stimuli of growth hormone (GH) release in the rat (24,30,31,68). Stimulation of lactation by morphine administration has provided the first indication of a stimulation of prolactin release by the opiate (44). This suggestion was later confirmed by direct measurement of plasma prolactin (PRL) levels (42).

Following reports of the presence of endogenous opiate activity in the brain (25,51,63), the pentapeptide H-Tyr-Gly-Gly-Phe-Met-OH (methionine-enkephalin) has been isolated from porcine (26) and calf (62) brain. The sequence of this peptide is the same as the N-terminus of the C-fragment (β-LPH$_{61\text{-}91}$, also called β-endorphin) of β-lipotropin first isolated from sheep pituitaries (37). The peptide called β-endorphin first isolated and characterized from camel pituitary glands (38) was shown to possess potent opiate activity when assayed *in vitro* (6,8,9,26,36,38,39,45) and *in vivo* (40).

These findings raised the possibility that methionine-enkephalin (met-enkephalin) and β-endorphin, in addition to their well-known analgesic effect (6,40) and their activity as behavior modulators (5), could be involved in the neuroendocrine control of PRL and GH secretion. The present chapter describes the stimulatory effect of met-enkephalin and β-endorphin on PRL and GH release in the rat. Moreover, when the opiate antagonist naloxone is used, the present data indicate a role of endorphins in the stimulation of prolactin release induced by stress and suckling in the rat as well as in the nocturnal rise of prolactin secretion in the human. Since recent evidence indicates that dopamine may be the main or even the only inhibitory substance of hypothalamic origin controlling prolactin secretion, we investigated the role of dopamine in the potent stimulatory action of opiates on prolactin secretion.

MATERIALS AND METHODS

Animals

Adult male and female Sprague-Dawley rats (obtained from Canadian Breeding Farms, St. Constant, Quebec) weighing 225 to 275 g on arrival, were kept in a sound-attenuated and temperature-controlled room (24 ± 2°C) and illuminated from 0500 to 1900 hr. Purina rat chow and water were available *ad libitum*.

Intraventricular Injections

In order to minimize stress-induced inhibition of GH release, animals were handled twice a day for 7 to 10 days before insertion of a catheter (Venocath No. 18, Abbott) into the right superior vena cava under thiamylal (Surital) (50 mg/kg, i.p.) anesthesia. The animals were then implanted stereotaxically with a metallic cannula (gauge 24) in the left lateral ventricle. The cannula was fixed to the skull with a polymerizing acrylate (Yates Flash Acrylic). This chronic technique permits a minimum of manipulations of the animal at the time of the experiment performed 2 days after implantation of the cannulas.

Animals were then injected intravenously through the intrajugular catheter with 0.2 ml of sheep somatostatin antiserum 5 min before injection of the peptides to be tested or the vehicle alone (40μl of 0.9% NaCl) over a 3-min period. Samples of 0.7 ml of blood were than withdrawn into heparinized syringes at the indicated time intervals. A volume of 0.7 ml of saline containing heparin was injected after each blood sampling to minimize extracellular volume changes. Plasma was separated by centrifugation at 1,200 × g for 40 min at 2 to 4°C and kept at −20°C until assayed.

Ether Stress

Male rats bearing a permanent cannula inserted into the jugular vein 2 days previously were injected subcutaneously with 10 mg/kg of naloxone 10 min before being placed for 1 to 2 min in an ether chamber. Blood samples (0.7 ml) were withdrawn in heparinized syringes at the indicated time intervals. After each blood sampling, 0.7 ml of 0.9% NaCl containing heparin was injected through the catheter to mantain blood volume.

Suckling

Two days after delivery, mothers were anesthetized with thiamylal (50 mg/kg, i.p.) and a permanent cannula was inserted into the jugular vein. Two days later, pups were separated from their mothers at 0800 hr. Six hours later, the animals received an intravenous injection of 5 mg/kg of naloxone 5 min before return of the pups. Blood samples were withdrawn at the time intervals indicated in Fig. 5.

Hormone Measurements

Rat plasma GH and PRL were measured in duplicate by double-antibody radioimmunoassays (2,49) using rat hormones (GH-1-2, PRL-I-1, GH-

RP-1, and PRL-RP-1) and rabbit antisera (anti-GH-S-2 and anti-PRL-S-2) kindly provided by Dr. A. F. Parlow for the National Institute of Arthritis and Metabolic Diseases, Rat Pituitary Hormone Program.

Calculations

Radioimmunoassay data were analyzed with a Hewlett-Packard desktop calculator using a program written in this laboratory and based on model II of Rodbard and Lewald (58). Data are expressed as mean ± SEM. Statistical significance was evaluated according to the multiple-range test of Duncan-Kramer (33).

RESULTS

Stimulatory Effect of β-Endorphin and Met-Enkephalin on PRL and GH Release

As illustrated in Fig. 1A, the intraventricular injection of 0.5 to 25 μg of β-endorphin (β-LPH$_{61-91}$) led to a rapid and important stimulation of PRL release in unanesthetized, freely moving rats. With the 0.5-μg dose, a sig-

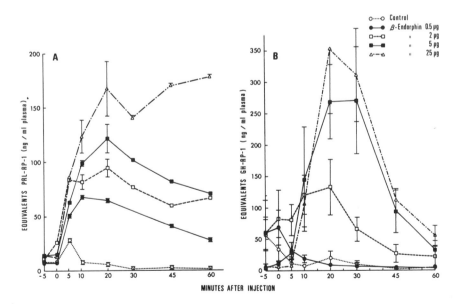

FIG. 1. Effect of increasing doses of β-endorphin on plasma PRL (A) and GH (B) levels in the rat. Male rats bearing intraventricular and intrajugular cannulas were injected intravenously with 0.2 ml of sheep somatostatin antiserum 5 min before the intraventricular injection of the indicated amounts of synthetic β-endorphin. PRL and GH concentrations were measured at the indicated time intervals after administration of β-endorphin to 8 to 10 animals per group. β-Endorphin was synthesized by solid-phase methods as described (10). Data are mean ± SEM.

nificant rise was already measured 5 min after injection of the peptide and a maximal stimulation (approximately sevenfold) was measured after 10 min with a slow decrease of plasma hormone levels at later time intervals. The higher doses of β-endorphin (2, 5, and 25 μg) led to a progressive increase of PRL release, a 30- to 60-fold increase being measured between 20 and 60 min after injection of 25 μg of the peptide.

Although inactive at 0.5 μg, doses of 2 μg and higher of β-endorphin led to a significant stimulation of plasma GH release. With the 2-μg dose, a 6- to 10-fold stimulation of the plasma GH concentration was measured 10 and 20 min after injection of β-endorphin, with a progressive decrease to basal levels reached at 45 min. The two higher doses (5 and 25 μg) of β-endorphin led to a 20- to 30-fold stimulation of plasma GH levels measured 20 and 30 min after injection of the peptide.

As shown in Fig. 2, met-enkephalin, the NH_2-terminal pentapeptide of β-endorphin, was much less potent than β-endorphin in stimulating PRL and GH release. In fact, at the 500- and 1,000-μg doses, met-enkephalin led to approximately four- and sixfold increases of plasma PRL levels, respectively. Maximal stimulation was measured 10 to 20 min after injection of the pentapeptide with a rapid return to basal levels between 30 and 45 min. It can be seen in Fig. 2B that stimulation of GH release was observed only at the 1,000-μg dose, thus indicating a greater sensitivity of the PRL than GH responses to the opioid peptide.

Specificity of the stimulatory effect of β-endorphin on PRL and GH re-

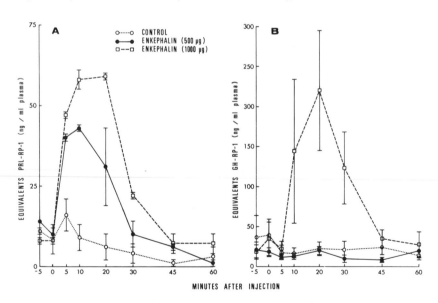

FIG. 2. Effect of 0.5 or 1.0 mg of met-enkephalin on plasma PRL (A) and GH (B) levels in the rat. The experiment was performed as described in Fig. 1. Met-enkephalin was synthesized by solid-phase methods as described (10).

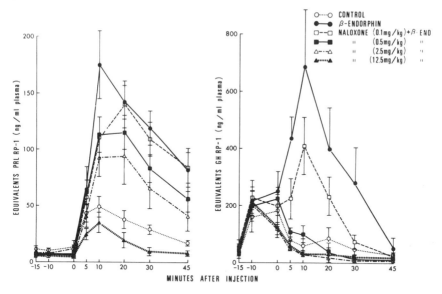

FIG. 3. Effect of increasing doses of naloxone on plasma PRL and GH release induced by intraventricular injection of 5 μg of β-endorphin in the rat. The experiment was performed as described in Fig. 1 except that naloxone was injected in the indicated groups 10 min before β-endorphin administration.

lease is illustrated in Fig. 3 where naloxone, a specific opiate antagonist, completely blocked the stimulation of GH release (B) at a dose of 0.5 mg/kg, whereas the highest dose of naloxone (12.5 mg) was required to completely abolish the rise of PRL secretion. This higher resistance of the PRL than GH response to naloxone might be due to a greater sensitivity of PRL than GH release to the stimulatory action of opiate peptides. This possibility is supported by the data of Figs. 1 and 2 where changes of PRL release were observed earlier and at lower doses compared to GH after β-endorphin and met-enkephalin injection. A similar preferential release of PRL has been observed after injection of β-endorphin into the cisterna magna of steroid-primed rats (56). It is also possible that these effects could be secondary to access of β-endorphin and/or naloxone to their sites of action on PRL and GH release.

The stimulatory effect of met-enkephalin on PRL and GH release is much lower than that of β-endorphin. In fact, the present data demonstrated that β-endorphin is 2,000 times more potent than met-enkephalin in stimulating prolactin and GH secretion. The analgesic action of met-enkephalin is also much weaker than that of β-endorphin when the agents are injected intracerebrally (8,39,40). This difference of biological activity is in marked contrast to the relative affinities of the two peptides for the opiate receptor; met-enkephalin shows a binding affinity for the opiate receptor approximately three times higher than β-endorphin (17). These data indicate that the higher potency of β-endorphin is probably due to its higher resistance to degradation.

It is of interest, in this connection, to mention that met-enkephalin is rapidly inactivated by plasma and brain tissue. Indeed, at 15 sec after i.v. injection of [³H]met-enkephalin, only 5% of total radioactivity co-migrated with intact met-enkephalin, whereas 74% of the radioactivity was eluted in the area corresponding to tyrosine (14). The long-lasting activity of [D-Ala²]met-enkephalin reported previously (11) indicates the importance of the Tyr-Gly amide bond for action of the degrading enzyme in plasma and various tissues. β-Endorphin and its [D-Ala²] analog displayed similar potency as stimulators of GH and PRL release when injected intraventricularly, but [D-Ala²]β-endorphin injected intravenously led to an increased duration of action of the peptide relative to the native molecule (35).

The stimulatory effect of morphine (21), β-endorphin (15,16), met-enkephalin (15,16), and the endorphin analogs (11) on GH release is observed in animals where circulating somatostatin should be neutralized by excess somatostatin antiserum, suggesting that the endogenous tetradecapeptide does not play an important role in the release of GH induced by opiates. Since opiate peptides cannot stimulate GH release from pituitary cells *in vitro,* it is more likely that the observed GH release is due to stimulated release of hypothalamic GH-releasing activity (GH-RH).

Role of Opiates in Stress- and Suckling-Induced Release of Prolactin in the Rat

Adult release of prolactin in the rat is well known to be induced by suckling (4,64) and a variety of stressful stimuli such as ether, surgery, restraint, nicotine injection, exposure to cold or heat, or simple venous puncture (3,18,28,47,53,67). Stress stimulates serum prolactin levels in the human, the response being higher in women than men (48). Moreover, suckling increases prolactin release in women (57). It was thus of interest to study the possible role of endorphins in the acute release of prolactin induced by stress and suckling. When the specific opiate antagonist naloxone is used, the present data provide evidence for such a role of endorphins.

Ether Stress

In agreement with previous data (47,66), it can be seen in Fig. 4 that exposure to ether vapor led to a rapid stimulation of plasma release. A maximal effect was already seen at 5 min with a progressive decrease toward control levels at 30 min. When the opiate antagonist naloxone (10 mg/kg) was injected 10 min before exposure to ether, the stimulation of prolactin release was completely abolished ($p < 0.01$).

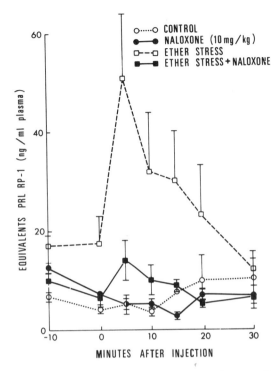

FIG. 4. Inhibitory effect of naloxone on prolactin release induced by ether stress. The experiment was performed as described in Materials and Methods. Data are mean ± SEM.

Suckling

As illustrated in a representative experiment shown in Fig. 5, a single injection of naloxone (5 mg/kg) 5 min before return of the pups led to a 50 to 95% inhibition of the marked rise of plasma prolactin induced by suckling up to the last time interval studied (90 min). In complementary experiments were naloxone was injected at −10, 45, and 90 min, plasma prolactin levels were still reduced from 600 ± 95 to 115 ± 40 ng/ml 2 hr after the start of suckling (data not shown).

The present data clearly indicate that endogenous opiate peptides could be involved as mediators of the stimulatory effect of stress and suckling on prolactin release in the rat. Since we have recently found that higher doses of naloxone than growth hormone were required to inhibit prolactin release induced by β-endorphin (Fig. 3), it is possible that the incomplete inhibition by naloxone of the suckling-induced rise of serum prolactin could be explained by the dose of the opiate antagonist used (5 mg/kg). In fact, in experiments where β-endorphin (5 μg) administration led to a rise of plasma prolactin similar to that observed after suckling, a 12.5-mg/kg dose of naloxone was required to completely abolish the prolactin rise whereas

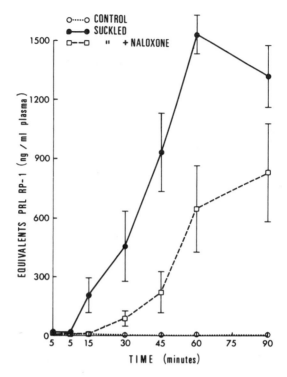

FIG. 5. Inhibitory effect of naloxone on prolactin release induced by suckling. The experiment was performed as described under Materials and Methods. Data are mean ± SEM.

growth hormone release was completely blocked after injection of only a 0.5-mg/kg dose of the opiate antagonist. As shown in Fig. 4, the relatively small stimulatory effect of ether stress on prolactin release was completely blocked by naloxone (10 mg/kg).

We have found that acute exposure to cold leads to a rapid but transient elevation of plasma prolactin levels accompanying the sustained rise of plasma TSH levels in male rats (28,29). These data could suggest that the increased TRH release presumably occurring during acute exposure to cold was responsible for increased prolactin release. It should, however, be mentioned that although TRH stimulates prolactin release in male rats treated with estrogens (12,13) or estrogens-progesterone (55) and in hypothyroid animals (65), the response to TRH is minimal or absent in intact male rats such as those used in the present experiments (13,55).

Moreover, although the transient increase of prolactin release following exposure to cold is accompanied by increased plasma TSH levels, the other stressful stimuli leading to acute prolactin release induce an inhibition of TSH secretion (22,29). These observations suggest that TRH is not involved in the acute prolactin response to stress. Similar conclusions could be deduced from experiments on the effects of pharmacological blockage to either ACTH or TSH secretion on the plasma prolactin responses to ether stress and acute exposure to cold (29).

That stress elevates plasma prolactin levels in both male and female rats except in the afternoon of proestrus or other conditions of high prolactin levels (47,54,69) suggests that inhibition of dopaminergic activity is involved in the response of prolactin to stress. We have in fact recently found that maximal doses of the antidopaminergic agent haloperidol have no effect on the already high prolactin levels found in the after-estrogen treatment (L. Ferland and F. Labrie, *unpublished observations*), thus suggesting that the afternoon peak of prolactin release occurring under the influence of estrogens is due to removal of the inhibitory dopaminergic influence on prolactin secretion. The observation of a lack of effect of stress under conditions of high prolactin secretion suggests that inhibition of dopaminergic activity is involved as mediator of the effect of stress.

A role of serotonin in the suckling-induced rise of prolactin release has been suggested by the finding of a blockage of suckling-induced prolactin release after inhibition of serotonin biosynthesis (32) or after administration of the serotonin antagonist methysergide (23). Suckling has also been found to be accompanied by decreased hypothalamic content of serotonin and increased levels of the serotonin metabolite 5-hydroxyindole acetic acid (45). Blockade of serotonergic receptors with methysergide has been shown to block the stress-induced release of prolactin in male rats (24), thus suggesting that serotonin is also involved in the prolactin response to stress. These data are in agreement with recent findings of a role of serotonin in the stimulatory effect of endorphins on prolactin release. Both endorphins and serotonin would then appear to be involved in the response of prolactin to stress and suckling in the rat.

Role of Opiates in the Nocturnal Rise of Serum Prolactin in the Human

Twenty-four hour studies of plasma PRL levels in the human show that this hormone is released episodically and that plasma concentrations of the hormone increase after the onset of sleep. The sleep-related increase in prolactin secretion is dependent on sleep itself and not related to clock time (50,59). In an attempt to gain a better understanding of the mechanisms involved in the increased release of this hormone during sleep, we have studied the effect of naloxone infusion on serum prolactin levels.

Six healthy postmenopausal women took part in this study after giving informed consent. Three milliliter blood samples were obtained at 20-min intervals through a long brachial intravenous catheter permitting sampling without disturbing the patient. A 24-hr basal study showed typical nyctohemeral secretory profile. In a subsequent 24-hr study, naloxone was infused continuously at the indicated doses between 2300 and 0700 hr. As illustrated

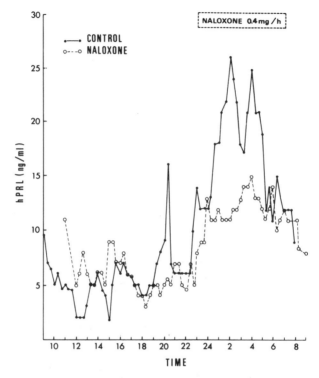

FIG. 6. Plasma PRL secretory pattern in postmenopausal woman, with and without infusion of naloxone (0.5 mg/hr). Blood sample (3 ml) was withdrawn every 20 min without disturbing the woman. Serum PRL concentrations were measured by RIA (27) using hPRL and anti-hPRL kindly supplied by Dr. H. Friesen. The sleep-related increase of PRL is well illustrated during the period of nocturnal sleep (2300–0700 hr).

in the representative cases shown in Figs. 6 and 7, the marked rise of serum prolactin levels occurring between 2400 and 0700 hr was 45 to 95% inhibited by naloxone infusion. As confirmed in other subjects, the inhibition by naloxone of serum prolactin levels is dose-dependent. No apparent change of sleeping pattern could be noticed during or after naloxone administration.

These data strongly suggest that endorphins are involved as mediators of the nocturnal rise of serum prolactin levels in the human. Coupled to our findings indicating a role of endogenous opiates in the stress- and suckling-induced release of prolactin in the rat (Figs. 4 and 5), the data obtained in the human give further support for a physiological role of endorphins in the control of prolactin secretion.

Role of Dopamine and Serotonin in the Opiate-Induced Stimulation of Prolactin Release in the Rat

Convincing evidence suggests that dopamine (DA) may be the main or even the only inhibitory substance of hypothalamic origin controlling pro-

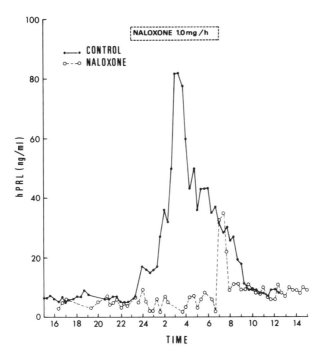

FIG. 7. Plasma PRL secretory pattern in postmenopausal woman with and without infusion of naloxone (1 mg/hr). The study was performed as described in Fig. 6 except that the dose of naloxone was 1 mg/hr. Infusion of naloxone suppressed completely the rise of plasma PRL concentrations induced by nocturnal sleep.

lactin secretion (34,43). In fact, the prolactin release-inhibiting activity contained in purified hypothalamic extracts could be accounted for by their catecholamine content (62), and preincubation of hypothalamic extracts with aluminium oxide or monoamine oxidase led to a complete loss of prolactin release-inhibiting activity (60). In agreement with a physiological role of DA in the control of prolactin secretion, DA has been measured in the portal blood (1) and typical dopaminergic receptors have been characterized in the anterior pituitary gland (7,34).

It thus appeared important to study the role of DA in the potent stimulatory effect of opiates on prolactin secretion. In order to minimize possible interference by changes of TRH secretion, we used adult male rats which show no or little prolactin response to TRH (13,55). The interest of such study was strengthened by the recent findings that intraventricular injection of met-enkephalin led to a marked inhibition of DA turnover in the tuberoinfundibular neurons (19). The present data indicate that the stimulatory effect of opiates on prolactin secretion is secondary to a decreased dopaminergic activity partly mediated by serotonin.

In order to avoid interference by stress or anesthesia, we performed all

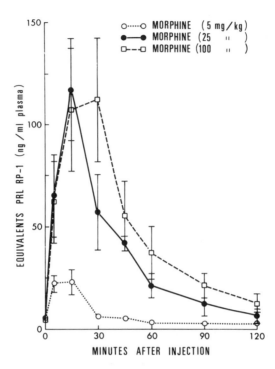

FIG. 8. Effect of increasing doses of morphine on plasma prolactin levels in the male rat. The indicated doses of morphine sulfate in 0.5 ml 0.9% NaCl were injected in freely moving, unanesthetized animals through an intrajugular catheter inserted 2 days previously. Plasma samples were taken at the indicated time intervals for measurement of prolactin by RIA. Data are expressed as mean ± SEM of duplicate determinations from 8 to 10 animals per group.

studies in unanesthetized, freely moving rats bearing an intrajugular cannula inserted 2 days previously. It can be seen in Fig. 8 that a maximal stimulatory effect of morphine injected s.c. on plasma prolactin levels is obtained at a dose of 25 to 100 mg/kg body weight. Maximal stimulation of plasma prolactin levels was measured 15 to 30 min after injection of the opiate with a progressive decrease toward basal levels at later time intervals.

That the potent stimulatory effect of morphine on prolactin release is secondary to inhibition of dopaminergic activity is indicated by the observation that the acute response (up to 30 min) of plasma prolactin induced by a maximal dose of morphine (40 mg/kg) was not further increased by simultaneous administration of a high dose of haloperidol (1 mg/kg) (Fig. 9). It can also be seen in Fig. 9 that the acute release of prolactin induced by the first injection of morphine is followed by a refractory period since no change of plasma prolactin levels is observed when the same dose of morphine is administered 30 and 60 min later. On the other hand, when haloperidol is injected during this refractory period to morphine (45 min

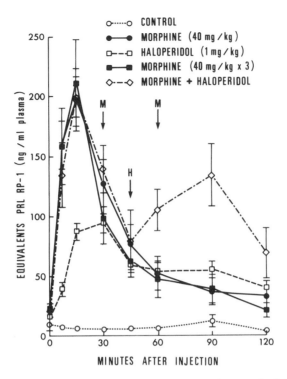

FIG. 9. Effect of haloperidol or repeated injection of morphine on plasma prolactin levels in male rats after already treated with morphine. Morphine was injected as a single dose or given at times 0, 30, and 60 min. In another group, haloperidol was injected 45 min after morphine.

after the injection of the opiate), a marked stimulation of prolactin release is observed, thus suggesting that the rapid decrease of plasma prolactin levels following acute stimulation by morphine is due to a return of inhibitory dopaminergic activity.

Since a role of serotonin has been proposed in the stimulation of prolactin secretion induced by stress (24) and suckling (23) and evidence has been recently obtained for a role of endorphins in stress- and suckling-induced rise of prolactin release (20,67; Labrie et al., *this volume*), we next used an inhibitor (parachlorophenylalanine) and a precursor (5-hydroxytryptophan) of serotonin biosynthesis to study a possible role of serotonin in the stimulatory effect of endorphins on prolactin release.

Inhibition of serotonin biosynthesis with parachlorophenylalanine (PCPA) reduced by 40 to 45% the rise of plasma prolactin levels induced by morphine in the absence (Fig. 10A) or presence (Fig. 10B) of simultaneous treatment with 5-hydroxytryptophan (5-HTP). Treatment with PCPA alone had no significant effect on the already low plasma levels of prolactin in control animals. It is of interest that the marked rise of prolactin secretion

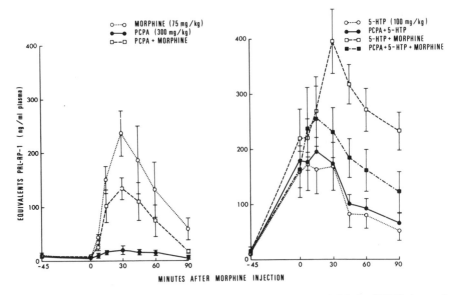

FIG. 10. Effect of morphine, 5-hydroxytryptophan (5-HTP) or parachlorophenylalanine (PCPC) alone or in combination on plasma prolactin levels in the rat. Morphine was injected s.c. at time 0, whereas 5-HTP was injected s.c. 45 min before the experiment and PCPA was injected i.p. 48 and 24 hr before time 0.

induced by 5-HTP was superimposable in control and PCPA-treated rats (Fig. 10B), thus indicating that lowering of endogenous serotonin by PCPA does not affect the sensitivity of the serotonergic response mechanisms.

The present data clearly indicate that the acute release of prolactin induced by morphine can be accounted for by an inhibition of the inhibitory hypothalamic dopaminergic influence on prolactin secretion. This is well illustrated by the absence of further increase of prolactin release by a high dose of haloperidol in animals already treated with morphine (Fig. 9). These data are in agreement with the findings of an inhibition of dopamine turnover in the medial palisade zone of the median eminence in rats injected intraventricularly with met-enkephalin (19). These effects are probably due to the activation of presynaptic inhibitory opiate receptors located on tuberoinfundibular dopaminergic nerve endings.

Coupled to the previous observations that (a) the prolactin release-inhibiting activity contained in hypothalamic extracts could be accounted for by catecholamines (60,62); (b) DA is present in hypothalamopituitary portal system (1); (c) typical dopaminergic receptors are present in anterior pituitary tissue (7,34); and (d) the control of prolactin release at the anterior pituitary level is typically dopaminergic (34), the present data add strong support for a predominant role of DA in the control of prolactin secretion. In fact, a 5- to 20-fold stimulation of plasma prolactin levels in the male rat after injection of a dopamine antagonist or of morphine indicates that, under basal conditions, prolactin release is 80 to 95% inhibited by dopamine.

Evidence has previously been obtained for a role of serotonin in the rise of prolactin secretion induced by stress or suckling. Treatment with methysergide, a serotonergic antagonist, has been found to inhibit the stress (24) and suckling (23,32) induced rise of plasma prolactin levels. Moreover, serotonin given intraventricularly (52) and treatment with 5-HTP (41), a precursor of serotonin biosynthesis, are well known to stimulate prolactin secretion. Since recent data support a role of endorphins in the rise of plasma prolactin induced by stress and suckling (20,67; Labrie et al., *this volume*), the present findings of a partial inhibition of the stimulatory effect of morphine on prolactin secretion after treatment with PCPA are in perfect agreement and extend the previous data indicating a role of serotonin in the control of prolactin secretion.

The present observations suggest that presynaptic inhibitory opiate receptors are present on dopaminergic neurons of the tuberoinfundibular system. Since the stimulatory effect of morphine on prolactin secretion is partly inhibited after inhibition of serotonin biosynthesis with PCPA, it is also possible that presynaptic stimulatory opiate receptors are present on serotonergic nerve endings in contact with the tuberoinfundibular dopaminergic system. It is also possible that effects of opiates on dopaminergic and serotonergic activity are not direct but are instead mediated by other neurotransmitter(s).

REFERENCES

1. Ben-Jonathan, M., Oliver, C., Weiner, H. J., Mical, R. A., and Porter, J. C. (1977): Dopamine in hypophyseal portal plasma of the rat during the estrous cycle and throughout pregnancy. *Endocrinology,* 100:452–458.
2. Birge, W. D., Rayford, P. L., Mariz, I. K., and Daughaday, W. H. (1967): Radioimmunoassayable growth hormone in the rat pituitary gland: Effects of age, sex and hormone state. *Endocrinology,* 81:195–200.
3. Blake, C. A. (1974): Stimulation of pituitary prolactin and TSH release in lactating and proestrus rat. *Endocrinology,* 94:503–508.
4. Blake, C. A., and Sawyer, C. H. (1972): Nicotine blocks the suckling-induced rise in circulating prolactin in lactating rats. *Science,* 177:619–621.
5. Bloom, F., Segal, D., Ling, N., and Guillemin, R. (1976): Endorphins: Profound behavioral effects in rats suggest new etiological factors in mental illness. *Nature,* 194:630–636.
6. Bradbury, A. F., Smyth, P. G., and Snell, C. R. (1976): C-fragment of lipotropin has a high affinity for brain opiate receptors. *Nature,* 260:793–805.
7. Caron, M. G., Beaulieu, M., Raymond, V., Gagné, B., Drouin, J., Lefkowitz, R. J., and Labrie, F. (1978): Dopamine receptors in the anterior pituitary gland: Correlation of [³H]dihydroergocryptine binding with the dopaminergic control of prolactin release. *J. Biol. Chem. (in press).*
8. Chang, J. K., Fong, B. T. W., Pert, A., and Pert, C. B. (1976): Opiate receptor affinities and behavioral effects of enkephalin: Structure-activity relationship of ten synthetic peptide analogs. *Life Sci.,* 18:1473–1482.
9. Cox, B. M., Goldstein, A., and Li, C. H. (1976): Opioid activity of peptide, beta-lipotropin (61–91), derived from beta-lipotropin. *Proc. Natl. Acad. Sci. USA,* 73:1821–1823.

10. Coy, D. H., Kastin, A. J., Schally, A. V., Morin, O., Caron, M. G., Labrie, F., Walker, J. M., Fertel, R., Bernston, G. G., and Sandman, C. A. (1976): Synthesis of opioid activity of stereoisomers and other D-amino acid analogs of methionine-enkephalin. *Biochem. Biophys. Res. Commun.,* 73:632–638.
11. Cusan, L., Dupont, A., Kledzik, G. S., Labrie, F., Coy, D. H., and Schally, A. V. (1977): Potent prolactin and growth hormone releasing activity of more analogues of met-enkephalin. *Nature,* 268:544–547.
12. De Léan, A., Garon, M., Kelly, P. A., and Labrie, F. (1977): Changes in pituitary thyrotropin-releasing hormone receptor level and prolactin response to TRH during the rat estrous cycle. *Endocrinology,* 100:23–28.
13. Drouin, J., De Léan, A., Rainville, D., Lachance, R., and Labrie, F. (1976): Characteristics of the interactions between TRH and somatostatin for thyrotropin and prolactin release. *Endocrinology,* 98:514–521.
14. Dupont, A., Cusan, L., Garon, M., Alvarado-U., G., and Labrie, F. (1977): Extremely rapid degradation of [³H]methionine-enkephalin by various rat tissues *in vivo* and in *vitro. Life Sci.,* 21:907–914.
15. Dupont, A., Cusan, L., Garon, M., Labrie, F., and Li, C. H. (1977): β-endorphin: Stimulation of growth hormone release *in vivo. Proc. Natl. Acad. Sci. USA,* 74:358–359.
16. Dupont, A., Cusan, L., Labrie, F., Coy, D. H., and Li, C. H. (1977): Stimulation of prolactin release in the rat by intraventricular injection of β-endorphin and methionine-enkephalin. *Biochem. Biophys. Res. Commun.,* 75:76–82.
17. Dupont, A., Cusan, L., Morin, O., Kledzik, G. S., Coy, D. H., Li, C. H., and Labrie, F. (1978): Stimulation of prolactin and growth hormone release by intraventricular injection of met-enkephalin, β-endorphin and endorphin and endorphin analogues in the rat. In: *Current Studies of Hypothalamic Functions, Part I (in press).*
18. Euker, J. S., Meites, J., and Riegle, G. D. (1975): Effects of acute stress on serum LH and prolactin in intact, castrated and dexamethasone-treated male rats. *Endocrinology,* 96:85–92.
19. Ferland, L., Fuxe, K., Eneroth, P., Gustafsson, J. A., and Skett, P. (1977): Effects of methionine-enkephalin on prolactin release and catecholamine levels and turnover in the median eminence. *Eur. J. Pharmacol.,* 43:89–90.
20. Ferland, L., Kledzik, G. S., Cusan, L., and Labrie, F. (1978): Evidence for a role of endorphins in stress- and suckling-induced prolactin release in the rat. *J. Mol. Cell. Endocrinol. (in press).*
21. Ferland, L., Labrie, F., Arimura, A., and Schally, A. V. (1977): Stimulated release of hypothalamic growth hormone releasing activity by morphine and pentobarbital. *J. Mol. Cell. Endocrinol.,* 2:247–252.
22. Fortier, C., Delgado, A., Du Commun, P., Ducommun, A., Dupont, A., Kraicer, J., MacIntosh-Hardt, B., Marceau, H., Mialhe, P., Mialhe-Voloss, C., Rerup, C., and VanRees, P. (1970): Functional interrelationships between the adenohypophysis, thyroid, adrenal cortex and gonads. *Can. Med. Assoc. J.,* 103:864–874.
23. Gallo, R. V., Rabii, J., and Moberg, G. P. (1975): Effect of methysergide, a blocker of serotonin receptors, in plasma prolactin levels in lactating and ovariectomized rats. *Endocrinology,* 97:1096–1105.
24. Goodman, G., Lawson, D. M., and Gala, R. R. (1976): The effect of neurotransmitter receptor antagonists on ether-induced prolactin release in ovariectomized estrogen-treated rats. *Proc. Soc. Exp. Biol. Med.,* 153:225–229.
25. Hughes, J. (1975): Isolation of an endogenous compound from the brain with pharmacological properties similar to morphine. *Brain Res.,* 88:295–308.
26. Hughes, J., Smith, T. W., Kosterlitz, H. W., Fothergill, L. A., Morgan, B. A., and Morris, H. R. (1975): Identification of two related pentapeptides from the brain with potent opiate activity. *Nature,* 258:577–579.
27. Hwang, P., Guyda, H., and Friesen, H. (1971): A radioimmunoassay for human prolactin. *Proc. Natl. Acad. Sci. USA,* 68:1902–1906.
28. Jobin, M., Ferland, L., Coté, J., and Labrie, F. (1975): Effect of cold exposure on hypothalamic TRH activity and plasma levels of TSH and prolactin in the rat. *Endocrinology,* 18:204–214.

29. Jobin, M., Ferland, L., and Labrie, F. (1976): Effect of pharmacological blockade of ACTH and TSH secretion on the stimulation of PRL release by cold exposure and ether stress. *Endocrinology,* 99:146–151.

30. Kokka, N., Garcia, J. F., and Elliot, H. W. (1973): Effect of acute and chronic administration of narcotic analgesics on growth hormone and corticotropin (ACTH) secretion in rats. *Prog. Brain Res.,* 39:347–360.

31. Kokka, N., and George, R. (1974): Effects of narcotic analgesics, anesthetics and hypothalamic lesions on growth hormone and adrenocorticotropic hormone secretion in rats. In: *Narcotics and the Hypothalamus,* edited by E. Zimmerman and R. George, pp.137–157. Raven Press, New York.

32. Kordon, C., Blake, C. A., Terkel, J., and Sawyer, C. H. (1973): Participation of serotonin-containing neurons in the suckling-induced rise in plasma prolactin levels in lactating rats. *Neuroendocrinology,* 13:213–223.

33. Kramer, C. Y. (1976): Extension of multiple-range test to group means with unequal numbers of replications. *Biometrics,* 12:307–310.

34. Labrie, F., Beaulieu, M., Caron, M. G., and Raymond, V. (1978): The adenohypophyseal dopamine receptor: Specificity and modulation of its activity by estradiol. In: *Proceedings of the International Congress on Prolactin,* edited by C. Robyn and M. Harter. Elsevier-North Holland, Amsterdam (*in press*).

35. Labrie, F., Dupont, A., Cusan, L., Lissitzky, J. C., Lepine, J., Raymond, V., and Coy, D. H. (1977): Effects of endorphins and their analogues on prolactin and growth hormone secretion. In: *Endorphins in Mental Health Research,* San Juan, Puerto Rico (*in press*).

36. Lazarus, L. H., Ling, N., and Guillemin, R. (1976): Beta-endorphin as a prohormone for the morphinomimetic peptides endorphins and enkephalins. *Proc. Natl. Acad. Sci. USA,* 73:2156–2159.

37. Li, C. H., Barnafi, L., Chrétien, M., and Chung, D. (1965): Isolation and amino acid sequence of β-LPH from sheep pituitary gland. *Nature,* 208:1093–1094.

38. Li, C. H., and Chung, D. (1976): Isolation and structure of an untriakontapeptide with opiate activity from camel pituitary gland. *Proc. Natl. Acad. Sci. USA,* 73: 1145–1148.

39. Li, C. H., Lemaire, S., Yamashiro, D., and Doneen, B. A. (1976): The synthesis and opiate activity of β-endorphin. *Biochem. Biophys. Res. Commun.,* 71:19–21.

40. Loh, H. H., Tseng, L. F., Wei, E. I., and Li, C. H. (1976): β-Endorphin is a potent analgesic agent. *Proc. Natl. Acad. Sci. USA,* 73:2895–2898.

41. Lu, K. H., and Meites, J. (1973): Effects of serotonin precursors and melatonin on serum prolactin release in rats. *Endocrinology,* 93:152–155.

42. McCann, S. M., Ojeda, S. R., Libertun, C., Horms, P. G., and Krulich, L. (1974): Drug-induced alterations in gonadotropin and prolactin release in the rat. In: *Narcotics and the Hypothalamus,* edited by E. Zimmerman and R. George, pp. 121–136. Raven Press, New York.

43. MacLeod, R. M., and Lehmeyer, J. E. (1974): Studies on the mechanisms of the dopamine-mediated inhibition of prolactin secretion. *Endocrinology,* 94:1077–1085.

44. Meites, J. (1966): Control of mammary growth and lactation. In: *Neuroendocrinology,* edited by L. Martini and W. F. Ganong, pp. 669–707. Academic Press, New York.

45. Mena, F., Enjalbert, A., Carbonell, L., Priam, M., and Kordon, C. (1976): Effect of suckling on plasma prolactin and hypothalamic monoamine levels in the rat. *Endocrinology,* 99:445–450.

46. Morin, O., Caron, M. G., De Léan, A., and Labrie F. (1976): Binding of the opiate pentapeptide methionine-enkephalin to a particulate fraction from rat brain. *Biochem. Biophys. Res. Commun.,* 73:940–946.

47. Neill, J. D. (1970): Effect of "stress" on serum prolactin and luteinizing hormone levels during the estrous cycle of the rat. *Endocrinology,* 87:1192–1197.

48. Noel, G. L., Suh, H. R., Stone, G., and Frantz, A. G. (1972): Human prolactin and growth hormone release during surgery and other conditions of stress. *J. Clin. Endocrinol. Metab.,* 35:840–851.

49. Odell, W. D., Rayford, P. L., and Ross, G. T. (1967): Simplified partially auto-

mated method for radioimmunoassay of human thyroid-stimulating growth, luteinizing and follicle-stimulating hormone. *J. Lab. Clin. Med.*, 70:973–980.

50. Parker, D. C., Rossman, L. G., and Vander Loan, E. F. (1973): Sheep related
nythmerol and briefly episodic variation in human plasma prolactin concentrations.
J. Clin. Endocrinol. Metab., 36:1119–1124.

51. Pasternak, G. W., Goodman, R., and Snyder, S. H. (1975): An endogenous
morphine-like factor in mammalian brain. *Life Sci.*, 16:1765–1769.

52. Porter, J. C., Mical, R. S., and Cramer, O. M. (1971): Effect of serotonin and
other indoles on the release of LH, FSH and prolactin. *Gynecol. Invest.*, 2:13–22.

53. Raud, H. R., Kiddy, C. A., and Odell, W. D. (1971): The effect of stress upon the
determination of serum prolactin by radioimmunoassay. *Proc. Soc. Exp. Biol. Med.*,
136:689–693.

54. Riegle, G. D., and Meites, J. (1976): The effect of stress on serum prolactin in the
female rat. *Proc. Soc. Exp. Biol. Med.*, 152:441–448.

55. Rivier, C., and Vale, W. (1974): *In vivo* stimulation of prolactin secretion in the
rat by thyrotropin releasing factor, releated peptides and hypothalamic extracts.
Endocrinology, 95:978–983.

56. Rivier, C., Vale, W., Ling, W., Brown, M., and Guillemin, R. (1977): Stimulation
in vivo of the secretion of prolactin and growth hormone by β-endorphin. *Endocrinology*, 100:238–241.

57. Robyn, C., Delvoye, P., Nokin, J., Vekemans, M., Badawi, M., Perez-Lopez, F. R.,
and L'Hermite, M. (1973): Prolactin and human reproduction. In: *Human Prolactin*, edited by J. L. Pasteels and C. Robyn, p. 167. Excerpta Medica, Amsterdam.

58. Rodbard, D., and Lewald, J. E. (1970): Computer analysis of radioligand assay
and radioimmunoassay data. In: *2nd Karolinska Symposium on Research Methods
in Reproductive Endocrinology*, edited by E. Diczfalusy, pp. 79–103. Karolinska
Institute, Geneva.

59. Sassin, J. F., Frantz, A. G., Kapen, S., and Weitzman, E. D. (1973): The nocturnal
rise of human prolactin is dependent on sleep. *J. Clin. Endocrinol. Metab.*, 37:436–
440.

60. Shaar, C. J., and Clemens, J. A. (1974): The role of catecholamines in the release of anterior pituitary prolactin *in vitro*. *Endocrinology*, 95:1202–1212.

61. Simantov, R., and Snyder, S. (1976): Morphine-like peptides in mammalian brain:
Isolation, structure, elucidation and interactions with the opiate receptor. *Proc. Natl.
Acad. Sci. USA*, 73:2515–2519.

62. Takahara, J., Arimura, A., and Schally, A. V. (1974): Suppression of prolactin
release by a purified porcine PIF preparation and catecholamine-infused into a rat
hypophysial portal vessel. *Endocrinology*, 96:462–465.

63. Terenius, L., and Wahlstrom, A. (1975): Research for an endogenous ligand for
opiate receptor. *Acta Physiol. Scand.*, 94:74–81.

64. Terkel, J., Blake, C. A., Hoover, V., and Sawyer, C. H. (1973): Pup survival and
prolactin levels in nicotine-treated lactating rats. *Proc. Soc. Exp. Biol. Med.*, 143:
1131–1135.

65. Vale, W., Blackwell, R., Grant, G., and Guillemin, R. (1973): TRF and thyroid
hormones on prolactin secretion by rat anterior pituitary cells in *vitro*. *Endocrinology*, 93:26–33.

66. Valverde, R. C., Chieffo, V., and Reichlin, S. (1973): Failure of reserpine to
block ether-induced release of prolactin: Physiological evidence that stress-induced
prolactin release is not caused by acute inhibition of PIF secretion, Part 1. *Life
Sci.*, 12:327–335.

67. Van Vugt, D. A., Bruni, J. F., and Meites, J. (1978): Naloxone inhibition of stress-
induced increase in prolactin secretion. *Life Sci.*, 22:85–90.

68. Wakabayashi, I., Arimura, A., and Schally, A. V. (1971): Effects of dexamethasone
and pentobarbital on plasma growth hormone levels in rats. *Neuroendocrinology*,
8:340–346.

69. Wuttke, W., and Meites, J. (1970): Effect of ether and pentobarbital on serum prolactin and LH levels in proestrus rats. *Proc. Soc. Exp. Biol. Med.*, 135:648–652.

Central Nervous System Effects of Hypothalamic Hormones and Other Peptides, edited by Collu et al. Raven Press, New York © 1979.

Role of Serotonergic Pathways in Hormonal Changes Induced by Opioid Peptides

Y. Taché, G. Charpenet, M. Chrétien, and R. Collu

Centre de Recherche Pédiatrique, Hôpital Sainte-Justine and Institut de Recherche Clinique, Université de Montréal, Montréal, Canada

In past years, much interest has been focused on the involvement of serotonergic pathways in the pharmacological effects of acute opiate administration. A vast amount of evidence indicates that the hypoactivity, hypothermia, and analgesia following morphine injection are closely associated with the integrity and normal functioning of the brain serotonergic system. These conclusions are based in part on observations which show that when the ascending serotonergic system is lesioned or pharmacological procedures [p-chlorophenylalanine (PCPA), 5,6-dihydroxytryptamine, cyproheptadine, reserpine] are used the resulting depletion of brain serotonin (5-HT) antagonizes morphine-induced hypoactivity (2,16,40), hypothermia (26,39,41,49,58), and analgesia (20,23,31,46,48,55,57,59), although there is some conflicting data in this latter case (2,3,25). Correlatively, the increase in serotonergic activity obtained by administration of 5-HT, 5-hydroxytryptophan, or specific inhibitors of 5-HT reuptake potentiated the hypothermic (18), analgesic (31,56), or catatonic (36) response to opiates.

In contrast to the vast number of papers dealing with the involvement of 5-HT in the behavioral and hypothermic effects of morphine, the participation of serotonergic pathways in the hormonal response to opiates has heretofore received little attention (34). Morphine and opioid peptides (β-endorphin, leucine-enkephalin, methionine-enkephalin) have been shown to stimulate GH and PRL secretion (1,4,8,12–14,17,33,47,54, and *this volume*). Since there is evidence that 5-HT plays a role in the hypothalamic regulation of GH (9,10,35,51) and PRL (6,9,21,35) release and that opiate alkaloids increase 5-HT turnover (22,27,50,60,61), it is possible that opiates exert at least part of their hormonal effects through activation of serotonergic pathways.

To test this hypothesis, we studied whether brain 5-HT depletion, induced by PCPA, affects the hormonal response to opioid peptides and whether β-endorphin modifies the activity of tryptophan hydroxylase.

MATERIALS AND METHODS

Male Charles River CD^R rats (Canadian Breeding Farms & Laboratories Ltd., St. Constant, Quebec) weighing 200 to 220 g were maintained *ad libitum* on Purina laboratory chow (J. Mondou Inc., Montreal, Quebec) and tap water. They were housed under conditions of controlled temperature (22 to 23°C) and illumination (from 0600 to 1800 hr). A chronic cannula was placed into the right lateral brain ventricle under pentobarbital anesthesia (50 mg/kg i.p.) according to the method of Hayden et al. (28), and the experiments were performed 48 hr later according to the same time schedule (0900 to 1100 hr), unless otherwise stated. The accuracy of the implantation was confirmed macroscopically after each experiment by injection of methylene blue dye.

Effects of Opiates, β-LPH, and β-MSH on Plasma GH, PRL, and LH Levels

Saline (10 μl), morphine sulfate, β-lipotropin hormone (β-LPH), β-melanotropic hormone (β-MSH), β-endorphin, met-enkephalin, and D-Ala²-met-enkephalin, freshly dissolved in saline, were injected intraventricularly (i.v.t.) at various dose levels. Blood was collected by decapitation 15 min after drug administration. Individual plasma samples were frozen for subsequent determination of GH, LH, and PRL concentrations.

Effect of PCPA on Hormonal Changes Induced by Opiates and β-LPH

Rats pretreated with saline or PCPA (31.6 mg/100 g body weight i.p., −72 hr and −48 hr) were given i.v.t. saline or 50 μg morphine or peptides and blood was collected by decapitation 15 min later. Plasma was frozen until determination of PRL, GH, and LH plasma levels.

Effect of β-Endorphin on Tryptophan Hydroxylase Activity in Raphe Nuclei

Rats were injected i.v.t. with saline or β-endorphin (50 μg) and decapitated 15 min later. Their brains were immediately removed, frozen on dry ice, and cut at 400 μm thickness in a refrigerated microtome. Using the microdissection technique of Palkovits (42) for isolating individual nuclei, we isolated raphe dorsalis and raphe centralis by punching out cylinders of tissue with hollow metal needles having an inner diameter of 900 μm. Individual rat nuclei were sonicated (15 sec) in 30 μl 0.05 M Tris-acetate (pH 7.6). The homogenate was centrifuged for 2 min at 7000 × g, and the supernatant was stored frozen at −20°C for tryptophan hydroxylase assay using the isotopic method of Gàl and Patterson (19), as modified by one of us (G.C.).

Taking into consideration the diurnal changes in 5-HT synthesis (29), we have established, under our experimental conditions, the nyctohemeral

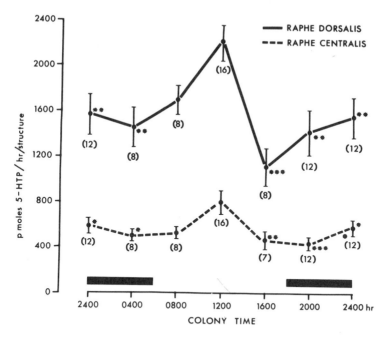

FIG. 1. Nyctohemeral variations of tryptophan hydroxylase activity in the raphe nuclei of adult male rats. Circles represent the means of animals (number in parentheses), and vertical lines the SEM. The degree of significance is shown as $*p < 0.05$; $**p < 0.01$; and $***p < 0.001$ as compared with 1200 hr.

variations of tryptophan hydroxylase activity (Fig. 1) and performed our experiments at 1600 hr, which corresponds to the end of midday stimulation of enzyme activity.

HORMONE ASSAYS

Plasma PRL and GH were measured in duplicate using specific double-antibody radioimmunoassay kits provided by the National Pituitary Agency of the National Institute of Arthritis, Metabolic and Digestive Diseases, and plasma LH levels were determined according to the method of Niswender et al. (38). The results are expressed in monograms per milliliter of their respective NIAMDD-Rat-RP-1 standards.

DRUGS

The drugs employed in this study were morphine sulfate (Demers Laboratories, Quebec, Quebec), synthetic human β-endorphin, D-Ala²-met-enkephalin, met-enkephalin (Peninsula Laboratories, Inc., San Carlos, Ca.), DL-*p*-chlorophenylalanine methyl-ester hydrochloride (Brickman and Co., Montreal, Que.). Sheep β-LPH and pig β-MSH were isolated and purified essentially by the method of Li et al. (32). Drugs in powder form were dissolved in 0.45 or 0.9% saline and injected i.v.t. or i.p. in a volume of 10 μl or 0.5 ml, respectively.

STATISTICAL EVALUATION

Statistical probabilities were calculated by one-way analysis of variance or Student's t-test.

RESULTS

Effects of Opiates, β-LPH, and β-MSH on Plasma GH, PRL, and LH Levels

Table 1 shows the plasma GH, PRL, and LH responses to opiates and β-LPH (50 μg) 15 min after i.v.t. injection. β-LPH and β-endorphin caused

TABLE 1. *Effects of opiates on plasma GH, PRL, and LH levels in male rats*

Treatment[a]	No. of rats	GH[b]	PRL[b]	LH[b]
Saline	25	33 ± 10	26 ± 7	19 ± 2
Morphine	8	15 ± 6 ns	170 ± 50[c]	44 ± 9 ns
β-Lipotropin	11	204 ± 62[c]	95 ± 32[d]	237 ± 57[c]
β-Endorphin	13	241 ± 54[c]	145 ± 23[c]	202 ± 33[c]
D-Ala²-met-enkephalin	9	234 ± 73[e]	145 ± 22[c]	15 ± 3 ns
Met-Enkephalin	11	98 ± 43 ns	17 ± 2 ns	21 ± 2 ns

nS, not significant.
[a] Adult male rats were injected with saline (10 μl) or the test materials (50 μg/rat) and decapitated 15 min later.
[b] Values, ng/ml; mean ± SE.
[c] $p < 0.001$ as compared with saline-treated controls.
[d] $p < 0.05$.
[e] $p < 0.01$.

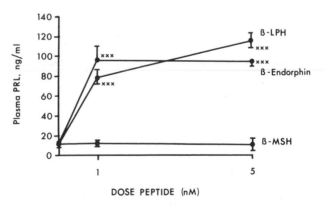

DOSE PEPTIDE (nM)

FIG. 2. Plasma PRL levels in rats 15 min after i.v.t. injection of β-LPH, β-endorphin, or β-MSH (1 or 5 nM). Circles represent the means of seven rats. ***$p < 0.001$ as compared with saline-treated controls.

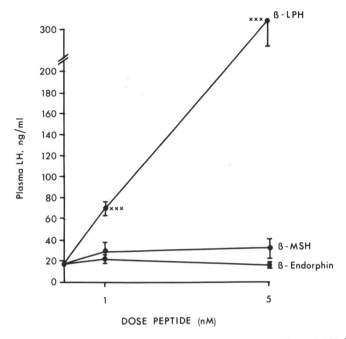

FIG. 3. Plasma LH levels in rats 15 min after i.v.t. injection of β-LPH, β-endorphin, or β-MSH (1 or 5 nM). For other details, see legend to Fig. 2.

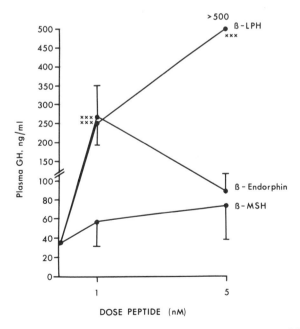

FIG. 4. Plasma GH levels in rats 15 min after i.v.t. injection of β-LPH, β-endorphin, or β-MSH (1 or 5 nM). For other details, see legend to Fig. 2.

a marked increase in plasma GH (6- to 7-fold), PRL (4- to 6-fold), and LH (10- to 12-fold). D-Ala²-met-enkephalin significantly elevated plasma PRL and GH values (around 6- to 7-fold), whereas morphine stimulated only PRL secretion and met-enkephalin did not affect antehypophyseal hormone release.

Since β-LPH and β-endorphin (β-LPH 61–69) were very potent stimulators of GH, PRL, and LH release, we further evaluated on a molar basis (1 and 5 nM) their hormonal effects as well as those of β-MSH, which consists of amino acid residues 41–58 of β-LPH (5).

As illustrated in Fig. 2, plasma PRL levels were significantly increased by β-LPH and β-endorphin, whereas β-MSH was ineffective. Maximal stimulation of PRL release by β-LPH and β-endorphin was observed at dose levels of 5 and 1 nM, respectively. Plasma LH concentrations were significantly enhanced by β-LPH in a dose-related manner, whereas β-endorphin and β-MSH given at 1 or 5 nM produced no such alterations (Fig. 3). Dose-

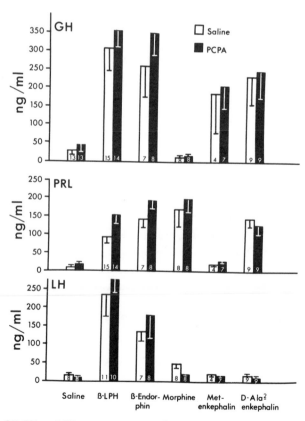

FIG. 5. Plasma GH, PRL, and LH response to opiates (50 µg, i.v.t.) in saline (*white column*) or PCPA (*black column*) pretreated rats. The columns represent the means ± SE. The number of animals in each group is shown at the base of each column.

dependent elevations of plasma GH titers were noted following injection of β-LPH (1 and 5 nM), whereas β-endorphin was effective only at the lower dose level (1 nM). β-MSH did not modify GH release (Fig. 4).

Effect of PCPA on Hormonal Changes Induced by Opiates and β-LPH

Figure 5 shows that PCPA pretreatment did not alter basal plasma GH, PRL, and LH levels and did not affect the antehypophyseal response to β-LPH or opiates, injected i.v.t. in 50-μg doses.

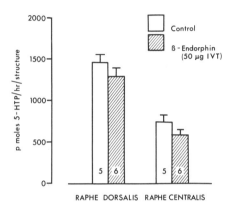

FIG. 6. Tryptophan hydroxylase activity in raphe centralis and raphe dorsalis 15 min after intraventricular injection of saline (*white columns*) or β-endorphin (50 μg; *dashed columns*). For other details, see legend to Fig. 5.

Effect of β-Endorphin on Tryptophan Hydroxylase Activity in Raphe Nuclei

The activity of tryptophan hydroxylase in raphe nuclei remained unchanged, as measured 15 min after β-endorphin injection (50 μg i.v.t.) (Fig. 6).

DISCUSSION

In the present study, we demonstrated that β-endorphin and D-Ala^2-met-enkephalin, injected i.v.t. at 50-μg dose levels, are potent stimulants for PRL and GH release. The increase of GH and PRL secretion by opiate receptor activators (β-endorphin, met-enkephalin, D-Ala^2-met-enkephalin) has been investigated by other laboratories under various experimental conditions: estrogen priming (47), urethane anesthesia (4), and anti-SRIF pretreatment (4,12–14,17). The absence of PRL- and GH-releasing effects of met-enkephalin under our conditions is not surprising since the minimal effective i.v.t. dose is reportedly 400 μg in anti-SRIF-pretreated rats (12), whereas the analog D-Ala^2-met-enkephalin is about 1,000 to 2,000 times more potent in that respect than met-enkephalin (12).

Morphine increased PRL levels but did not raise GH concentrations, as compared with saline-treated controls. Chihara et al. (4) recently reported that in urethane-anesthetized rats morphine sulfate 10^{-8} M caused a significant elevation of both GH and PRL 10 to 60 min after i.v.t. injection, whereas at 10^{-9} M it stimulated only PRL secretion. A greater sensitivity of the PRL response to met-enkephalin and β-endorphin has also been observed (12,13). These data suggest that the stimulatory threshold for PRL release may be lower than that of GH. In agreement with other reports (4,12,13,47), our data show that, on a molar basis, β-endorphin is the most potent among the peptide and alkaloid opiates tested for GH and PRL release.

Data on the effects of opiates on LH secretion are not very numerous, and the findings are not as consistent as those reported for PRL or GH. In our study, morphine sulfate, met-enkephalin, and D-Ala^2-met-enkephalin did not modify LH release, whereas β-endorphin significantly increased plasma LH but only at 50-μg dose levels (14 nM). Under other experimental conditions, acute injection of morphine sulfate (2 or 10 mg/kg but not 15 mg) or met-enkephalin (5 mg/kg) is reported to reduce LH concentrations in male rats (1,7). Morphine, given to females of these species in a single large dose (50 to 100 mg/kg) at the onset of the critical period on the afternoon of proestrus, abolished the LH, FSH, and PRL surges (37,43), whereas a 10 mg/kg dose induced an apparent stimulation of LH release, which was reversed by naloxone (43). The reason for these discrepancies is unclear, but it has already been observed in the rat that morphine could exert biphasic effects on thermoregulation (39) and motor activity (2), depending on the dose and time of administration.

Our results also indicate that sheep pituitary β-LPH preparation—which had a very weak morphine-like activity as assayed on electrically stimulated mouse vas deferens or on stereospecific brain opiate binding (5)—exerted a marked dose-related enhancing effect on PRL, LH, and GH release comparable or even superior on a molar basis to that of β-endorphin. However, β-MSH (amino acid sequence 41–58 of β-LPH) did not modify plasma GH, PRL, or LH levels. To the best of our knowledge, the hormonal variations induced by these peptides have not been evaluated so far. A slight cross-reactivity ($< 2\%$) between ovine β-LPH preparation and LH has been observed in our heterologous LH RIA system which, however, could not totally account for the surge of LH observed after β-LPH administration. Moreover, the results could not be attributed to a stressor action of the drug since PRL and LH secretions, induced by acute stress, are always associated with an inhibition of GH release (15,53). In addition, the fact that β-LPH (5 nM) and β-endorphin (14 nM) are almost equally potent in stimulating PRL, GH, and LH release suggests that β-LPH *per se* must induce plasma hormonal variations, and a possible enzymatic cleavage to β-endorphin could not explain the effects observed. Pelletier et al. (44; *this volume*) have described the presence of β-LPH in the rat and human hypothalamus. The significance of morphological and pharmacological data with regard to a possible physiological involvement of β-LPH in the release of pituitary hormones remains to be established.

The precise mechanisms through which opiates exert their hormonal effects are still unclear, although several possibilities have been explored. Some authors have reported that met-enkephalin or morphine stimulated prolactin release *in vitro* (24,33) and that morphine slightly but significantly increased LH secretion by the pituitary (7). By contrast, Rivier et al. (47) have failed to observe any GH and PRL stimulatory effect of morphine, β-endorphin, or met-enkephalin *in vitro*. These data suggest a central nervous system site of action for opiates which could be exerted through releasing or inhibiting factors and through biogenic amines. Recent studies have clearly shown that the rise of plasma GH and PRL levels in response to opiates did not involve an inhibition of somatostatin secretion since neutralization of endogenous somatostatin by specific antiserum did not alter the stimulatory effect of opioid peptides or morphine (4,12–14,17). It is possible therefore that the stimulatory effect is exerted through activation of a GH-RF.

We explored the possibility that part of the hormonal effects of opiates is mediated through serotonergic pathways. The results of the present experiments do not support this hypothesis. PCPA, an inhibitor of serotonin synthesis at the tryptophan hydroxylase step (30) known to produce a marked depletion of cerebral 5-HT (2), did not alter the hormonal changes induced by opioid peptides, suggesting that the integrity of the serotonergic system is not necessary for the hormonal response to opioid peptides.

By contrast, Scampino et al. (52) have recently reported a possible mediation of PRL release induced by enkephalins via the brain 5-HT system, based on inhibition by 5-HT receptor blockers (methysergide and metergoline) of met-enkephalin-induced PRL release. A dichotomy of effects between methysergide and PCPA has already been observed: methysergide but not PCPA has been shown to inhibit PRL release elicited by stress, by α-methyl-*p*-tyrosine, or by blockade of dopamine receptors (11). Moreover, it has been indicated that the inhibiting effect of methysergide on PRL release may be due not to its antiserotonergic properties but rather to a dopamine receptor agonist type of action (11; Labrie et al., *this volume*), suggesting that results obtained with this compound must be interpreted with caution.

From these experiments it also appears that tryptophan hydroxylase activity in raphe nuclei is not modified 15 min after β-endorphin treatment (50 μg i.v.t.), when the hormonal variations are significantly increased. Although it is possible that the effects of opioid peptides on the enzyme activity occur in other 5-HT cell bodies or in 5-HT nerve terminals and at a time other than those examined, these results show a lack of correlation between modifications of an enzyme of serotonin synthesis in the main 5-HT cells bodies and the hormonal response to opiates. Acute treatment with morphine has been reported to increase the turnover of 5-HT (22,27,50,60, 61) and the activity of tryptophan-hydroxylase (45) in the forebrain and to a lesser degree in the brainstem. In addition, morphine-induced GH release can be enhanced by pretreatment with PCPA (Collu and Taché, *this volume*). To what extent the discrepancies observed between the effects of morphine and those of opiate peptides are related to differences in experimental conditions or correspond to intrinsic differences between opiate peptides and opiate alkaloids remains to be further investigated.

In conclusion, we have noted that β-endorphin and D-Ala^2-met-enkephalin given at 50-μg dose levels stimulated PRL and GH secretion in male rats. β-Endorphin, under these conditions but not at lower doses, also activated LH release as measured 15 min after injection. β-LPH induced a dose-dependent increase of plasma PRL, GH, and LH levels, whereas β-LPH-41–58 (β-MSH) had no such effect. Moreover, in contrast to the fact that the behavioral and hypothermic effects of opiates are closely associated with the integrity and normal functioning of the brain serotonergic system, the unchanged hormonal response to opiate peptides following depletion of brain 5-HT levels by PCPA and the lack of significant alterations in tryptophan hydroxylase activity in raphe nuclei suggest that the serotonergic system is not primarily involved in the hormonal changes induced by opioid peptides. However, further experiments need to be performed to exclude this possibility altogether.

ACKNOWLEDGMENTS

This work was supported in part by the Medical Research Council of Canada (MA-4691) and the Conseil de la Recherche en Santé du Québec. The authors thank Dr. A. F. Parlow of the National Pituitary Agency, NIAMDD, and Dr. G. D. Niswender for donating the materials used in the radioimmunoassay of GH, LH, and PRL. The technical assistance of Miss F. Dionne, Mrs. H. Guillet, and O. Rebouco as well as the secretarial work of Mrs. Denyse Drouin are gratefully acknowledged.

REFERENCES

1. Bruni, J. F., Van Vugt, D., Marshall, S., and Meites, J. (1977): Effects of naloxone, morphine and methionine enkephalin on serum prolactin, luteinizing hormone, follicle stimulating hormone, thyroid stimulating hormone and growth hormone. *Life Sci.*, 21:461–466.
2. Buxbaum, D. M., Yarbrough, G. G., and Carter, M. E. (1973): Biogenic amines and narcotic effects. I. Modification of morphine-induced analgesia and motor activity after alteration of cerebral amine levels. *J. Pharmacol. Exp. Ther.*, 185: 317–327.
3. Cheney, D. L., and Golstein, A. (1971): The effect of p-chlorophenylalanine on opiate-induced running, analgesia, tolerance and physical dependence in mice. *J. Pharmacol. Exp. Ther.*, 177:309–315.

4. Chihara, K., Arimura, A., Coy, D. H., and Schally, A. V. (1978): Studies on the interaction of endorphins, substance P, and endogenous somatostatin in growth hormone and prolactin release in rats. *Endocrinology,* 102:281–290.
5. Chrétien, M., Seidah, N. G., Benjannet, S., Dragon, N., Routhier, R., Motomatsu, T., Crine, P., and Lis, M. (1977): A β-LPH precursor model: Recent developments concerning morphine-like substances. *Ann. N. Y. Acad. Sci.,* 297:84–107.
6. Clemens, J. A., Sawyer, B. D., and Cerimele, B. (1977): Further evidence that serotonin is a neurotransmitter involved in the control of prolactin secretion. *Endocrinology,* 100:692–698.
7. Cicero, T. J., Badger, T. M., Wilcox, C. E., Bell, R. D., and Meyer, E. R. (1977): Morphine decreases luteinizing hormone by an action on the hypothalamic pituitary axis. *J. Pharmacol. Exp. Ther.,* 203:548–555.
8. Cocchi, D., Santagostino, A., Gil-Ad, I., Ferri, S., and Müller, E. E. (1977): Leu-enkephalin-stimulated growth hormone and prolactin release in the rat: Comparison with the effect of morphine. *Life Sci.,* 20:2041–2046.
9. Collu, R. (1977): Role of central cholinergic and aminergic neurotransmitters in the control of anterior pituitary hormone secretion. In: *Clinical Neuroendocrinology,* edited by L. Martini and G. M. Besser, pp. 43–65. Academic Press, New York.
10. Collu, R., Fraschini, F., Visconti, P., and Martini, L. (1972): Adrenergic and serotonergic control of growth hormone secretion in adult male rats. *Endocrinology,* 90:1496–1501.
11. Coppings, R. J., Giachetti, A., and Krulich, L. (1978): Inhibition of prolactin secretion by a direct effect of methysergide on pituitary lactotrophs in the rat. *Fed. Am. Soc. Exp. Biol.,* 37:637.
12. Cusan, L., Dupont, A., Kledzik, G. S., and Labrie, F. (1977): Potent prolactin and growth hormone releasing activity of more analogues of met-enkephalin. *Nature,* 268:544–547.
13. Dupont, A., Cusan, L., Labrie, F., Coy, D. H., and Li, C. H. (1977): Stimulation of prolactin release in the rat by intraventricular injection of β-endorphin and methionine-enkephalin. *Biochem. Biophys. Res. Commun.,* 75:76–82.
14. Dupont, A., Cusan, L., Garon, M., Labrie, F., and Li, C. H. (1977): β-Endorphin: Stimulation of growth hormone release in vivo. *Proc. Natl. Acad. Sci. USA,* 74:358–359.
15. Du Ruisseau, P., Taché, Y., Brazeau, P., and Collu, R. (1978): Pattern of adenohypophyseal hormone change induced by various stressors in male and female rats. *Neuroendocrinology* (in press).
16. Eidelberg, E., and Schwartz, A. S. (1970): Possible mechanism of action of morphine on brain. *Nature,* 222:1152–1153.
17. Ferland, L., Labrie, F., Arimura, A., and Schally, A. V. (1977): Stimulated release of hypothalamic growth hormone-releasing activity by morphine and pentobarbital. *Mol. Cell. Endocrinol.,* 6:247–252.
18. Fuller, R. W., and Baker, J. C. (1974): Further evidence for serotonin involvement in thermoregulation following morphine administration from studies with an inhibitor of serotonin uptake. *Res. Commun. Chem. Pathol. Pharmacol.,* 8:715–718.
19. Gal, E. M., and Patterson, K. (1973): Rapid nonisotopic assay of tryptophan-5-hydroxylase activity in tissues. *Anal. Biochem.,* 52:625–629.
20. Genovese, E., Zonta, N., and Mantegazza, P. (1973): Decreased antinociceptive activity of morphine in rats pretreated intraventricularly with 5,6-dihydroxytryptamine, a long-lasting selective depletor of brain serotonin. *Psychopharmacologia,* 32:359–364.
21. Gil-Ad, I., Zambotti, F., Carruba, M. O., Vicentini, L., and Müller, E. E. (1978): Stimulatory role for brain serotoninergic system on prolactin secretion in the male rat. *Proc. Soc. Exp. Biol. Med.,* 151:512–518.
22. Goodlet, I., and Sugrue, M. F. (1974): Effects of acutely administered analgesic drugs on rat brain 5-hydroxytryptamine turnover. *Eur. J. Pharmacol.,* 29:241–248.
23. Görlitz, B.-D., and Frey, H. H. (1972): Central monamines and antinociceptive drug action. *Eur. J. Pharmacol.,* 20:171–180.

24. Hall, T. R., Advis, J. P., Smith, A. F., and Meites, J. (1976): Stimulation of prolactin release by morphine and enkephalins. *IRCS Med. Sci.*, 4:559.
25. Harvey, J. A., Schlosberg, A. J., and Yunger, L. M. (1974): Effect of p-chlorophenylalanine and brain lesions on pain sensitivity and morphine analgesia in the rat. *Adv. Biochem. Psychopharmacol.*, 10:233–245.
26. Haubrich, D. R., and Blake, D. E. (1971): Modification of the hypothermic action of morphine after depletion of brain serotonin and catecholamines. *Life Sci.*, 10:175–180.
27. Haubrich, D. R., and Blake, D. E. (1973): Modification of serotonin metabolism in rat brain after acute or chronic administration of morphine. *Biochem. Pharmacol.*, 22:2753–2759.
28. Hayden, J. F., Johnson, L. R., and Maickel, R. P. (1966): Construction and implantation of a permanent cannula for making injection into the lateral ventricle of the rat brain. *Life Sci.*, 5:1509–1515.
29. Kan, J. P., Chouvet, G., Hery, F., Debilly, G., Mermet, A., Glowinski, J., and Pujol, J. F. (1977): Daily variations of various parameters of serotonin metabolism in the rat. I. Circadian variations of tryptophan-5-hydroxylase in the raphe nuclei and the striatum. *Brain Res.*, 123:125–136.
30. Koe, W. B., and Weissman, A. (1966): p-Chlorophenylalanine: A specific depletor of brain serotonin. *J. Pharmacol. Exp. Ther.*, 154:499–516.
31. Lee, R. L., Sewell, R. D. E., and Spencer, P. S. J. (1978): Importance of 5-hydroxytryptamine in the antinociceptive activity of the leucine-enkephalin derivative, D-Ala²-Leu⁵-enkephalin (BW 180C), in the rat. *Eur. J. Pharmacol.*, 47:251–253.
32. Li, C. H., Barnafi, L., Chrétien, M., and Chung, D. (1965): Isolation and structure of β-LPH from sheep pituitary gland. *Excerta Med. Int. Congr.*, 112:349–364.
33. Lien, E. L., Fenichel, R. L., Garsky, V., Sarantakis, D., and Grant, N. H. (1976): Enkephalin-stimulated prolactin release. *Life Sci.*, 19:837–840.
34. Martin, J. B., Audet, J., and Saunders, A. (1975): Effects of somatostatin and hypothalamic ventromedial lesions on GH release induced by morphine. *Endocrinology*, 96:839–847.
35. Martin, J. B., Durand, D., Gurd, W., Faille, G., Audet, J., and Brazeau, P. (1978): Neuropharmacological regulation of episodic growth hormone and prolactin secretion in the rat. *Endocrinology*, 102:106–113.
36. Motomatsu, T., Lis, M., Seidah, N., and Chrétien, M. (1977): Cataleptic effect of 61–91 beta-lipotropic hormone in rat. *Can. J. Neurol. Sci.*, 1:49–52.
37. Muraki, T., Tokunaga, Y., and Makino, T. (1977): Effects of morphine and naloxone on serum LH, FSH and prolactin levels and on hypothalamic content of LH-RF in proestrus rats. *Endocrinol. Jpn.*, 24:313–315.
38. Niswender, G. D., Rees Midgley, A., Jr., Monroe, S. E., and Reichert, L. E., Jr. (1968): Radioimmunoassay for rat luteinizing hormone with antiovine LH serum and ovine LH¹³¹. *Proc. Soc. Exp. Biol. Med.*, 128:807–811.
39. Oka, T. (1977): Role of 5-hydroxytryptamine in morphine-, pethidine-, and methadone-induced hypothermia in rats at low ambient and room temperature. *Br. J. Pharmacol.*, 60:323–330.
40. Oka, T., and Hosoya, E. (1976): Effects of humoral modulators and naloxone on the morphine-induced changes in the spontaneous locomotor activity of the rat. *Psychopharmacologia*, 47:243–248.
41. Oka, T., Nozaki, M., and Hosoya, E. (1972): Effects of p-chlorophenylalanine and cholinergic antagonists on body temperature changes induced by the administration of morphine to non tolerant and morphine-tolerant rats. *J. Pharmacol. Exp. Ther.*, 180:136–143.
42. Palkovits, M. (1973): Isolated removal of hypothalamic or other brain nuclei of the rat. *Brain Res.*, 59:449–450.
43. Pang, C. N., Zimmermann, E., and Sawyer, C. H. (1977): Morphine inhibition of the preovulatory surges of plasma luteinizing hormone and follicle stimulating hormone in the rat. *Endocrinology*, 101:1726–1732.
44. Pelletier, G., Désy, L., Labrie, F., and Li, C. H. (1978): Immunohistochemical localization of β-LPH in the human hypothalamus. *Life Sci. (in press)*.

45. Pérez-Cruet, J., Thoa, N. B., and Ng, L. K. Y. (1976): Acute effects of heroin and morphine on newly synthesized serotonin in rat brain. *Life Sci.,* 17:349–362.
46. Proudfit, H. K., and Anderson, E. G. (1975): Morphine analgesia: Blockade by raphe magnus lesions. *Brain Res.,* 98:612–618.
47. Rivier, C., Vale, W., Ling, N., Brown, M., and Guillemin, R. (1977): Stimulation *in vivo* of the secretion of prolactin and growth hormone by β-endorphin. *Endocrinology,* 100:238–341.
48. Samanin, R., Gumulka, W., and Valzelli, L. (1970): Reduced effect of morphine in midbrain lesioned rats. *Eur. J. Pharmacol.,* 10:339–343.
49. Samanin, R., Kon, S., and Garatini, S. (1972): Abolition of the morphine effect on body temperature in midbrain raphe lesioned rats. *J. Pharm. Pharmacol.,* 24:374–377.
50. Sawa, A., and Oka, T. (1976): Effects of narcotic analgesia on serotonin metabolism in the brain of rats and mice. *Jpn. J. Pharmacol.,* 26:599–605.
51. Smythe, G. S., Brandstater, J. F., and Lazarus, L. (1975): Serotoninergic control of rat growth hormone secretion. *Neuroendocrinology,* 17:245–257.
52. Scampino, S., Locatelli, V., Cocchi, D., Bajusz, S., Ferri, S., and Müller, E. E. (1978): Involvement of brain serotonin in the prolactin-releasing effect of opiate peptides. International Symposium on Central Nervous System Effects of Hypothalamic Hormones and Other Peptides, Montréal (abstr.)
53. Taché, Y., Du Ruisseau, P., Selye, H., Taché, J., and Collu, R. (1976): Shift in adenohypophyseal activity during chronic intermittent immobilization of rats. *Neuroendocrinology,* 22:325–336.
54. Taché, Y., Lis, M., and Collu, R. (1977): Effects of thyrotropin-releasing hormone on behavioral and hormonal changes induced by β-endorphin. *Life Sci.,* 21:841–846.
55. Tenen, S. S. (1968): Antagonism of the analgesic effect of morphine and other drugs by p-chlorophenylalanine, a serotonin depletor. *Psychopharmacologia,* 12:278–285.
56. Tulunay, F. C., Yano, I., and Takemori, A. E. (1976): The effect of biogenic amine modifiers on morphine analgesia and its antagonism by naloxone. *Eur. J. Pharmacol.,* 35:285–292.
57. Vogt, M. (1974): The effect of lowering the 5-hydroxytryptamine content of the rat spinal cord on analgesia produced by morphine. *J. Physiol.,* 236:483–498.
58. Warwick, R. O., Blake, D. E., Miya, T. S., and Bousquet, N. F. (1973): Serotonin involvement in thermoregulation following administration of morphine to nontolerant and morphine-tolerant rats. *Res. Commun. Chem. Pathol. Pharmacol.,* 6:19–32.
59. Yaksh, T. L., Plant, R. L., and Rudy, T. A. (1977): Studies on the antagonism by raphe lesions of the antinociceptive action of systemic morphine. *Eur. J. Pharmacol.,* 41:399.
60. Yarbrough, G. G., Buxbaum, D. M., and Sanders-Bush, E. (1971): Increased serotonin turnover in the acutely morphine treated rats. *Life Sci.,* 10(1):977–983.
61. Yarbrough, G. G., Buxbaum, D. M., and Sanders-Bush, E. (1973): Biogenic amines and narcotic effects. II. Serotonin turnover in the rat after acute and chronic morphine administration. *J. Pharmacol. Exp. Ther.,* 185:328–335.

LH-RH–SRIF–PLG

*Central Nervous System Effects of Hypothalamic
Hormones and Other Peptides*, edited by Collu et al.
Raven Press, New York © 1979.

Structure-Function Studies and Prediction of Conformational Requirements for LH-RH

David H. Coy, Janos Seprodi, Jesus A. Vilchez-Martinez,
Escipion Pedroza, Joseph Gardner, and Andrew V. Schally

*Department of Medicine, Tulane University School of Medicine, and
Veterans Administration Hospital, New Orleans, Louisiana 70112*

Although luteinizing hormone-releasing hormone (LH-RH) is widely distributed in a number of central nervous system (CNS) regions, its behavioral effects remain ill-defined. Analog studies have, therefore, been aimed primarily at elucidating chemistry of action, improving therapeutic properties for the treatment of various conditions of male and female infertility, and developing competitive inhibitors that could be used to disrupt the reproductive cycle. The really important discoveries which have resulted in a better understanding of the mechanism of action of LH-RH and in the design of clinically interesting compounds have been made possible by the synthesis of well over 500 analogs by a number of research groups. Some of the more critical results are discussed here.

ANALOG STUDIES AND RELATIONSHIPS TO POSSIBLE CONFORMATION

In terms of the role of individual amino acid residues in the LH-RH decapeptide (Fig. 1), histidine and tryptophan appear to take part in the chemical mechanism activating adenyl cyclase after binding to pituitary membranes. This appears to be linked in some way to the acid-base characteristics of the imidazole group of histidine (3) and to the electron-donating capacity of the indole nucleus of tryptophan (1). Of the remaining amino acids, modifications to pyroglutamic acid in position 1 and glycine in positions 6 and 10 have yielded the most information on the binding requirements of the molecule and its biologically active conformation.

The substitution of glycine in position 6 by D-amino acids (10), particularly those with large side chains (5), results in analogs up to 15 times more active than LH-RH for gonadotropin release. It was suggested (10) that this was the result of the stabilization of a β-bend conformation in the center of the molecule for which glycine acts as a kind of hinge. Much later this proposition was supported by free-energy calculations on favorable pGLU-HIS-TRP-SER-TYR-GLY-LEU-ARG-PRO-GLY-NH$_2$

1 2 3 4 5 6 7 8 9 10

FIG. 1. Amino acid sequence of LH-RH.

conformations of LH-RH (8,9). Structure-activity studies (11) on pyro-glutamic acid at the N-terminus suggested to us that a principal function of this amino acid was to undergo hydrogen bonding between the pyrrolidone carbonyl group and some other part of the molecule, one possibility being the glycinamide NH$_2$ group at the other end of the molecule. In this way, the β-bend conformation of the molecule could be stabilized. Such an inter-action, requiring close proximity between the N- and C-termini, can quite easily be embodied in a model proposed by Momany (9), and was further supported by the synthesis of two N-C terminally cyclized analogs (Fig. 2) of the hormone which retained significant LH-RH activity despite the com-plete lack of activity of the linear precursor molecules.

If the glycinamide residue in position 10 is replaced by simple alkylamine groups (6), then again gonadotropin-releasing activity is increased to a limit of about five times the activity of LH-RH. This cannot be explained by increased resistance to peptidases since the plasma half-lives of this class of peptides are not increased. Also, at first sight, this result appears strange because any possibility of hydrogen bonding between pGlu and glycinamide is lost. To explain this, we propose that a second hydrogen bond may be formed between the proline peptide bond C$=$O group and a peptide bond NH group located somewhere toward the N-terminus. From observations with molecular models and from structure-activity considerations that are discussed subsequently, one possibility is that the histidine peptide bond NH group could be involved. Electron-releasing alkyl groups adjacent to Pro would be expected to increase the strength of this hydrogen bond, resulting in increased stability of the required conformation. These position 6 and 10 substitutions would, therefore, have the same overall conformational conse-

NH-CH$_2$CH$_2$CH$_2$CH$_2$CH$_2$CO-HIS-TRP-SER-TYR-D-ALA-LEU-ARG-PRO-GLY

LH-releasing activity = 0.65% (0.48–0.89)

NH-CH$_2$CH$_2$CO-HIS-TRP-SER-TYR-D-ALA-LEU-ARG-PRO-GLY

LH-releasing activity = 1.20% (0.92–1.56)

FIG. 2. Cyclic analogs of LH-RH.

quences and an ideal situation should be attainable which cannot be improved on by these approaches. This has been shown (5) to be the case with analogs containing both the position 6 and 10 alterations within the same peptide, the best ones of which have limiting gonadotropin releasing activities in the region of 20 times that of LH-RH in the rat. More polar, and therefore less electron-donating, groups at the C-terminus generally result (2) in loss of activity which is expected from loss of hydrogen bonding at Pro. There is, however, a problem with the theory because the substitution of electron-withdrawing fluoroalkylamine groups for glycinamide unexpectedly results (4) in even more biological activity. An explanation for this might be hydrogen bonding between fluorine and a suitable proton. The substitution of D-amino acid amides such as D-alanine or proline (Table 1) for glycinamide results in almost complete loss of activity. Possibly the altered stereochemistry at the C-terminus does not allow hydrogen bonding between the ends of the molecule to occur.

The histidine and tryptophan residues can be altered in a number of ways to give analogs with almost no gonadotropin releasing activity which still retain much affinity for LH-RH receptors. In general, antagonist activity can be greatly increased by the D-amino acid-6 substitutions, particularly D-Phe and D-Trp. However, in contrast to the agonists, the C-terminal alkylamide modifications have deleterious effects on inhibitory activity possibly due to the loss of hydrogen bonding capability between histidine, which is either deleted or, much more effectively, replaced by D-phenylalanine in most antagonists, and proline.

This complex interaction between the ends of the LH-RH peptide chain is manifested in several other ways. For instance, although [D-pGlu^1]-LH-RH (7) has only 10% LH releasing activity, antagonists containing D-pGlu, such as those shown in Table 2, are more active than the corresponding L-pGlu-peptides in the standard blockade of ovulation assay in the rat. Similarly, [D-Ala^{10}]-LH-RH has very low LH-releasing activity, whereas

TABLE 1. Comparison of LH-RH agonists and antagonists modified in position 10

LH-RH analog		% LH-releasing activity
D-Ala^{10}		0.21
D-Pro^{10}		0.16
	Dose (mg)	% Blockade of ovulation
D-Phe^2,D-Trp^3,D-Phe^6,D-Ala^{10}	1.5	80
	0.5	0
D-Phe^2,D-Trp^3,D-Phe^6,D-Phe^{10}	1.5	0
D-Phe^2,D-Trp^3,D-Phe^6,desGly^{10}	1.5	0

TABLE 2. Comparison of L- and D-pGlu^1 inhibitors of LH-RH

LH-RH analog	Dose (mg)	% Blockade of ovulation
D-Phe^2,D-Trp^3,D-Phe^6	1.0	90
	0.5	0
D-pGlu^1,D-Phe^2,D-Trp^3,D-Phe^6	1.0	100
	0.5	80
D-Phe^2,D-Trp^3,D-Lys^6	1.5	0
D-pGlu^1,D-Phe^2,D-Trp^3,D-Lys^6	1.5	80

[D-Phe^2, D-Trp^3, D-Phe^6, D-Ala^{10}]-LH-RH retains essentially full inhibitory activity (Table 1). The corresponding D-Phe^{10}-antagonist has no inhibitory activity at a comparable dose level (Table 1), presumably because of steric effects associated with the large aromatic side chain. Deletion of glycinamide in [D-Phe^2, D-Trp^3, D-Phe^6, desGly-NH$_2$^{10}]-LH-RH (Table 1) also eliminates inhibitory activity, which is not surprising since the possibility of N-C terminal hydrogen bonding is removed.

One approach for investigating structural requirements of the side chains of the position 6 D-amino acids, other than the substitution of a variety of D-amino acids, was to introduce various moieties by reaction with a suitable functional side group in this position (12). [D-Phe^2, D-Trp^3, D-Lys^6]-LH-RH was chosen for this purpose (Table 3). The introduction of large aromatic groups onto the E-amino group of the D-Lys residue resulted in no increase in antiovulatory activity. However, the branched-chain peptide [D-Phe^2, D-Trp^3, N$^\epsilon$-(pGlu-D-Phe-Trp-Ser-Tyr)-D-Lys^6]-LH-RH had far greater inhibitory activity than [D-Phe^2, D-Trp^3, D-Lys^6]-LH-RH on a weight basis,

TABLE 3. N$^\epsilon$ compounds of D-Phe^2,D-Trp^3,D-Lys^6-LH-RH—blockade of ovulation

$$\overset{\displaystyle X}{\underset{\displaystyle |}{}}$$
pGlu-D-Phe-D-Trp-Ser-Tyr-D-Lys-Leu-Arg-Pro-Gly-NH$_2$

Peptide, X=	Dose (mg)	No. rats ovulating	% Blockade of ovulation
H	1.5	7 (7)	0
Benzoyl	1	8 (9)	10
Indomethacinyl	1	8 (8)	0
Acetylsalicylyl	1	8 (9)	10
pGlu-D-Phe-D-Trp-Ser-Tyr	1	3 (11)	73
(pGlu-D-Phe-D-Trp-Ser-Tyr)$_2$-D-Lys	1	7 (9)	22
pGlu-His	1	4 (5)	10
Succ-Leu-Arg-Pro-Gly-NH$_2$	1	8 (9)	11
Succ-D-p-Cl-Phe-Leu-Arg-Pro-Gly-NH$_2$	1	9 (9)	0
Control	—	11 (11)	0

despite its higher molecular weight. It is possible to attribute this increased activity to the presence of two N-termini in one molecule which could interact with and block two receptor sites simultaneously. However, this effect is peculiar to the N-terminus since branched-chain peptides with an extra C-terminal portion did not have increased inhibitory activity (Table 3). A peptide with three N-termini also had much decreased activity presumably due to steric problems between chains.

We extended this approach to full dimers and trimers of [D-Phe^2, D-Trp^3, D-Lys^6]-LH-RH and were able to derive some even more potent inhibitors. The best of the series (Table 4) were the isophthaloyl followed by the succinoyl dimers of the D-Lys^6-peptide. Thus the relative orientations of the peptide chains have a dramatic effect on inhibitory activity which would be expected if interactions with more than one receptor were taking place. In every instance, trimeric molecules were inactive and it appeared that the steric constraints imposed by the close proximity of three large decapeptide chains were too great.

The corresponding agonist series (Table 5) of branched-chain and dimeric peptides were based on [D-Lys^6, desGly-NH$_2$^{10}]-LH-RH ethylamide, which has very high LH-releasing activity. Unlike the results with the inhibitors, the corresponding agonists all had lower LH-releasing activities than their

TABLE 4. N^ϵ-*Polymeric compounds of D-Phe^2,D-Trp^3,D-Lys^6-LH-RH—blockade of ovulation*

pGlu-D-Phe-D-Trp-Ser-Tyr
D-Lys$_n$X
NH$_2$-Gly-Pro-Arg-Leu

Peptide, X=	Dose (mg)	No. rats ovulating	% Blockade of ovulation
HO$_2$CCH$_2$CO$_2$H	1	2 (10)	80
	0.5	6 (10)	40
HO$_2$CCH$_2$CHCO$_2$HCH$_2$CO$_2$H			
n = 3	1	9 (9)	0
n = 2	1	2 (11)	78
CO$_2$H / CO$_2$H	1	1 (9)	89
	0.5	8 (8)	0
HO$_2$C / CO$_2$H	1	10 (10)	100
	0.5	4 (10)	60
HO$_2$C / CO$_2$H / CO$_2$H	1	11 (11)	0

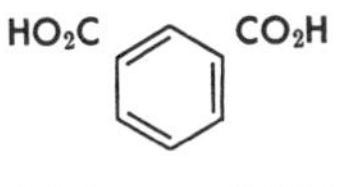

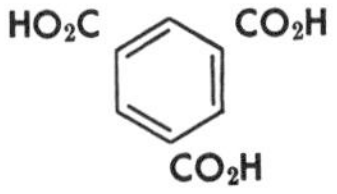

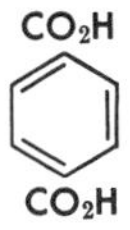

TABLE 5. Agonist activities of branched-chain and dimeric derivatives of [D-Lys^6,desGly-NH$_2^{10}$]-LH-RH ethylamide (EA)

LH-RH analog	% LH releasing activity
[D-Lys^6,desGly-NH$_2^{10}$]-LH-RH EA	1,600
N$^\alpha$,N$^\epsilon$-(pGlu-His-Trp-Ser-Tyr)-D-Lys^6, desGly-NH$_2^{10}$-LH-RH EA	800
Succinoyl-bis[(D-Lys^6,desGly-NH$_2^{10}$)-LH-RH EA]	500
p-Phthaloyl-bis[(D-Lys^6,desGly-NH$_2^{10}$)-LH-RH EA]	110

precursor, the least active being the *p*-phthaloyl and succinoyl dimers which were among the most active in the inhibitory series. Here again, an obvious conformational difference between agonists and antagonists is revealed. It seems that the stereochemistry of the agonist chains, which of course differ considerably from the antagonists at the N-terminus, does not allow two chains to be in such close proximity without tending to destroy binding affinity.

CONCLUSIONS

The complex problems of establishing a mechanism of action and a three-dimensional shape for the biologically active form of LH-RH appear to be yielding to the pressure of information derived from the synthesis and testing of many hundreds of analogs. Similarly, the challenge of developing increasingly more powerful antagonists of the hormone is being met. A combination of several of the inhibitor design approaches described here can be expected to yield analogs of sufficient potency to enable extensive trials to take place and eventually for more convenient routes of administration such as nasal spray to be used.

ACKNOWLEDGMENTS

This work was supported by NIH Contract NICHD 6–2841 and the Veterans Administration.

REFERENCES

1. Coy, D. H., Coy, E. J., Hirotsu, Y., Vilchez-Martinez, J. A., Schally, A. V., van Nispen, J. W., and Tesser, G. I. (1974): Investigation of the role of tryptophan in LH-RH. *Biochemistry*, 13:3550–3553.
2. Coy, D. H., Coy, E. J., Schally, A. V., and Vilchez-Martinez, J. A. (1975): Synthesis and biological activity of LH-RH analogs modified at the carboxy terminus. *J. Med. Chem.*, 18:275–277.
3. Coy, D. H., Hirotsu, Y., Redding, T. W., Coy, E. J., and Schally, A. V. (1975):

Synthesis and biological properties of the 2-L-β-(pyrazolyl-1) alanine analogs of LH-RH and TRH. *J. Med. Chem.*, 18:948–949.

4. Coy, D. H., Vilchez-Martinez, J. A., Coy, E. J., Nishi, N., Arimura, A., and Schally, A. V. (1975): Polyfluoroalkylamine derivatives of LH-RH. *Biochemistry*, 14:1848–1851.

5. Coy, D. H., Vilchez-Martinez, J. A., Coy, E. J., and Schally, A. V. (1976): Analogs of LH-RH with increased biological activity produced by D-amino acid substitutions in position 6. *J. Med. Chem.*, 19:423–425.

6. Fujino, M., Kobayashi, S., Obayashi, M., Shinagawa, S., Fukada, T., Kitada, C., Nakayama, R., Yamakazi, I., White, W. F., and Rippel, R. H. (1972): Structure-activity relationships in the C-terminal part of LH-RH. *Biochem. Biophys. Res. Commun.*, 60:863–869.

7. Hirotsu, Y., Coy, D. H., Coy, E. J., and Schally, A. V. (1974): Stereoisomers of LH-RH. *Biochem. Biophys. Res. Commun.*, 59:277–282.

8. Momany, F. A. (1976): Conformational energy analysis of the molecule, LH-RH. 1. Native decapeptide. *J. Am. Chem. Soc.*, 98:2990–2996.

9. Momany, F. A. (1976): Conformational energy analysis of the molecule, LH-RH. 2. Tetrapeptide and decapeptide analogues. *J. Am. Chem. Soc.*, 98:2996–3000.

10. Monahan, M. W., Amoss, M. S., Anderson, H. A., and Vale, W. (1973): Synthetic analogs of hypothalamic LRF with increased agonist or antagonist properties. *Biochemistry*, 12:4616–4620.

11. Nikolics, K., Coy, D. H., Vilchez-Martinez, J. A., Coy, E. J., and Schally, A. V. (1977): Synthesis and biological activity of position 1 analogs of LH-RH. *Int. J. Peptide Protein Res.*, 9:57–62.

12. Seprodi, J., Coy, D. H., Vilchez-Martinez, J. A., Pedroza, E., and Schally, A. V. (1978): Branched-chain analogues of LH-RH. *J. Med. Chem.*, 21:276–280.

Central Nervous System Effects of Hypothalamic Hormones and Other Peptides, edited by Collu et al. Raven Press, New York © 1979.

Distribution of LH-RH and SRIF in the Central Nervous System

Michael J. Brownstein

Laboratory of Clinical Science, National Institute of Mental Health, Bethesda, Maryland 20014

Two techniques have been used to elucidate the anatomy of peptidergic neurons in the central nervous system. The first of these involves either gross dissection or microdissection of the brain followed by analysis of the peptide content of the resulting tissue samples. The second is based on immuno-histochemical visualization of the peptides. A review dealing with the immunocytochemical localization of luteinizing hormone-releasing hormone (LH-RH) and somatotropin release-inhibiting factor (SRIF) appears elsewhere in this volume. Therefore, in the following paragraphs I shall comment only on studies in which LH-RH and SRIF were measured in tissue homogenates.

Both bioassays and radioimmunoassays have been used to quantitate LH-RH and SRIF in brain extracts. Neither type of assay is absolutely specific; both may detect "big" forms of the hormones, or metabolites. Furthermore, unrelated agents can mimic or antagonize LH-RH and SRIF in the bioassay systems and interfere with radioimmunoassays. Thus the terms "LH-RH" and "SRIF" should be understood to mean LH-RH- and SRIF-like in the context of this chapter.

LH-RH

In 1960 McCann (14) demonstrated that the hypothalamus contains a substance which releases LH from the anterior pituitary, and he set out to find more precisely where it was located. First, he prepared extracts of the stalk median eminence, ventral hypothalamus, dorsal hypothalamus, and suprachiasmatic hypothalamus and measured LH-releasing activity in these extracts. Most of the releasing factor seemed to be present in the stalk and median eminence, although some activity was found in the basal hypothalamus (14). Next, McCann and his co-workers measured LH-releasing activity in serial sections of the preoptic area and hypothalamus. They showed that it was present in a region that extended from the preoptic area through the suprachiasmatic area to the area of the median eminence and arcuate nuclei (13). Subsequently, Wheaton et al. (23) measured LH-RH in brain slices by means of radioimmunoassay. The distribution of LH-RH measured in this way agrees well with the distribution reported earlier.

Rather than assaying LH-RH in brain slices, Palkovits et al. (16) assayed the peptide in discrete hypothalamic nuclei, which were punched out (15) of serial frozen frontal sections of the rat hypothalamus (Table 1). The amount of LH-RH in each tissue sample was determined by radioimmunoassay. A high concentration of LH-RH was found in the median eminence (see ref. 10); moderate levels were detected in the arcuate nucleus; small amounts were present in the suprachiasmatic and preoptic regions. In the preoptic area, the bulk of the LH-RH seems to reside in the supraoptic crest, a vascular organ that forms part of the rostral tip of the third ventricle (19). The supraoptic crest and the other circumventricular organs are quite rich in LH-RH (9) (Table 2).

LH-releasing activity in the medial basal hypothalamus of the rat fell after lesions were made in the suprachiasmatic area (18). Moreover, surgical isolation of the medial basal hypothalamus or rostral deafferentation of this region caused LH-RH to decrease by about 80% there, but did not cause the level of LH-RH to change in the supraoptic crest (4,5,22). Apparently, the LH-RH in the supraoptic crest must be made by neurons located outside of the posterior two-thirds of the hypothalamus. Much—but not all—of the LH-RH in the medial basal hypothalamus, however, seems to be made either by cells rostral to this region or by cells whose synthesis or storage of the peptide is regulated by more rostral neurons. The remaining LH-RH (20%) is endogenous to the hypothalamus; presumably it is made in cells of the arcuate nucleus.

TABLE 1. *Distribution of LH-RH and somatostatin (SRIF) among nuclei of the hypothalamus (3,11,16)*

Nuclei	LH-RH	SRIF
	(ng/mg protein)	
Medial preoptic	0.15	10.4
Periventricular		23.7
Suprachiasmatic	0.05–0.1	8.0
Supraoptic	0.05–0.1	3.2
Anterior hypothalamic		8.6
Lateral anterior		4.9
Paraventricular		4.4
Retrochiasmatic area		56.0
Arcuate	2.9	44.6
Ventromedial	0.6	14.6
Dorsomedial		5.4
Perifornical		3.8
Lateral posterior		3.5
Ventral premammillary		17.3
Dorsal premammillary		4.3
Posterior hypothalamic	0.05–0.1	3.8

TABLE 2. *LH-RH and SRIF in the circumventricular organs of the rat brain (3,9,16,17)*

	LH-RH	SRIF
	(ng/mg protein)	
Median eminence	24.1	309.1
Subfornical organ	4.2	9.8
Subcommissural organ	5.9	17.7
Area postrema	10.2	14.7
Organum vasculosum	14.0	21.0

SRIF

SRIF is found both in the central nervous system and in the periphery, where it is present in the gut and pancreas (20). It has been detected in the brains of several mammals, the pigeon, the frog, the catfish, and the hagfish (19).

Using biological (21) and immunological (3,11) techniques, a number of workers have shown that SRIF is concentrated in the median eminence (Table 2). Other hypothalamic regions that are relatively rich in immunoassayable SRIF include the arcuate, ventromedial, ventral premammillary, periventricular, and medial preoptic nuclei (Table 1). Of these, the ventromedial nucleus was alone in being devoid of biological activity, possibly because of the presence of a growth hormone-releasing factor in this area (21).

Surgical isolation of the medial basal hypothalamus resulted in a marked decrease in its somatostatin content (2,7). Similarly, lesions in the anterior hypothalamic area and ventral medial preoptic area caused decreases in SRIF in the median eminence of 90 and 80%, respectively (7). The above data indicate that the SRIF in the median eminence is present in processes of

TABLE 3. *Regional distribution of somatostatin (SRIF) in the rat brain (3)*

Region	Weight (mg)	SRIF	
		ng/mg wet wt	ng/region
Olfactory bulb	51.9	0.02	1.0
Septum and preoptic area	38.6	0.64	24.7
Hypothalamus	18.5	2.12	39.3
Thalamus	116.4	0.15	17.5
Midbrain	158.5	0.06	9.5
Brainstem	195.7	0.05	9.8
Cerebellum	226.7	0.02	4.5
Striatum	64.8	0.05	3.2
Cortex	1,000	0.03	30.0
		Total	139.5

TABLE 4. *Somatostatin-like material in selected areas of the rat brain*[a]

	Protein (ng/mg)
Cortical areas	
Amygdala	3.9
Parietal cortex	2.4
Hippocampus	1.1
Cingulate cortex	0.7
Entorhinal cortex	1.6
Olfactory tubercle	6.3
Septum	1.9
Preoptic area	4.3
Caudate-putamen	0.6
Diencephalon	
Anterior hypothalamus	2.7
Medial basal hypothalamus	73.1
Posterior hypothalamus	2.5
Thalamus	0.5
Habenula	1.3
Pineal gland	0.5
Brainstem-mesencephalon	
Substantia nigra	0.9
Interpeduncular nucleus	1.0
Central gray	3.3
Dorsal raphe	1.1
Pons	0.9
Medulla	2.4
Cervical spinal cord	2.4

[a] From refs. 3 and 11.

neurons whose perikarya are in the anterior hypothalamus and ventral preoptic area. Such a population of somatostatin-containing neurons has been visualized immunocytochemically in the anterior periventricular area (1, 6,8).

SRIF has been found in the brain outside of the hypothalamus as well as inside of it (Tables 3 and 4). In fact, only about one-third of the SRIF in the brain is present in the hypothalamus. The septum and preoptic area have fairly high somatostatin levels, as do the circumventricular organs (Table 2). Recently, Speiss and Vale (*personal communication*) have succeeded in demonstrating that most of the extrahypothalamic somatostatin has the same amino acid composition as the material present in the hypothalamus.

DISCUSSION

A great deal remains to be learned about LH-RH and SRIF. Relatively little is known yet about the cells which manufacture these peptides or about their mode of manufacture. Immunocytochemical and microanalytical methods should continue to be brought to bear on these problems.

REFERENCES

1. Alpert, L. C., Brawer, J. R., Patel, Y. C., and Reichlin, S. (1976): Somatostatinergic neurons in anterior hypothalamus: Immunohistochemical localization. *Endocrinology*, 98:255–258.
2. Brownstein, M. J., Arimura, A., Fernandez-Durango, R., Schally, A. V., Palkovits, M., and Kizer, J. S. (1977): The effect of hypothalamic deafferentation on somatostatin in the rat brain. *Endocrinology*, 100:246–249.
3. Brownstein, M., Arimura, A., Sato, H., Schally, A. V., and Kizer, J. S. (1975): The regional distribution of somatostatin in the rat brain. *Endocrinology*, 96:1456–1461.
4. Brownstein, M. J., Arimura, A., Schally, A. V., Palkovits, M., and Kizer, J. S. (1976): The effect of surgical isolation of the hypothalamus on its luteinizing hormone-releasing hormone content. *Endocrinology*, 98:662–665.
5. Brownstein, M. J., Palkovits, M., and Kizer, J. S. (1975): On the origin of luteinizing hormone-releasing hormone (LH-RH) in the supraoptic crest. *Life Sci.*, 17:679–682.
6. Elde, R. P., and Parsons, J. A. (1975): Immunocytochemical localization of somatostatin in cell bodies of the rat hypothalamus. *Am. J. Anat.*, 144:541–548.
7. Epelbaum, J., Willoughby, J. O., Brazeau, P., and Martin, J. B. (1977): Effects of lesions and hypothalamic deafferentation on somatostatin distribution in the brain. *Endocrinology*, 101:1495–1502.
8. Hökfelt, T., Efendic, S., Hellerstrom, C., Johansson, O., Luft, R., and Arimura, A. (1975): Cellular localization of somatostatin in endocrine-like cells and neurons of the rat with special references to the A_1-cells of the pancreatic islets and to the hypothalamus. *Acta Endocrinol.*, (Kbh.), 80: Suppl 200.
9. Kizer, J. S., Palkovits, M., and Brownstein, M. (1976): Releasing factors in the circumventricular organs of the rat brain. *Endocrinology*, 98:309–315.
10. Kizer, J. S., Palkovits, M., Tappaz, M., Kebabian, J., and Brownstein, M. (1976): Distribution of releasing factors, biogenic amines, and related enzymes in the bovine median eminence. *Endocrinology*, 98:649–659.
11. Kobayashi, R., Brown, M., and Vale, W. (1977): Regional distribution of neurotensin and somatostatin in rat brain. *Brain Res.*, 126:584–588.
12. Martini, L., Fraschini, F., and Motta, M. (1968): Neural control of anterior pituitary functions. *Recent Prog. Horm. Res.*, 24:439–485.
13. McCann, S. M. (1962): A hypothalamic luteinizing-hormone-releasing factor. *Am. J. Physiol.*, 202:395–400.
14. McCann, S. M., Taleisnik, S., and Friedman, H. M. (1960): LH-releasing activity in hypothalamic extracts. *Proc. Soc. Exp. Biol. Med.*, 104:432–434.
15. Palkovits, M. (1973): Isolated removal of hypothalamic or other brain nuclei of the rat. *Brain Res.*, 59:449–450.
16. Palkovits, M., Arimura, A., Brownstein, M. J., Schally, A. V., and Saavedra, J. M. (1974): Luteinizing hormone-releasing hormone (LH-RH) content of the hypothalamic nuclei in rat. *Endocrinology*, 96:554–558.
17. Palkovits, M., Brownstein, M., Arimura, A., Sato, H., Schally, A. V., and Kizer, J. S. (1976): Somatostatin content of the hypothalamic ventromedial and arcuate nuclei and the circumventricular organs in the rat. *Brain Res.*, 109:430–434.
18. Schneider, H. P. B., Crighton, D. B., and McCann, S. M. (1969): Suprachiasmatic LH-releasing factor. *Neuroendocrinology*, 5:271–280.
19. Vale, W., Ling, N., Rivier, C., Rivier, J., Villarreal, J., and Brown, M. (1976): Anatomic and phylogenetic distribution of somatostatin. *Metabolism*, 25:1491–1494.
20. Vale, W., Rivier, C., and Brown, M. (1977): Regulatory peptides of the hypothalamus. *Annu. Rev. Physiol.*, 39:473–527.
21. Vale, W., Rivier, C., Palkovits, M., Saavedra, J. M., and Brownstein, M. J. (1974): Ubiquitous brain distribution of inhibitors of adenohypophyseal secretion. *Endocrinology*, 94:A 128.
22. Weiner, R. I., Pattou, E., Kerdelhue, B., and Kordon, C. (1975): Differential

effects of hypothalamic deafferentation upon luteinizing hormone-releasing hormone in the median eminence and organum vasculosum of the lamina terminalis. *Endocrinology,* 97:1597–1600.

23. Wheaton, J. E., Krulich, L., and McCann, S. M. (1975): Localization of luteinizing hormone-releasing hormone in the preoptic area and hypothalamus of the rat using radioimmunoassay. *Endocrinology,* 97:30–38.

Central Nervous System Effects of Hypothalamic
Hormones and Other Peptides, edited by Collu et al.
Raven Press, New York © 1979.

Immunohistochemical Localization of Hypothalamic Hormones and Other Peptides in the Central Nervous System

Georges Pelletier

Medical Research Council Group in Molecular Endocrinology,
Le Centre Hospitalier de l'Université Laval, Quebec, Canada

During the last few years, the characterization and chemical synthesis of two hypothalamic releasing hormones and one release-inhibiting hormone (1,2,5,7–9) have led to the production of specific antibodies against these hormones. The use of these antibodies for immunohistochemical localization has been revealed as a powerful tool to identify the cellular elements containing these hormones as well as to determine the precise distribution of the positive nervous structures throughout the brain. Moreover, immunoelectron microscopy can provide information about the intracellular storage and the mode of release of the hormones. The ultrastructural localization can also clearly establish the identity of the neurons involved in the production of peptides (31).

In addition to the hypothalamic regulatory hormones, several peptides found in the pituitary gland, such as β-lipotropin (β-LPH), β-endorphin, adrenocorticotropin (ACTH), and α-melanocyte-stimulating hormone (α-MSH) have also been observed in the central nervous system. These peptides which play a role in behavior and neuroendocrine function (4,6,10,12, 15,16,21,43) have been recently localized in the brain by radioimmunoassay and light microscopic immunohistochemical techniques.

In the present chapter we will discuss the most recent findings about the immunohistochemical localization of luteinizing hormone-releasing hormone (LH-RH), somatostatin, α-MSH, ACTH, and β-LPH. Our immunohistochemical studies have been performed at both light and electron microscopic levels with the help of techniques involving use of the peroxidase-antiperoxidase complex (40).

LH-RH

In many species, LH-RH was consistently observed in the external zone of the median eminence (2,18,28,34,37–39; Fig. 1). By immunoelectron

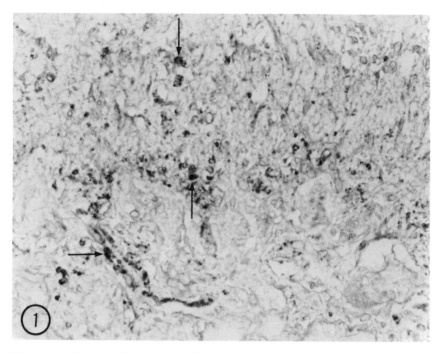

FIG. 1. Immunohistochemical localization of LH-RH in a coronal section through the median eminence of an human hypothalamus. Numerous immunostained fibers (→) are present in the neurovascular zone. ✕420.

microscopy studies, we have been the first to show that LH-RH is present in the secretory granules (75 to 95 nm in diameter) of a few nerve endings (Fig. 2) located in the external zone of the median eminence, in proximity of the capillaries of the pituitary portal plexus (28,33,34). This ultrastructural localization of LH-RH confirmed the hypothesis that hypothalamic hormones are stored in nerve endings and released into the capillaries of the portal plexus under appropriate stimulation.

Many investigators have been unable to detect immunostained cell bodies in the hypothalamus (2,18,34,37). In guinea pigs previously injected with colchicine, Barry et al. (3), using immunofluorescence, observed a few LH-RH-positive cell bodies scattered in a large area extending from the preoptic area to the caudal part of the tuber. More recently, Setalo et al. (38) described LH-RH-containing cell bodies in the rat suprachiasmatic area.

Somewhat surprisingly, LH-RH was also found in the periventricular organs. At the light microscope level, LH-RH was localized in the organum vasculosum of the lamina terminalis (OVLT) in many species (3,18,28–35,39). With the electron microscope, this hormone could clearly be detected in the secretory granules of a few endings located in close proximity to the

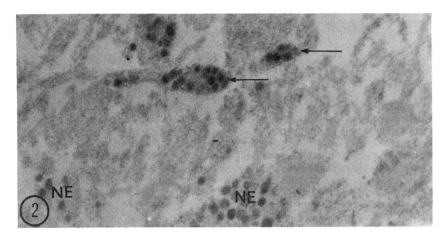

FIG. 2. Electron micrograph showing a section of the external zone of the rat median eminence. Nerve endings containing granules positive for LH-RH (→) can be observed. Other nerve endings (NE) are negative. ×31,000.

fenestrated capillaries of the organum vasculosum (28,34). These observations suggest that LH-RH is secreted from this organ into the general circulation.

In the other periventricular organs, namely, the subfornical organ, the subcommissural organ, and the area postrema, a common pattern for the distribution of LH-RH was observed: a diffuse reaction was present in the cytoplasm of the ependymal and subependymal cells (28,34). These findings have been confirmed by Kizer et al. (23) who have detected by radioimmunoassays the presence of LH-RH in the periventricular organs. The role of LH-RH in these organs remains to be elucidated. So far, LH-RH has not been detected in any other brain areas.

SOMATOSTATIN

In contrast with LH-RH which is mostly found in the hypothalamus, somatostatin is more largely distributed in the central nervous system. By immunocytochemistry, somatostatin-containing fibers were found to be concentrated in the external zone of the median eminence and were detected in a few hypothalamic nuclei, such as the ventromedial, the arcuate, and the periventricular nucleus (13,20,22,34,35). Positive fibers were also seen in the amygdala and the substantia gelatinosa of the spinal cord (19,20).

In the rat hypothalamus, immunostained cell bodies (Fig. 3) have been detected only in the periventricular nucleus (17,20,31). With the aid of immunoelectron microscopy, we have localized somatostatin within secretory

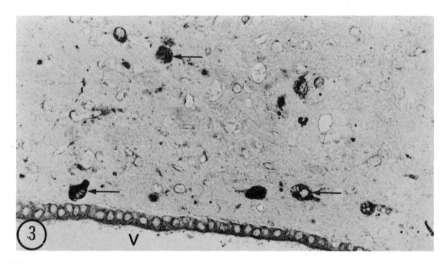

FIG. 3. Localization of somatostatin in the periventricular nucleus of the rat hypothalamus. Immunoreactive cell bodies (→) are located in proximity of the third ventricle (V). ×350.

granules of many nerve endings present in the external zone of the median eminence (32). The granules were slightly larger than those containing LH-RH (90 to 110 nm versus 75 to 95 nm). Very recently, we have also been able to demonstrate somatostatin within the cell bodies of the somatostatinergic neurons in the periventricular nucleus (Fig. 4). The immunohistochemical reaction was localized in most secretory granules present in the cytoplasm of positive neurons. As shown in Fig. 5, this cell type has all the characteristics of a secretory neuron. Thus these observations establish for the first time the identity of neurosecretory neurons involved in the regulation of adenohypophyseal secretion. The somatostatin system appears to have many characteristics in common with the magnocellular system involved in the production of vasopressin and oxytocin.

Somatostatin has also been detected in the periventricular organs (28, 33–35). In the OVLT, somatostatin was shown to be present in the secretory granules (90 to 120 nm in diameter) of many endings located close to the capillaries of the organum vasculosum (28,34). In the other periventricular organs, the reaction was similar to that observed for LH-RH, the reaction product being found dispersed in the cytoplasm of ependymal and subependymal cells.

In the human hypothalamus, somatostatin-containing perikarya were mostly localized in the anterior portion of the arcuate nucleus (11). Immunostained fibers were also detected in the neurovascular zone of the pituitary stalk, suggesting that somatostatin is released in that region to reach the capillaries of the pituitary portal plexus. In the periventricular nucleus, a large bundle of fibers extending from the anterior part of the paraventricular

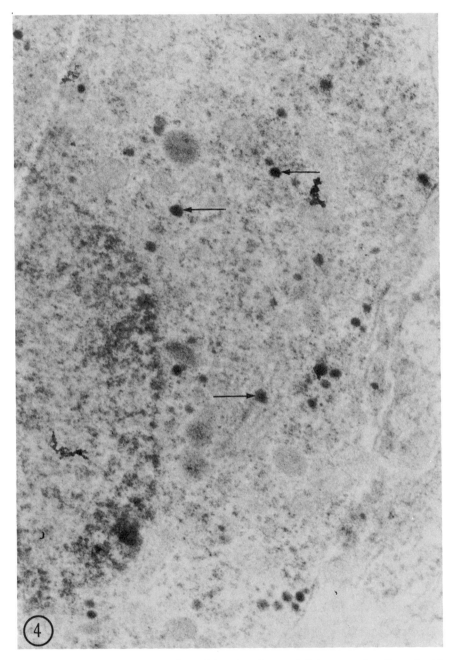

FIG. 4. Electron microscope immunohistochemical detection of somatostatin in a neuron from the periventricular nucleus. A positive reaction is present in most secretory granules (→). ×35,000.

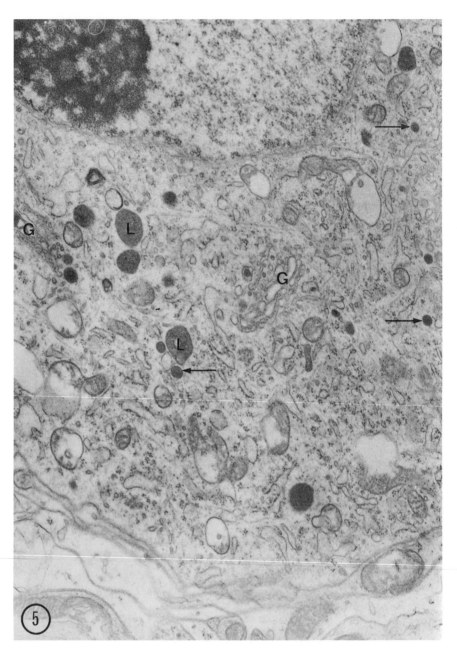

FIG. 5. Section of a somatostatinergic neuron treated for conventional ultrastructural studies. This neuron is characterized by the presence of a well-developed Golgi apparatus (G), secretory granules (→), and lysosomes (L). ×33,000.

nucleus up to the posterior portion of the mammillary body has also been detected. The role of these fibers still remains to be clarified.

α-MSH

α-MSH, a peptide known for its pigmentary effect on the skin of lower vertebrates, also plays a role in variety of adaptative mechanisms in mammals (10,12). Recently, α-MSH has been found by radioimmunoassays in many areas of the rat brain (27,41). With the help of immunohistochemistry, we have been able to clearly identify, for the first time, the nervous structures associated with α-MSH (14,30). Immunostained nerve fibers are found in the hypothalamus, thalamus, and midbrain. They are particularly abundant in the hypothalamus. Positive cell bodies were confined to the arcuate nucleus (Fig. 6). With the electron microscope, it was possible to determine that immunostaining was restricted to the vesicles (40 to 70 nm in diameter) of the α-MSH-containing fibers (Fig. 7). Since identical results were obtained in rats hypophysectomized 15 days previously, α-MSH-positive fibers must originate from the cell bodies contained in the hypothalamus. In the human hypothalamus, immunostained neuronal cell bodies were also found in the arcuate nucleus (Fig. 8). The localization of cells and nerve fibers containing α-MSH in wide regions of the brain strongly reinforces the suggested effects of α-MSH on mammalian central nervous functions.

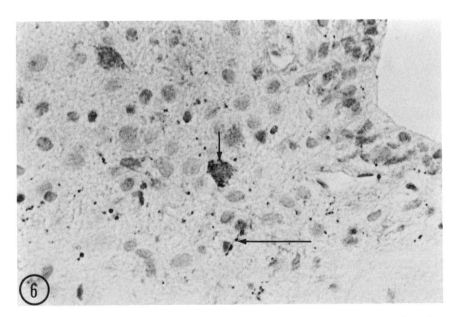

FIG. 6. Immunohistochemical detection of α-MSH in a coronal section through the arcuate nucleus of rat hypothalamus. Neuronal bodies (*short arrows*) as well as beaded fibers (*long arrows*) are immunoreactive. ×500.

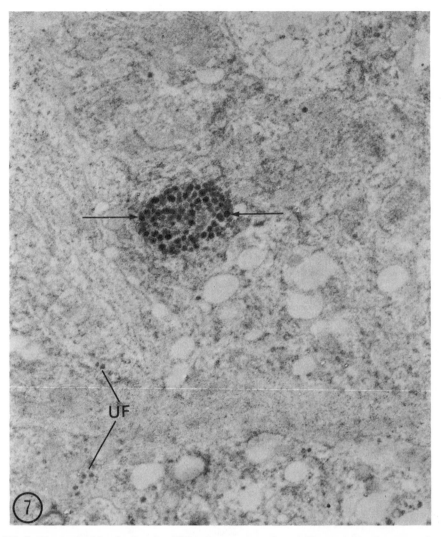

FIG. 7. Ultrastructural localization of α-MSH in the arcuate nucleus. A fiber containing immunoreactive dense core vesicles (→) can be observed. Unstained fibers (UF) are present in the same section. ×32,000.

β-LPH–ACTH SYSTEM

As α-MSH, ACTH is another pituitary hormone that seems to exert some action on the central nervous system of mammals including man (10,12,42). Recently, this peptide has been reported to be present in the brain of both normal and hypophysectomized rats as well as in the bovine central nervous system (24,25). So far, the morphological localization of ACTH in the central nervous system had not been reported. With the help of antibodies

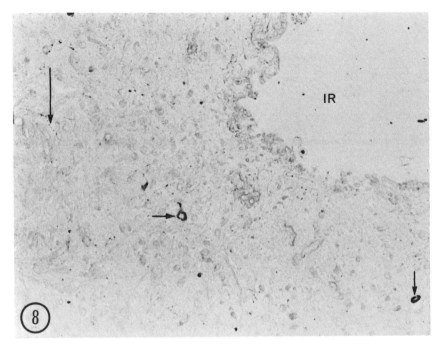

FIG. 8. Localization of α-MSH in the human hypothalamus. Positive cell bodies (*short arrows*) and fibers (*long arrows*) are present in the arcuate nucleus. IR; infundibular recess of the third ventricle. ×170.

specific to ACTH$^{1-39}$, it has been possible to identify the nervous structures containing ACTH in the central nervous system of the rat and man. In the rat brain, immunostained fibers were found in many brain areas (Fig. 9). They were abundant in most hypothalamic nuclei, particularly in the periventricular preoptic area and the periventricular and arcuate nuclei (Fig. 10). At the mesencephalic level, many positive fibers were seen in the periaqueductal gray. The positive perikarya were detected only in the caudal portion of the arcuate nucleus (Fig. 10). Hypophysectomy did not significantly affect immunostaining. In the human hypothalamus, the application of the same anti-ACTH serum produced staining of numerous fibers which were largely distributed throughout the hypothalamus. They were particularly abundant in the periventricular nucleus. As observed in the rat brain, immunoreactive cell bodies were found only in the arcuate nucleus.

At the electron microscope level, ACTH was localized within the dense core vesicles of nerve fibers or endings (Fig. 11). The diameter of the dense core was of 60 to 80 nm. This morphological localization of ACTH in neuronal cell bodies and fibers confirms the hypothesis that ACTH, or an ACTH-like molecule, is really produced by the central nervous system. Moreover, the presence of ACTH within dense core vesicles suggests that this peptide could possibly act as a neurotransmitter. Since both β-LPH and ACTH had

RAT BRAIN

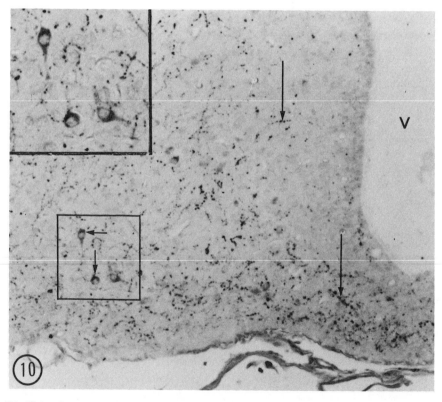

▲ FIBERS
● CELL BODIES

ACTH

FIG. 9. Diagram of the rat brain showing the distribution of neuronal cell bodies and fibers containing ACTH.

FIG. 10. Localization of ACTH in a coronal section through the arcuate nucleus of the rat hypothalamus. Immunostained cell bodies (*short arrows*) and fibers (*long arrows*) can be observed. V; third ventricle. ×200.

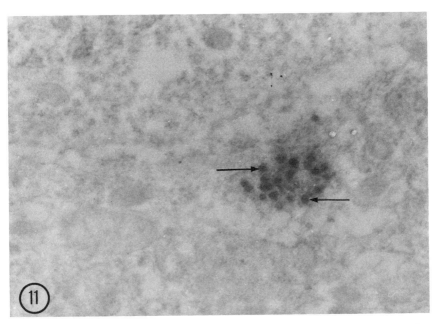

FIG. 11. Ultrastructural localization of ACTH in the arcuate nucleus. Positive dense core vesicle (→) are localized in a fiber. ×32,000.

been localized in the same pituitary cells in several species (36), it seemed important to know if these two peptides are also present in the same neurons.

Using an antiserum to human β-LPH (supplied by Dr. C. H. Li) which does not cross-react with ACTH, it has been possible to show that the pattern of distribution of β-LPH fibers was similar to that of ACTH fibers (29). When consecutive sections were alternatively stained with anti-β-LPH and anti-ACTH, is was demonstrated that ACTH fibers are more abundant than the β-LPH fibers and that these two peptides are contained in different neuronal cell bodies.

Since it has been recently demonstrated that ACTH and β-LPH originate from the same precursor molecule in mouse pituitary tumor cells AtT-20 (26), the present data strongly suggest that the processing of ACTH and β-LPH is markedly different in the pituitary and the central nervous system. Such a system would permit the transformation of the same peptide precursor into different active peptides according to the need of the particular cell type. It remains, however, possible that different biosynthetic mechanisms exist in the pituitary gland and central nervous system.

SUMMARY AND CONCLUSION

The application of immunohistochemical techniques to the localization of hypothalamic hormones and other peptides of biological importance has produced interesting observations leading to some generalization. In the hypothalamus, the hypothalamic regulatory hormones (LH-RH) and somatostatin) are produced by neurosecretory neurons which send their axons into the external zone of the median eminence. In the nerve endings, these hormones are stored in small secretory granules before being released into the fenestrated capillaries of the pituitary portal plexus. α-MSH, β-LPH, and ACTH have been found to be associated with typical neuronal structures in the rat and human brain. Whereas immunostained nerve fibers have been found to be largely distributed in the hypothalamus, thalamus, and midbrain, the cell bodies containing these peptides have been detected only in the arcuate nucleus. Although the pattern of distribution is similar for these three peptides, they are clearly produced by different neurons and thus belong to different systems. Recent observations at the electron microscope level strongly suggest that these peptides which are contained within dense core vesicles could act as neurotransmitters.

REFERENCES

1. Baba, Y., Matsuo, H., and Schally, A. V. (1971): Structure of the porcine LH- and FSH-releasing hormone. II. Confirmation of the proposed structure by conventional sequential analyses. *Biochem. Biophys. Res. Commun.*, 44:459–467.
2. Baker, B. L., Dermody, W. C., and Reel, J. R. (1974): Localization of luteinizing hormone-releasing hormone in the mammalian hypothalamus. *Am. J. Anat.*, 139:129–134.
3. Barry, J., Dubois, M. P., and Poulain, P. (1974): LRF producing cells of the mammalian hypothalamus. *Z. Zellforsch.*, 146:351–366.
4. Bloom, F., Segal, D., Ling, N., and Guillemin, R. (1976): Endorphins: Profound behavioral effects in rats suggest new etiological factors in mental illness. *Science*, 194:630–632.
5. Bøler, J., Enzman, F., Folkers, K., Bowers, C. Y., and Schally, A. V. (1969): The identity of chemical and hormonal properties of the thyrotropin-releasing hormone and pyroglutamyl-histidyl proline amide. *Biochem. Biophys. Res. Commun.*, 37:705–710.
6. Bradbury, A. F., Smyth, D. G., and Snell, C. R. (1976): Lipotropin: Precursor to two biologically active peptides. *Biochem. Biophys. Res. Commun.*, 69:950–956.
7. Brazeau, P., Vale, W., Burgus, R., Ling, N., Butcher, M., Rivier, J., and Guillemin, R. (1973): Hypothalamic polypeptide that inhibits the secretion of immunoreactive pituitary growth hormone. *Science*, 179:77–79.
8. Burgus, R., Butcher, M., Ling, N., Monahan, M., Rivier, J., Fellows, R., Amoss, M., Blackwell, R., Vale, W., and Guillemin, R. (1971): Structure moléculaire du facteur hypothalamique (LRF) d'origine ovine contrôlant la sécrétion de l'hormone gonadotrope hypophysaire de lutéinisation. *C. R. Acad. Sci. [D] (Paris)*, 273:1611–1613.
9. Burgus, R., Dunn, T. F., Desiderio, D., and Guillemin, R. (1969): Structure moléculaire du facteur hypothalamique TRF d'origine ovine: mise en évidence par spectrométrie de masse de la séquence PCA-His-Pro-NH₂. *C. R. Acad. Sci. [D] Paris*, 269:1870–1973.
10. Dattu, P. C., and King, M. G. (1977): Effects of melanocyte-stimulating hormone (MSH) and melanotin on passive avoidance and on an emotional response. *Biochem. Behav.*, 6:449–452.
11. Désy, L., and Pelletier, G. (1977): Immunohistochemical localization of somatostatin in the human hypothalamus. *Cell Tissue Res.*, 184:491–497.

12. De Wied, D., and Gispen, W. H. (1976): Behavioral effects of peptides. In: *Peptides in Neurobiology,* edited by H. Gainer, pp. 397–448. Plenum Press, New York.
13. Dubé, D., Leclerc, R., Pelletier, G., Arimura, A., and Schally, A. V. (1975): Immunohistochemical detection of growth hormone-releasing inhibiting hormone (somatostatin) in the guinea pig brain. *Cell Tissue Res.,* 161:385–392.
14. Dubé, D., Lissitsky, J. C., Leclerc, R., and Pelletier, G. (1978): Localization of alpha-melanocyte-stimulating hormone in the rat brain and pituitary. *Endocrinology,* 102:1283–1291.
15. Dupont, A., Cusan, L., Garon, M., Labrie, F., and Li, C. H. (1977): Beta-endorphin: Stimulation of growth hormone release in *vivo. Proc. Natl. Acad. Sci. USA,* 74:358–359.
16. Dupont, A., Cusan, L., Labrie, F., Coy, D. H., and Li, C. H. (1976): Stimulation of prolactin release in the rat by intraventricular injection of β-endorphin and methionine-enkephalin. *Biochem. Biophys. Res. Commun.,* 75:76–82.
17. Elde, R. P., and Parsons, J. A. (1975): Immunocytochemical localization of somatostatin in cell bodies of the rat hypothalamus. *Am. J. Anat.,* 144:541–548.
18. Gross, D. S. (1976): Distribution of gonadotropin-releasing hormone in the mouse brain as revealed by immunohistochemistry. *Endocrinology,* 98:1408–1417.
19. Hökfelt, T., Efendic, S., Hellerstrom, C., Johansson, O., Luft, R., and Arimura, A. (1975): Immunohistochemical evidence for separate populations of somatostatin-containing and substance P-containing primary afferent neurons in the rat. *Neuroscience,* 1:131–136.
20. Hökfelt, T., Efendic, S., Hellerstrom, C., Johansson, O., Luft, R., and Arimura, A. (1975): Cellular localization of somatostatin in endocrine-like cells and neurons of the rat with special references to the A₁-cells of the pancreatic islets and to the hypothalamus. *Acta Endocrinol. [Suppl.] (Kbh.),* 80:5–41.
21. Jacquet, Y. F., and Marks, N. (1976): The C-fragment of β-lipotropin: An endogenous neuroleptic or anti-psychotogen. *Science,* 194:632–635.
22. King, J. C., Gerall, A. A., Fishback, J. B., Elkind, K. E., and Arimura, A. (1975): Growth hormone-release inhibiting hormone (GH-RIH) pathway of the rat hypothalamus revealed by the unlabeled antibody peroxidase-antiperoxidase method. *Cell Tissue Res.,* 160:423–430.
23. Kizer, J. S., Palkovits, M., and Brownstein, M. J. (1976): Releasing factors in the circumventricular organs in the rat brain. *Endocrinology,* 98:311–316.
24. Krieger, D. T., Liotta, A., and Brownstein, M. J. (1977): Presence of corticotropin in brain of normal and hypophysectomized rats. *Proc. Natl. Acad. Sci. USA,* 74:648–652.
25. Krieger, D. T., Liotta, A., Sudo, T., Palkovits, M., and Brownstein, M. J. (1977): Presence of immunoassayable β-lipotropin in bovine brain and spinal cord: Lack of concordance with ACTH concentrations. *Biochem. Biophys. Res. Commun.,* 76:930–936.
26. Mains, R. E., Eipper, B. A., and Ling, N. (1977): Common precursor to corticotropins and endorphins. *Proc. Natl. Acad. Sci. USA,* 74:3014–3018.
27. Oliver, C., Barnea, A., Usategui, R., Mical, R. S., and Porter, J. C. (1976): Localisation et sécrétion de l'α-MSH chez le rat. *INSERM,* Rapp. no. 7:49–53.
28. Pelletier, G. (1976): Immunohistochemical localization of hypothalamic hormones at the electron microscope level. In: *Hypothalamus and Endocrine Functions,* edited by F. Labrie, J. Meites, and G. Pelletier, pp. 433–450. Plenum Press, New York.
29. Pelletier, G., Désy, L., Lissitzky, J. C., Labrie, F., and Li, C. H. (1978): Immunohistochemical localization of β-LPH in the human hypothalamus. *Life Sci,* 22:1799–1804.
30. Pelletier, G., and Dubé, D. (1977): Electron microscopic immunohistochemical localization of α-MSH in the rat brain. *Am. J. Anat.,* 150:201–205.
31. Pelletier, G., Dubé, D., and Puviani, R. (1977): Somatostatin: Electron microscope immunohistochemical localization in secretory neurons of rat hypothalamus. *Science,* 196:1469–1470.

32. Pelletier, G., Labrie, F., Arimura, A., and Schally, A. V. (1974): Electron microscopic immunohistochemical localization of growth hormone-release inhibiting hormone (somatostatin) in the rat median eminence. *Am. J. Anat.,* 140:445–450.
33. Pelletier, G., Labrie, F., Puviani, R., Arimura, A., and Schally, A. V. (1974): Immunohistochemical localization of luteinizing hormone-releasing hormone in the rat median eminence. *Endocrinology,* 95:314–317.
34. Pelletier, G., Leclerc, R., and Dubé, D. (1976): Immunohistochemical localization of hypothalamic hormones. *J. Histochem. Cytochem.,* 24:864–871.
35. Pelletier, G., Leclerc, R., Dubé, D., Labrie, F., Puviani, R., Arimura, A., and Schally, A. V. (1975): Localization of growth hormone-release-inhibiting hormone (somatostatin) in the rat brain. *Am. J. Anat.,* 142:397–401.
36. Pelletier, G., Leclerc, R., Labrie, F., Côté, J., Chretien, M., and Lis, M. (1977): Immunohistochemical localization of β-lipotropic hormone in the pituitary gland. *Endocrinology,* 100:770–776.
37. Setalo, G., Vigh, S., Schally, A. V., Arimura, A., and Flerko, B. (1974): LH-RH-containing neural elements in the rat hypothalamus. *Endocrinology,* 96:135–142.
38. Setalo, G., Vigh, S., Schally, A. V., Arimura, A., and Flerko, B. (1976): Immunohistochemical study of the origin of LHRH-containing nerve fibers of the rat hypothalamus. *Brain Res.,* 103:597–602.
39. Silverman, A. J., Antunes, J. L., Ferin, M., and Zimmerman, E. A. (1977): The distribution of luteinizing hormone-releasing hormone (LH-RH) in the hypothalamus of the rhesus monkey. Light microscopic studies using immunoperoxidase technique. *Endocrinology,* 101:134–142.
40. Sternberger, L. A. (1974): *Immunocytochemistry.* Prentice-Hall Inc., Englewood Cliffs, N.J.
41. Usategui, R., Oliver, C., Vaudry, H., Lombardi, G., Rozenberg, I., and Mourne, A. M. (1976): Immunoreactive α-MSH and ACTH levels in rat plasma and pituitary. *Endocrinology,* 98:189–196.
42. Van Riezen, H., Rigter, H., and De Wied, D. (1977): Possible significance of ACTH fragments for human mental performance. *Behav. Biol.,* 20:311–324.
43. Watson, S. J., Barchas, J. P., and Li, C. H. (1977): β-Lipotropin: Localization of cells and axons in rat brain by immunocytochemistry. *Proc. Natl. Acad. Sci. USA,* 74:5155–5158.

Central Nervous System Effects of Hypothalamic Hormones and Other Peptides, edited by Collu et al.
Raven Press, New York © 1979.

Effects of LH-RH on Sexual Activities in Animal and Man

Robert L. Moss, Peter Riskind, and Carol A. Dudley

*Physiology Department, University of Texas Health Science Center at Dallas,
Southwestern Medical School, Dallas, Texas 75235*

More than three decades ago, it was proposed that secretions of the anterior pituitary gland were regulated by substances generated in the hypothalamus (35). Firm support for this concept came later with the demonstration of the existence of a factor in the hypothalamus that caused luteinizing hormone (LH) to be released from the anterior pituitary gland (52). Subsequently, three hypothalamic factors or hormones were isolated, purified, structurally analyzed, and synthesized (11–13,49,75). These hypophysiotropic peptide hormones are thyrotropin-releasing hormone (TRH), luteinizing hormone-releasing hormone (LH-RH), and somatostatin. Today, despite many unanswered questions, the endocrine effects of these peptide hormones have clearly been established in animal and man (for recent reviews see 88,106). TRH, for example, can increase thyroid-stimulating hormone (TSH) and prolactin release. LH-RH releases both follicle-stimulating hormone (FSH) and luteinizing hormone. On the other hand, somatostatin appears to inhibit release of both growth hormone and TRH-induced TSH release.

Until recently, major emphasis was directed solely toward the endocrine effects of the hypothalamic hypophysiotropic hormones. However, and perhaps of even more far-reaching significance, these same hypothalamic peptide hormones have now been implicated in a variety of CNS activities from the cellular to the behavioral level. These CNS-dependent activities occur independently of the pituitary gland and include changes in neuronal excitability, general locomotive behavior, appetitive behavior, antidepressive and antisedative activities, and mating behavior (1,2,22,42,59,60,77,85,89). The present chapter summarizes the extra-pituitary behaviors associated with one of the hypothalamic hypophysiotropic hormones, namely, LH-RH, and its role in modulating sexual activities in both animal and man.

EFFECT OF LH-RH ON ANIMAL SEXUAL BEHAVIOR

Our interest in the action of LH-RH in the control of female sexual behavior evolved from two observations. The first observation was the existence of a temporal relationship between the LH-RH-induced spontaneous discharge of LH and the onset of sexual receptivity. For example, in the regular 4-day cyclic female rat a preovulatory surge of gonadotropins, presumably triggered by the release of LH-RH, occurs on the afternoon of proestrus (28,51). This unique endocrine event is followed 2 to 3 hr later by the onset of behavioral heat (10,76,99). This pronounced temporal association suggested that LH-RH, the gonadotropins, LH and FSH as well as the ovarian hormones, may be involved in the initiation of female sexual receptivity. Second, there appears to be an anatomical overlap of the neural tissue responsible for producing LH-RH, controlling gonadotropin secretion, and regulating mating behavior. It is thought that the hypophysiotropic area of the hypothalamus, which now includes the medial preoptic area as well as the medial basal hypothalamus, produces LH-RH. The LH-RH reaches the anterior pituitary gland by way of the hypothalamic-hypophyseal portal system (33,35,36). As seen in Fig. 1, LH-RH has been localized in a band of tissue extending from the rostral medial preoptic area to the arcuate nucleus–median eminence complex (4,27,40,45,46,79,107).

The second observation is that the primary CNS site concerned with female mating behavior also appears to be the medial preoptic area, since lesions in the area facilitate whereas electrical stimulation inhibits mating activities (73,84,102). Other CNS sites involved in regulating mating behavior are anterior hypothalamus (47,102), arcuate-ventromedial region (47), and midbrain (34). It is presumed that all the neurons that project to the median eminence are hypophysiotropic neurons which inhibit or stimulate anterior pituitary gland secretion(s) via the releasing and inhibiting hormones. How-

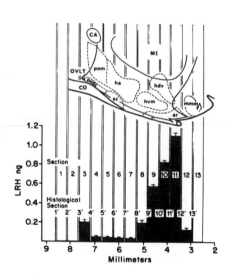

FIG. 1. The bars of the histogram represent the means of the immunoassayable LRH contained in extracts of 400 μm thick frontal sections (1–13). The vertical line above each bar gives the SEM. A thin section (1'–13') was cut before each 400-μm section and was used for histological study. The millimetric scale of the abscissa corresponds to the stereotaxic coordinate used in König and Klippel's *Rat Brain Atlas*. Frontal sections are diagrammatically projected through an outline of a parasagittal section. Abbreviations used for this figure: ar, n. arcuatus; ha, n. anterior (hypothalamic); hdv, n. dorsomedialis (hypothalamic); hpv, n. periventricularis (hypothalamic); hvm, n. ventromedialis (hypothalamic); pom, n. preopticus medialis; posc, n. preopticus, pars suprachiasmatica; mmm, n. mammillaris medialis, para medialis; sc, n. suprachiasmaticus; CA, commissura anterior; CO, chiasma opticum; F, columna fornicis; I, infundibulum; ME, median eminence; OVLT, organum vasculosum lamina terminalis; MI, massa intercalata; TD, tractus diagonalis; VIII, third ventricle. (Taken from ref. 107.)

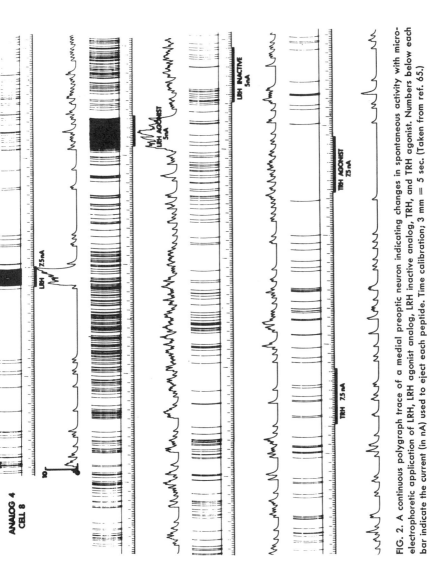

FIG. 2. A continuous polygraph trace of a medial preoptic neuron indicating changes in spontaneous activity with micro-electrophoretic application of LRH, LRH agonist analog, LRH inactive analog, TRH, and TRH agonist. Numbers below each bar indicate the current (in nA) used to eject each peptide. Time calibration; 3 mm = 5 sec. (Taken from ref. 65.)

ever, some of the medial preoptic neurons, and possibly arcuate neurons, that do not project to median eminence may be responsive to LH-RH and subsequently mediate extrapituitary behaviors such as mating. Support of this concept has come from neurophysiological experiments in which LH-RH has been microelectrophoresed, in small quantities, onto the membrane of nerve cells (25,43,44,58,59,65,67–69,83,90,92,93,103). Figure 2 shows a typical response to the microelectrophoresis of LH-RH, LH-RH agonist analog [D-Trp^6, Pro^9-NHEt-LH-RH, agonist analog (LH-RH+)], LH-RH inactive analog [des-Pro^9-Gly^{10}-LH-RH, inactive analog (LH-RH°)], TRH, and TRH agonist analog [3 Me-His^2-TRH, agonist analog (TRH+)] on a single medial preoptic neuron that was electrophysiologically determined not to project to the median eminence. As observed in this illustration, LH-RH and LH-RH agonist analog initiated marked excitation whereas TRH agonist caused an inhibition. Interestingly, LH-RH responsive neurons have been found throughout the medial preoptic area, septum, medial basal hypothalamus, and the midbrain central gray region. The medial preoptic and basal hypothalamic neurons that do not project to the median eminence are just as responsive and in some cases more responsive to LH-RH than those that do project to the median eminence and are presumably involved in gonadtropin secretion. This indicates that the CNS sites regulating gonadotropin secretions and mating behavior overlap and that some of the neurons contained within these CNS sites are responsive to LH-RH independent of whether their axons terminate in the median eminence. Based on the aforementioned data which emphasized (a) the temporal relationship between gonadotropin release and sexual receptivity, (b) the overlapping CNS sites regulating both reproductive activities, and (c) the presence of LH-RH-responsive neurons in these reproductive sites, it was considered of particular interest to evaluate the action of LH-RH on sexual behavior in the female rat.

Female Rat

Investigation of LH-RH in animals has offered the most direct evidence thus far of a central action of hypothalamic polypeptides. LH-RH has been demonstrated to have a specific action on mating behavior in the rat. The initial series of experiments demonstrated that subcutaneous injections of 500 ng of LH-RH potentiated mating behavior as measured by the lordosis response in estrone-primed ovariectomized female rats (62,70,71). The potentiation of lordosis behavior has been found to be specific to LH-RH, in that the administration of estrone alone or estrone in combination with TRH, LH, or FSH was ineffective in enhancing mating behavior (Fig. 3). In addition, LH-RH was found to potentiate lordosis behavior in estrone-primed ovariectomized, adrenalectomized (57,62,71,72), and in estradiol benzoate-

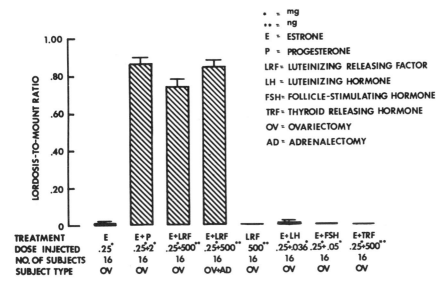

FIG. 3. Effect of gonadotropins, ovarian hormones, and releasing factors on lordosis behavior in the ovariectomized female rat. (Taken from ref. 71.)

primed ovariectomized, hypophysectomized rats (81). The LH-RH-induced mating behavior thus appears to be independent of the gonadotropins and the pituitary-adrenal axis. Supportive experiments have demonstrated that activation of lordosis responsiveness by vaginal stimulation is independent of anterior and posterior pituitary gland hormones (95). Interestingly, mating behavior in the ovariectomized female rat has been thought to be a consequence of the synergistic interaction between estrogen and progesterone (5,9). The present findings suggest that LH-RH may be substituted for progesterone in the estrogen-progesterone paradigm for the induction of sexual receptivity. However, it should be mentioned that as studied so far (70,71,81) LH-RH does not have as great an effect on lordosis behavior as progesterone (53).

The most effective dose and time course for the LH-RH response has been established (71). A dose of 150 ng given subcutaneously was determined to be the minimal dose of LH-RH needed to potentiate lordosis in estrone-primed, ovariectomized female rats, whereas the maximum response was observed with 500 ng. The first appearance of a potentiation of mating behavior occurred approximately 2 to 3 hr following a single injection of 500 ng LH-RH. The maximum response was observed 5 to 7 hr postinjection and the total time of the LH-RH-induced heat period was approximately 8 hr. Thus LH-RH, which has a half-life in circulation of minutes, potentiates mating behavior several hours after administration and this behavior is maintained for 8 hr. It should be noted that the period of sexual receptivity in the 4-day cyclic female rat follows shortly (3 to 5 hr) after the preovulatory release of

LH and persists for a period of 8 to 10 hr. This is very similar to the afore-mentioned data for LH-RH potentiation of mating behavior.

LH-RH also has been shown to facilitate sexual behavior in mice (48). However, except for the rat and the mouse, the species generality of the potentiation effect of LH-RH has not been clearly demonstrated. Administration of LH-RH initiated only slight lordosis facilitation in the estradiol benzoate-primed guinea pig (14), and no response in the estrogen-primed hamster (14). In the estrogen-primed hamster, neither systemic nor intraventricular administration (14) of LH-RH induced a potentiation of lordosis behavior (14). In another more recent study, a long-acting analog of LH-RH was administered to adult male chimpanzees. The hormonal responses were normal, but LH-RH did not initiate any change in sexual behavior (C. H. Doering, P. R. McGinnis, G. W. Kraemer, and D. A. Hamburg, *personal communication*). At the present time, no explanation is apparent to explain these negative findings.

The positive findings demonstrating an LH-RH facilitatory action on mating are certainly suggestive of the possibility that the decapeptide may be acting directly on neural tissue to bring about the reported changes. To test the notion that LH-RH has a neural action in facilitating lordosis behavior in estrone-primed, ovariectomized female rats, a series of experiments was conducted in which small quantities (50 ng) of LH-RH, TRH, as well as saline were infused via cannulas into the medial preoptic area, arcuate nucleus, lateral hypothalamic area, or the cerebral cortex (30,31,66,69). As shown in Fig. 4, medial preoptic and arcuate microinfusions of LH-RH, but not TRH, potentiated lordosis behavior (30,31,39,66). TRH infusions resulted in decreased mating behavior as compared to that obtained with control infusions. Similar infusion of LH-RH and TRH into the lateral hypothalamus and cerebral cortex resulted in no change in the mating behavior pattern.

Interestingly, increases, although slightly significant, in lordosis behavior were observed in the control groups, that is, in the vehicle (sham, saline), neural site (lateral hypothalamic area, cerebral cortex), and peptide (TRH) controls (Fig. 4). These increases in mating were not as large as those observed with LH-RH infusions into the medial preoptic area and arcuate nucleus. The control increases were attributed to the animal being "twice mated," that is, being mated prior to and following infusion. This increase in mating also occurs in noncannulated ovariectomized and ovariectomized, adrenalectomized female rats. The increase in the lordosis behavior as a result of being twice mated is an extremely interesting finding especially since coitus has been shown to be a sufficient stimulus to release LH, presumably by initiating LH-RH release (20,57,61,64). Thus LH-RH has been shown to potentiate mating and mating has been shown to amplify LH release which is dependent on LH-RH. Therefore, mating can probably potentiate mating by a facilitation of the release of LH-RH (57,59,60).

In subsequent medial preoptic and arcuate-ventromedial microinfusion ex-

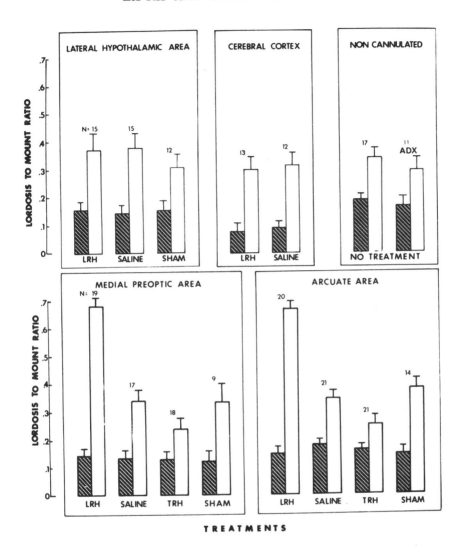

FIG. 4. Effects of LH-RH, TRH, saline, and sham infusions upon mating behavior in ovariectomized, estrone-primed female rats cannulated in the medial preoptic area, arcuate area, lateral hypothalamic area, and cerebral cortex as compared to mating behavior in noncannulated, ovariectomized and ovariectomized-adrenalectomized (ADX), estrone-primed female rats. N, number of animals; I, SEM; stippled bars, preinfusion mating; open bars, postinfusion mating. (Taken from ref. 31.)

periments, LH or TRH but not LH-RH inhibited sexual receptivity in animals given a high dose of estrone to ensure a high preinfusion mating activity (32). The addition of either TRH or LH solutions to LH-RH infusates diminished the decapeptides' facilitation of sexual behavior (32). The infusion of FSH or the addition of FSH to LH-RH infusates neither enhanced nor depressed the mating behavior. The aforementioned data are summarized in Table 1.

TABLE 1. *Behavioral responses to intrahypothalmic infusions*

Pharmacological agent	Behavioral response (change in receptivity)						
	Low preinfusion receptivity model			High preinfusion receptivity model		LRH blockade model	
	MPOA	ARC—VM	LHA	MPOA	ARC—VM	MPOA	ARC—VM
LRH	+	+	0	0	0	(+)	(+)
TRH	0	0	0	—	—	—	—
LH	0	0	0	—	—	—	—
FSH	0	0	0	0	0	0	0

+ = Facilitation; — = suppression; 0 = no effect. (From ref. 32)

The inhibitory effects of medial preoptic area and arcuate-ventromedial region infusions of LH on lordotic behavior observed are in agreement with the previous proposals that LH may suppress mating behavior in male and female rats (18,80). These inhibitory effects of LH on sexual behavior correlated with the inhibitory effects observed on hypothalamic multiunit activity (87,104), single-unit activity (98), oxidative metabolism (54), and RNA transcription (41). These inhibitory effects also parallel the inhibitory effects of LH described for LH-RH secretion (16,17,19,23,55,87,105). The parallelisms in LH suppression of neuronal activity and endocrine and behavioral responses indicate that LH may feed back on hypothalamic neurons involved in the coordination of both reproductive responses. Further, the LH blockade of LH-RH effects suggests that LH may act on LH-RH-responsive neurons within the medial preoptic and arcuate-ventromedial regions.

The findings of the microinfusion experiments are indicative of a facilitative action of LH-RH and an inhibitory action of TRH on mating behavior. This suggests that peptide hormones may be acting directly on neural tissue to potentiate or depress lordotic behavior in the female rat. These excitatory and inhibitory actions have corroborated neurophysiological observations of LH-RH excitation and TRH depression of neuronal activity within the septum, medial preoptic area, and arcuate-ventromedial complex (25,58,59,63, 65,69,90,92,93). Furthermore, LH-RH has been shown to excite single-cell activity of neurons that were inhibited by TRH (59). These neurons did not project to or terminate in the median eminence, thus suggesting a hypothalamic pathway whose neurons are responsive to LH-RH and TRH. Interestingly, an LH-RH hypothalamic-mesencephalic pathway has been recently proposed (3,101). Moreover, as shown in Fig. 5, LH-RH infusions into the midbrain central gray region of estrone-primed, ovariectomized female rats initiated a significantly higher magnitude of lordosis behavior than that observed with TRH and saline infusions (94). Recently, LH-RH has been localized by radioimmunoassay in a similar region around the midbrain central gray (Samson and McCann, *personal communication*). Electrophysiological

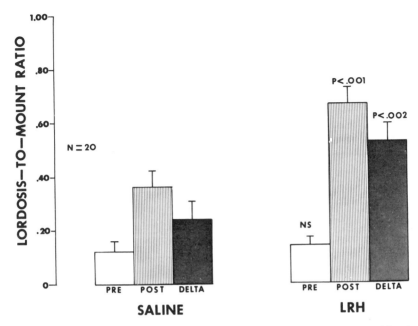

FIG. 5. Effects of LH-RH and saline on lordosis behavior in the estrone-primed ovariectomized female rats cannulated in the midbrain (ventral lateral) central gray region. Open bars represent preinfusion mating; striped bars represent postinfusion mating, cross-hatched bars represent the delta, that is, the difference between preinfusion and postinfusion mating. (Taken from ref. 94.)

experiments have also shown LH-RH- and TRH-responsive neurons in the midbrain (Moss, Dudley, and Chud, *unpublished observations*).

Further support of the involvement of LH-RH in the mediation of sexual receptivity has come from experiments testing the influence of substances known to induce release of LH-RH. The prostaglandins (PGs), in particular PGE_2, have been shown to facilitate LH-RH release (78). Systemic injections, as shown in Fig. 6, or intracerebral infusion of PGE_2 to ovariectomized (OVX) or OVX-adrenalectomized, estrogen-primed animals resulted in facilitation of sexual receptivity (24,37,96). PGE_2 has recently been shown to facilitate lordosis responding in ovariectomized rats even without estrogen priming (97). Neurophysiological data suggest that PGE_2 might have the capacity to modulate firing of preoptic-hypothalamic LH-RH neurons (82) implicated in the control of mating behavior as well as gonadotropin secretion. It has thus been proposed (24) that PGE_2 acts indirectly, via the release of LH-RH, to facilitate mating behavior.

Perhaps the most convincing evidence to date in support of an LH-RH neural system mediating lordosis behavior comes from a study utilizing anti-LH-RH antibody, a substance that competes with LH-RH for binding sites. Infusions of this antibody into the third ventricle of ovariectomized, estrogen-progesterone-primed females resulted in suppression of lordosis behavior

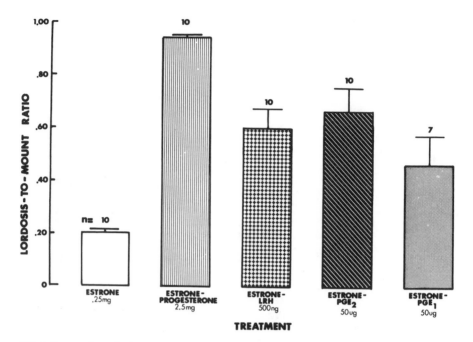

FIG. 6. Mean and standard of the lordosis-to-mount ratio in 5 groups of animals primed with 0.25 mg estrone and then mated, or estrogen primed and subsequently injected with 2.5 mg progesterone, 500 ng LH-RH, 50 μg prostaglandin E_2 (PGE₂) or 50 μg prostaglandin E_1 (PGE₁) before mating. Number of rats in each group in parentheses. (Taken from ref. 24.)

(46). This study is the first to indicate that LH-RH may have a physiological role in the initiation of sexual receptivity. The antibody appears to act directly on the brain and subsequently inhibit mating behavior, presumably by inactivating the animal's endogenous LH-RH levels.

In summary, the aforementioned findings are indicative of a facilitative action of LH-RH and an inhibitory action of TRH on female mating behavior. LH-RH- and TRH-sensitive sites appear to be confined to the medial preoptic area, arcuate-ventromedial nucleus, and midbrain central gray; the peptides were not active when infused into either the lateral hypothalamus or the cerebral cortex. However, the results with the decapeptide, in conjunction with the decreased receptivity following the infusion of antibody to LH-RH into the third ventricle, suggest that this peptide hormone may be acting directly on neural tissue in these areas to potentiate female lordotic behavior, independent of the pituitary and adrenal gland.

Male Rat

The evidence described thus far is based largely on the effects of LH-RH in estrone-primed, ovariectomized female rats. However, LH-RH also affects sexual behavior in male rats. In one series of experiments, the effect of LH-RH on sexual behavior in the intact male rat was investigated (62). All intact males were sexually experienced and tested under two conditions, namely, under the influence of saline and LH-RH. Synthetic LH-RH or saline was injected subcutaneously into male rats 2 hr prior to the mating test. There was no significant difference in the number of mounts or intromissions observed during the 15-min testing period between the saline- and LH-RH-treated animals. However, as shown in Fig. 7, the mean latency to the first mount and first ejaculation was significantly lower in LH-RH-treated males than in the saline-treated controls. These findings appear to be comparable to the observations obtained in the ovariectomized, estrone-LH-RH-primed female rats.

In other experiments, sexually experienced male rats were castrated and treated daily with testosterone propionate in doses (10 μg) too low to initiate good and consistent copulatory behavior. Following 3 weeks of testosterone therapy, the castrated male rats were injected with either saline or 500 ng of LH-RH. Administration of a single injection of synthetic LH-RH was found to decrease significantly the time needed to achieve ejaculation, whereas a single injection of saline had no effect. No other significant differences in the data recorded were observed. Thus LH-RH facilitated the time to intromission and ejaculation in the intact male, and time to ejaculation in the testosterone propionate-primed castrated male rat. It should be noted that castrated male rats treated with saline in combination with LH-RH (but without testosterone propionate) displayed little or no copulatory behavior.

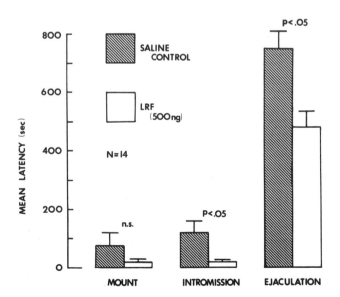

FIG. 7. Paired comparison of mean latency to first mount, first intromission, and first ejaculation under saline and LH-RH treatments (modified from ref. 57). (Taken from ref. 62.)

Like the female, the male rat was affected by PGE_2. Intracerebral infusion of PGE_2 facilitated copulatory behavior in castrated male rats when given daily systemic injections of testosterone propionate (50 μg) (15). It is interesting to note that LH-RH-induced copulatory behavior in the female and male is dependent on the presence of estrogen and testosterone, respectively.

EFFECTS OF LH-RH ON HUMAN SEXUAL BEHAVIOR

It is obvious from the aforementioned data that the hypothalamic-releasing hormones exert brain effects apart from their actions on the anterior pituitary gland. LH-RH facilitates mating behavior in both the male and female rat. A direct CNS stimulatory action of LH-RH on sexual behavior, possibly by activating neurons in the medial preoptic area, arcuate nucleus, and midbrain, has been proposed (59). A key question arises as to whether there is a similar LH-RH action on human sexual behavior. Following the initial reports of LH-RH potentiation of mating in animals (70,71,81), a few clinical investigators privately reported the remarkable side effects of LH-RH in increasing libido. However, only recently have a number of studies appeared in the

TABLE 2. *Summary of LH-RH effects on sexual activity in man*

Reference	Subjects	Route of administration	Result
Mortimer et al., 1974	Hypogonadal men (N = 12)	s.c. (500 μg/inj.) q 8hr	Increased potency (In 6 men, potency ↑ before 17-OHA ↑ to normal)
Doering et al. (personal communication)	Normal adult men	Injection	Increased sexual interest
Benkert et al., 1975	Sexually impotent men[a] (N = 20)[b]	Nasal spray (1.0 mg/day)	Increased sexual activity 4–6 weeks following injections
Schwarzstein et al., 1975	Hypogonadal men (N = 4)	i.m. (500 μg/inj.)	Increased libido and sexual potency following 1 month of treatment
Ehrensing and Kastin, 1976	Normal adult men (N = 3)[a] (N = 3)[b]	a. i.v. (700 μg) b. i.v. (1,250–3,000 μg/wk)	No effect
Moss et al., (unpublished) 1976	Sexually impotent men[a] (N = 8)	s.c. (500 μg/inj.)	Increased sexual activity immediately following injection in masturbators

[a] No clinical endocrinological pathology was evident.
[b] Reduced erection capability during intercourse regardless of level of libido.

literature. A summary chart of these studies is presented in Table 2. Initially, Mortimer and associates (56) reported that long-term (several weeks) treatment with LH-RH (500 μg every eight hr, self-administered by subcutaneous injections) may provide an efficient means of treating patients with hypogonadotropic hypogonadism. It was noted that LH-RH therapy restored potency and fertility in some of these hypogonadal men. A second study on hypogonadal men reported a slight increase in libido during 1 month of continuous treatment with LH-RH (100).

The concept of continuous administration of the active LH-RH agent over a number of weeks has received some support. In a double blind crossover study of sexually impotent male patients in whom no clinical endocrinological pathology was evident, it was demonstrated that 4 to 6 weeks following cessation of LH-RH treatment a significant increase in libido and sexual behavior was observed as compared to placebo (7). In subsequent experiments, LH-RH has also been administered via nasal spray (see Fig. 8 for a summary of the results). It should be noted that TRH (see Table 3) and somatostatin have been shown to have no effect on human sexual behavior (6,8). In a recent collaborative study (Moss and associates, *unpublished observations;* 74) an increase in sexual activity was observed in some impotent males in whom no clinical endocrinological pathology was evident.

As shown in Fig. 9, the preliminary data analysis showed an LH-RH-induced increase in the total number of erections, masturbations, and intercourse in patients that had displayed some pre-test masturbatory activity. Psychogenically impotent (secondary) patients with little or no pre-test masturbatory activity did not display any consistent LH-RH-induced increase in sexual behavior. Unfortunately, the smaller number of subjects precluded

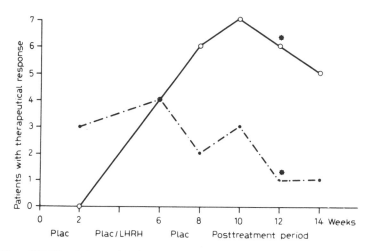

FIG. 8. Effect of LH-RH and placebo (Plac) in 18 patients with sexual impotence. Each group consisted of 9 patients. The therapeutic effects reported apply to the preceding 2 weeks treatment or post-treatment. 0, LH-RH; ●, placebo, *p = 0.024. (Taken from ref. 7.)

TABLE 3. *Therapeutic effect of placebo and TRH[a] in 12 impotent patients*

Placebo (4 wk)	TRF (4 wk)	N (6)
0	0	1
+	0	1
0	+	2
+	+	2
TRH (4 wk)	**Placebo (4 wk)**	**N (6)**
0	0	0
+	0	3
0	+	2
+	+	1

Symbols: +, beneficial effect within the period; 0, no beneficial effect within the period (investigator rating). (From ref. 6.)

[a] 40 mg daily for 4 weeks.

any statistical analysis. Although such reports are extremely subjective, one patient experienced not only an increase in frequency of sexual intercourse following LH-RH administration but also a complete change in mood and emotional outlook on life. Interestingly, a recent study (50) demonstrated that LH-RH had a definite psychological (mood) action but only a modest behavior effect. Changes were observed in aggression, anxiety, and fatigue. Thus a number of experiments utilizing a variety of routes of administration from nasal spray (intravenous infusions, intramuscular injections) to subcutaneous injections have demonstrated an LH-RH-induced increase in sexual activity (libido and/or behavior) in normal adults and in hypogonadal and impotent men. However, the LH-RH increase has not been marked. In fact, a number of experiments have demonstrated negative findings. For example, intravenous injection of LH-RH in three normal adult men resulted in no measurable change in sexual activity (26), and subcutaneous administration every 8 hr for 1 month resulted in no improvement in libido in sexually impotent patients (21). The latter study indicated that LH-RH had no obvious clinical effect on the sexual performance or mental well-being of men suffering from secondary impotence. However, it was emphasized that statistical analysis did show that LH-RH had improved libido, but the treatment effect was rather small and unlikely to be of clinical significance.

Quite obviously, the clinical usefulness of LH-RH in the treatment of male and female sexual dysfunction remains to be ascertained. Negative data do not prove that LH-RH normally has no influence on sexual behavior in man since the psychological factors in the impotent patients may have been powerful enough to suppress any stimulant effects. The positive evidence presented attesting to LH-RH's ability to enhance human sexual potency is suggestive,

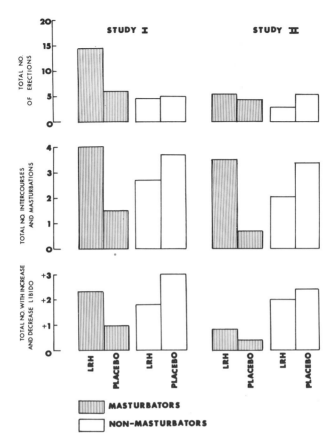

FIG. 9. LH-RH and placebo tests in 8 patients suffering from secondary sexual impotency. Study I consisted of double-blind crossover study with 10 days of LH-RH and placebo. Study II consisted of 1 week of placebo, 2 weeks of LH-RH, and 1 week of no treatment.

at best. Firm support of this concept will be accomplished only by rigorously controlled clinical studies conducted on a large number of patients.

CONCLUDING REMARKS

A variety of findings from the laboratory and clinic suggest that LH-RH exerts a direct brain effect at the cellular and behavioral level. Unlike the other hypothalamic hypophysiotropic hormones, the LH-RH CNS effects appear to be specific and of physiological importance. For instance, only LH-RH and its precursors potentiate mating behavior in the male and female rat. TRH, LH, and FSH do not facilate sexual behavior. Even more important, anti-LH-RH antibody suppresses LH-RH-induced behavior. The mechanisms by which LH-RH exerts such effects on the CNS are largely unknown. However, evidence of CNS localization of LH-RH in neurons

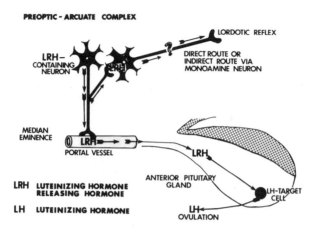

FIG. 10. Theoretical model of the mechanism of action for LH-RH (LRH) enhancement of sexual behavior. (Taken from ref. 60.)

(4,107,110), its identification in synaptosome fractions of the hypothalamus (86), and finally its direct action on nerve cell membranes (58,59,63,89) are suggestive of the following concept illustrated in Fig. 10 for the mechanism of action of LH-RH in the potentiation of mating behavior. LH-RH which is synthesized within specialized nerve cells in the preoptic-hypothalamic region exerts one influence by being released into the hypothalamohypophyseal portal system, where it initiates the release of LH and FSH. These same specialized nerve cells may exert a second influence on the brain itself by a system of collateral connections on arcuate neurons. These collateral fibers could project to various hypothalamic and extrahypothalamic areas where LH-RH could modulate sexual performance, either directly or indirectly, through a catecholamine system (18,29). Interestingly, arcuate neurons have been shown to contain collaterals as indicated by several recent electrophysiological studies (38,89,91,108,109). In addition, some evidence for recurrent facilitation and recurrent inhibition has also been shown in these arcuate neurons, suggesting transmitter and/or modulatory roles for the hypothalamic peptides.

Complex interactions between the peptide hormones, other substances affected by these hormones (i.e., catecholamines), and endogenous hormone levels seem to be involved in the control of mating behavior. These interactions must finally effectuate changes in neuronal excitability at hypothalamic and extrahypothalamic sites, and subsequently lead to a change in sexual receptivity. In light of the firm evidence implicating LH-RH in animal sexual behavior, it seems probable that the investigation of LH-RH brain action will substantially contribute to better understanding of the neural mechanisms mediating sexual behavior in animals and man.

ACKNOWLEDGMENTS

Research from the senior author's laboratory referred to in this manuscript was supported by the National Institutes of Health Research Grant NIH-USPHS-10434 END and the National Science Foundation Grant NSF-GB-43494. R. L. M. is recipient of USPHS-NIH Career Development Award K04-HD-00146.

The authors express their appreciation to Donna King for typing the manuscript. Synthetic luteinizing hormone-releasing hormone and its agonist analog D-Ala^6, des Gly^{10} LRH ethylamide were generously provided by Drs. M. Götz and R. Deghenghi of Ayerst Research Laboratories, Montreal, Canada; estrone and progesterone were obtained through the kindness of Dr. Preston of Parke-Davis, Ann Arbor, Michigan; and the prostaglandins were supplied through the courtesy of Dr. Pike of the Upjohn Company, Kalamazoo, Michigan. Thyrotropin-releasing hormone was supplied by Drs. J. Dorn and J. Weinstein and Mr. C. Flanagan of Abbot Laboratories, North Chicago, Illinois; and Dr. Rivier of the Salk Institute at San Diego supplied the LRH analog peptides (a) D-Trp^6, Pro^9-NHET-LRH, agonist analog (LRH+), (b) D-Phe^2, D-Trp^6-LRH, antagonist analog (LRH-), and (c) des-Pro^9-Gly^{10}-LRH inactive analog (LRH°), and [(τ-ME-His^2) TRH].

REFERENCES

1. Barker, J. L. (1976): Peptides: Roles in neuronal excitability. *Physiol. Rev.,* 56(2):435–452.
2. Barker, J. L. (1977): Physiological roles of peptides in the nervous system. *Peptides in Neurobiology,* edited by Harold Gainer, pp. 295–343. Plenum Press, New York.
3. Barry, J., and Dubois, M. P. (1976): Immunoreactive LRH neurosecretory pathways in mammals. *Acta Anat. (Basel),* 94:497–503.
4. Barry, J., Dubois, M. P., and Carette, B. (1974): Immunofluorescent study of the preoptic-infundibular LRH neurosecretion pathway in normal, castrated or testosterone-treated male guinea-pig. *Endocrinology,* 95:1416–1423.
5. Beach, F. A. (1947): A review of physiological and psychological studies of sexual behavior in mammals. *Physiol. Rev.,* 27:240–307.
6. Benkert, O., Horn, K., Pickardt, C. R., and Schmid, D. (1976): Sexual impotence: Studies of the hypothalamic-pituitary-thyroid axis and the effect of oral thyrotropin-releasing factor. *Arch. Sex. Behav.,* 5(4):275–281.
7. Benkert, O., Jordan, R., Dahlen, H. G., Schneider, H. P. G., and Gammel, G. (1975): Sexual impotence: A double-blind study of LHRH nasal spray versus placebo. *Neuropsychobiology,* 1:203–210.
8. Besser, G. M., Thorner, M. O., Wass, J. A. H., Mortimer, C. H., and Yeo, T. (1977): Therapeutic use of bromocriptine and growth hormone release inhibiting hormone. *Prog. Reprod. Biol.,* 2:261–278.
9. Boling, J. L., and Blandau, R. J. (1939): The estrogen-progesterone induction of mating responses in the spayed female rat. *Endocrinology,* 25:359–364.
10. Boling, J. L., Blandau, R. J., and Young, W. C. (1941): The length of heat in the albino rat as determined by the copulatory response. *Anat. Rec.,* 79:453–463.
11. Brazeau, P., Rivier, J., Vale, W., and Guillemin, R. (1974): Inhibition of growth

hormone secretion in the rat by synthetic somatostatin. *Endocrinology*, 94:184–187.

12. Burgus, R., Butcher, M., Amoss, M., Ling, N., Monahan, M., Rivier, J., Fellows, R., Blackwell, R., Vale, W., and Guillemin R. (1972): Primary structure of the hypothalamic luteinizing hormone-releasing factor (LRH) of ovine origin. *Proc. Natl. Acad. Sci. USA*, 69:278–282.

13. Burgus, R., Dunn, T. F., Deisiderio, D., Ward, D. N., Vale, W., and Guillemin, R. (1970): Characterization of the hypothalamic hypophysiotropic TSH-releasing factor (TRF) of ovine origin. *Nature*, 226:321–325.

14. Carter, C. S., and Davis, J. M. (1977) Biogenic amines, reproductive hormones and female sexual behavior: A review. *Biobehav. Rev.*, 1:213–224.

15. Clemens, L. G., and Gladue, B. A. (1977): The effect of prostaglandin E₂ on masculine sexual behavior in the rat. *J. Endocrinol.*, 75:383–389.

16. Corbin, A. (1966): Pituitary and plasma LH of ovariectomized rats with median eminence implants of LH. *Endocrinology*, 78:893–896.

17. Corbin, A., and Cohen, A. I. (1966): Effect of median eminence implants of LH on pituitary LH of female rats. *Endocrinology*, 78:41–46.

18. Crowley, W. R., Feder, H. H., and Morin, L. P. (1976): Role of monoamines in sexual behavior of the female guinea pig. *Biochem. Behav.*, 4:67–71.

19. David, M. A., Fraschini, F., and Martini, L. (1966): Control of LH secretion: Role of a "short" feedback mechanism. *Endocrinology*, 78:55–60.

20. Davidson, J. M., Smith, E. R., and Bowers, C. Y. (1973): Effects of mating on gonadotropin release in the female rat. *Endocrinology*, 93:1185.

21. Davies, T. F., Mountjoy, C. Q., Gomez-Pan, A., Watson, M. J., Hanker, J. P., Besser, G. M., and Hall, R. (1977): Reduced gonadotrophin: Response to releasing hormone after chronic administration to impotent men. *Clin. Endocrinol.*, 5(6).

22. Deniker, P., Ginestet, D., Loo, H., Zarifian, E., and Cottereau, M. J. (1974): Etude preliminaire de l'action de la thyreostimuline hypothalamique (thyrotropine releasing hormone ou T.R.H.) dans les etats depressifs. *Ann. Med. Psychol.* 1:249–255.

23. Docke, F., and Glaser, D. (1971): Internal feedback of luteinizing hormone in cycling female rats. *J. Endocrinol.*, 51:403–404.

24. Dudley, C. A., and Moss, R. L. (1976): Prostaglandin E₂: Facilitatory action on the lordotic response. *J. Endocrinol.*, 71:457–458.

25. Dyer, R. G., and Dyball, R. E. J. (1974): Evidence for a direct effect of LRF and TRF on single unit activity in the rostral hypothalamus. *Nature*, 252:486–488.

26. Ehrensing, R. H., and Kastin, A. J. (1976): Clinical investigations for emotional effects of neuropeptide hormones. *Pharmacol. Biochem. Behav.*, 5(1):89–93.

27. Elde, R., and Hokfelt, T. (1978): Distribution of hypothalamic hormones and other peptides in the brain. In: *Frontiers in Neuroendocrinology*, edited by L. Martini and W. F. Ganong, pp. 1–33. Raven Press, New York.

28. Everett, J. W. (1964): Central neural control of reproductive functions of the adenohypophysis. *Physiol. Rev.*, 44:373–431.

29. Everitt, B. J., Fuxe, K., Hokfelt, T., and Jonsson, G. (1975): Role of monoamines in the control by hormones of sexual receptivity in the female rat. *J. Comp. Physiol. Psychol.*, 89:556–572.

30. Foreman, M. M., and Moss, R. L. (1975): Enhancement of lordotic behavior by intrahypothalamic infusion of luteinizing hormone-releasing hormone. *Neuroscience Abstracts*, Society for Neuroscience, 5th Annual Meeting, New York City.

31. Foreman, M. M., and Moss, R. L. (1977): Effects of subcutaneous injection and intrahypothalamic infusion of releasing hormones upon lordotic response to repetitive coital stimulation. *Horm. Behav.*, 8:219–234.

32. Foreman, M. M., and Moss, R. L. (1978): Roles of gonadotropins and releasing hormones in the hypothalamic control or lordotic behavior in the ovariectomized-estrogen primed female rat. (*Submitted for publication*)

33. Friedgood, H. B. (1936): Hypophysiotropic hormones in portal vessel blood. In:

Hypophysiotropic Hormones of the Hypothalamus: Assay and Chemistry, edited by J. Meites, pp. 282–297. Williams & Wilkins Co., Baltimore.

34. Gorski, R. A. (1976): The possible neural sites of hormonal facilitation of sexual behavior in the female rat. *Psychoneuroendocrinology*, 1:371–387.
35. Green, J., and Harris, G. W. (1947): The neurovascular link between the neuro-hypophysis and adenohypophysis. *J. Endocrinol.*, 5:136–146.
36. Halasz, B., Pupp, L., and Uhlarik, S. (1962): Hypophysiotropic area in the hypothalamus. *J. Endocrinol.*, 25:147–154.
37. Hall, N. R., Luttge, W. G., and Berry, R. B. (1975): Intracerebral prostaglandin E_2: Effect upon sexual behavior, open activity and body temperature in ovari-ectomized female rats. *Prostaglandins*, 10:877–888.
38. Harris, M., and Sanghera, M. (1974): Projection of medial basal hypothalamic neurones to the preoptic anterior hypothalamic areas and the paraventricular nucleus in the rat. *Brain Res.*, 81:401–411.
39. Herrenkohl, R. L., and Verhalst, I. M. (1975): Intracerebral infusions of luteinizing hormone-releasing factor induce lordosis in rats. Society for Neuro-science, 5th Annual Meeting, New York (Abst.).
40. Hoffman, G. E., Melnyk, V., Hayes, T., Bennett-Clarke, C., and Fowler, E. (1978): Immunocytology of LH-RH neurons. Brain-endocrine interaction III. *Neural Hormones and Reproduction*, pp. 67–82. 3rd International Symposium, Wurzburg.
41. Ifft, J. D. (1965): Further evidence on an internal feedback from the adeno-hypophysis to the hypothalamus. *Neuroendocrinology*, 1:350–357.
42. Kastin, A. J., Plotnikoff, N. P., Schally, A. V., and Sandman, C. A. (1976): Endocrine and CNS effects of hypothalamic peptides and MSH. In: *Reviews in Neuroscience*, pp. 111–148. Raven Press, New York.
43. Kawakami, K., and Sakuma, Y. (1974): Responses of hypothalamic neurons to the microiontophoresis of LH-RH, LH and FSH under various levels of circulatory ovarian hormones. *Neuroendocrinology*, 15:290–307.
44. Kawakami, K., and Sakuma, Y. (1976): Electrophysiological evidences for pos-sible participation of periventricular neurons in anterior pituitary regulation. *Brain Res.*, 101:79–94.
45. King, J. C., Elkind, K. E., Gerall, A. A., and Millar, R. P. (1978): Investigation of the LH-RH system in the normal and neonatally steroid-treated male and female rat. Brain endocrine interaction III. *Neural Hormones and Reproduction*, pp. 97–107. 3rd International Symposium, Wurzburg.
46. Kozlowski, G. P., and Hostetter, G. (1978): Cellular and subcelluar localization and behavioral effects of gonadotropin-releasing hormone (Gn-RH) in the rat. Brain endocrine interaction III. *Neural Hormones and Reproduction*, pp. 138–153. 3rd International Symposium, Wurzburg.
47. Law, O. T., and Meagher, W. (1958): Hypothalamic lesions and sexual behavior in the female rat. *Am. J. Physiol.*, 203:1626–1627.
48. Luttge, W. G., and Sheets, C. S. (1977): Further studies on the restoration of estrogen-induced sexual receptivity in ovariectomized mice treated with di-hydrotestosterone: Effects of progesterone, dihydroprogesterone and LH-RH. *Pharmacol. Biochem. Behav.*, 7:563–566.
49. Matsueo, H., Baba, Y., Nair, R. M. G., Arimura, A., and Schally, A. V. (1971): Structure of the porcine LH- and FSH-releasing hormone. I. The proposed amino acid sequence. *Biophys. Res. Commun.*, 43:1334–1339.
50. McAdoo, B. C., Doering, C. H., Kraemer, H. C., Dessert, N. J., Brodie, H. K. H., and Hamburg, D. A. (1978): A study of the effects of gonadotropin-releasing hormone on human mood and behavior. *Psychosom. Med. (in press)*.
51. McCann, S. M., and Porter, J. C. (1969): Hypothalamic pituitary stimulating and inhibiting hormones. *Physiol. Rev.*, 49:240–284.
52. McCann, S. M., Taleisnik, S., and Friedman, H. M. (1960): LH-releasing activity in hypothalamic extracts. *Proc. Soc. Biol. Med.*, 104:432–434.
53. Modianos, D., and Pfaff, D. (1976): Steroid and peptide hormones, and the neural mechanisms for reproductive behavior. Proceedings of the V International

Congress of Endocrinology, Hamburg. *Excerpta Medica Int. Cong. Ser.* 402:67–71.

54. Moguilevsky, J. A. (1971): Effects gonadotropins on the oxidative metabolism of hypothalamus. In: *Influence of Hormones on the Nervous System, Proceedings of the International Society of Psychoneuroendocrinology*, edited by D. H. Ford, pp. 366–377. S. Karger, Basel.

55. Molitch, M., Edmonds, E., Jones, E. E., and Odell, W. D. (1976): Short loop feedback control of luteinizing hormone in the rabbit. *Am. J. Physiol.*, 230:907–910.

56. Mortimer, C. H., McNeilly, A. S., Fisher, R. A., Murray, M. A. F., and Besser, G. M. (1974): Gonadotrophin-releasing hormone therapy in hypogonadal males with hypothalamic or pituitary dysfunction. *Br. Med. J.*, 14:617–621.

57. Moss, R. L. (1974): Relationship between the central regulation of gonadotropins and mating behavior in female rats. *Reprod. Behav.*, edited by W. Montagna and W. Sandler, pp. 55–76. Plenum Press, New York.

58. Moss, R. L. (1976): Unit responses in preoptic and arcuate neurons related to anterior pituitary function. In: *Frontiers in Neuroendocrinology*, edited by L. Martini and W. F. Ganong, pp. 95–128. Raven Press, New York.

59. Moss, R. L. (1977): Role of hypophysiotropic neurohormones in mediating neural and behavioral events. *Fed. Proc.*, 36:1978–1983.

60. Moss, R. L. (1978): Effects of hypothalamic peptides on sex behavior in animal and man. *Psychopharmacology: A Generation of Progress*, edited by M. A. Lipton, A. DiMascio, and K. F. Killam, pp. 431–440. Raven Press, New York.

61. Moss, R. L., and Cooper, K. J. (1973): Temporal relationship of spontaneous and coitus-induced release of luteinizing hormone in the normal cycling rat. *Endocrinology*, 92:1748–1753.

62. Moss, R. L., Dudley, C. A., Foreman, M. M., and McCann, S. M. (1975): Synthetic LRF: A potentiator of sexual behavior in the rat. In: *Hypothalamic Hormones*, edited by M. Motta, P. G. Crosignani, and L. Martini, pp. 269–278. Academic Press, London.

63. Moss, R. L., Dudley, C. A., and Kelly, M. (1978): Hypothalamic polypeptide releasing hormone: Modifiers of neuronal activity. *Neuropharmacology*, 17:87–93.

64. Moss, R. L., Dudley, C. A., and Schwartz, N. B. (1977): Coitus-induced release of luteinizing hormone in the proestrous rat: Fantasy or fact? *Endocrinology*, 100(2):394–397.

65. Moss, R. L., Dudley, C. A., and Vale, W. (1978): Hypothalamic peptides: Putative modulators of neural activity. In: *Brain Endocrine Interaction. III. Neural Hormones and Reproduction*, pp. 313–326. Karger, Basel.

66. Moss, R. L., and Foreman, M. M. (1976): Potentiation of lordosis behavior by intrahypothalamic infusion of synthetic luteinizing hormone-releasing hormone (LRH). *Neuroendocrinology*, 20:176–181.

67. Moss, R. L., Kelly, M. and Dudley, C. A. (1975): Responsiveness of medial-preoptic neurons to releasing hormones and neurohumoral agents. *Fed. Proc.*, 34:219.

68. Moss, R. L., Kelly, M., and Dudley, C. A. (1976): Effects of peptide hormones on extracellular electrical activities of preoptic-hypothalamic neurons. *Neurosci. Abstr.*, 2(2):652.

69. Moss, R. L., Kelly, M., Foreman, M. M., and Dudley, C. A. (1975): Luteinizing hormone-releasing hormone (LRH) regulation of neural events controlling mating behavior. *Physiologist*, 18:326.

70. Moss, R. L., and McCann, S. M. (1973): Induction of mating behavior in rats by luteinizing hormone-releasing factor. *Science*, 181:177–179.

71. Moss, R. L., and McCann, S. M. (1975): Action of luteinizing hormone-releasing factor (LRF) in the initiation of lordosis behavior in the estrone-primed ovariectomized female rat. *Neuroendocrinology*, 17:309–318.

72. Moss, R. L., McCann, S. M., and Dudley, C. A. (1975): Releasing hormones and sexual behavior. *Prog. Brain Res.* 42:36–46.

73. Moss, R. L., Paloutzian, R. F., and Law, O. T. (1974): Electrical stimulation of

forebrain structures and its effect on copulatory as well as stimulus-bound behavior in ovariectomized hormone-primed rats. *Physiol. Behav.,* 12:997–1004.
74. Moss, R. L., Riskind, P., McCann, S. M., Danhof, I., and Rochefort, G. (1978): *(Manuscript in preparation).*
75. Nair, R. M. G., Barrett, J. F., Bowers, C. Y., and Schally, A. V. (1970): Structure of porcine thyrotropin releasing hormone. *Biochemistry,* 9:1103–1106.
76. Nequin, L. G., Alvarez, J., and Schwartz, N. B. (1975): Steroid control of gonadotropin release. *J. Steroid Biochem.,* 6:1007–1012.
77. Nicoll, R. A. (1976): Promising peptides. *Soc. Neurosci. Symp.,* 1:99–122.
78. Ojeda, S. R., Wheaton, J. R., and McCann, S. M. (1975): Prostaglandin E₂ induced release of luteinizing hormone-releasing factor (LRF). *Neuroendocrinology,* 17:283–287.
79. Pelletier, G., Labrie, F., Puviani, R., Arimura, A., and Schally, A. V. (1974): Electron microscopic localization of luteinizing hormone releasing hormone in the rat median eminence. *Endocrinology,* 95:314–315.
80. Pfaff, D. W. (1970): Mating behavior of hypophysectomized rats. *J. Comp. Physiol. Psychol.,* 72:45–50.
81. Pfaff, D. W. (1973): Luteinizing hormone-releasing factor (LRF) potentiates lordosis behavior in hypophysectomized ovariectomized female rats. *Science,* 182:1148–1149.
82. Poulain, P., and Carette, B. (1974): Iontophoresis of prostaglandins on hypothalamic neurons. *Brain Res.,* 79:311–314.
83. Poulain, P., and Carette, B. (1978): Septal afferents to the arcuate-median eminence region in the guinea pig: Microiontophoretically-applied LRF effects. *Brain Res.,* 137:154–157.
84. Powers, B. J., and Valenstein, E. S. (1972): Sexual receptivity: Facilitation by medial preoptic lesions in female rats. *Science,* 175:1003–1005.
85. Prange, A. J., Jr., Nemeroff, C. B., and Lipton, M. A. (1978): Behavioral effects of peptides: Basic and clinical studies. *Psychopharmacology: A Generation of Progress,* edited by M. A. Lipton, A. DiMascio, and K. F. Killam, pp. 441–458. Raven Press, New York.
86. Ramirez, V. D., and Kordon, C. (1975): Studies on luteinizing hormone-releasing hormone (LH-RH): In: *Hypothalamic Hormones,* edited by M. Motta, P. G. Crosignani, and L. Martini, pp. 57–74. Academic Press, London.
87. Ramirez, V. D., and Sawyer, C. H. (1965): Fluctuations of hypothalamic luteinizing hormone-releasing factor during the estrous cycle. *Endocrinology,* 76:282–289.
88. Reichlin, S., Saperstein, R., Jackson, I. M. D., Boyd, A. E., III, and Patel, Y. (1976): Hypothalamic hormones. *Annu. Rev. Physiol.,* 38:389–424.
89. Renaud, L. P. (1978): Peptides as neurotransmitters or neuromodulators. In: *Psychopharmacology: A Generation of Progress,* edited by M. A. Lipton, A. DiMascio, and K. F. Killam, pp. 423–430. Raven Press, New York.
90. Renaud, L. P., and Martin, J. B. (1975): Thyrotropin releasing hormone (TRH): Depressant action on central neuronal activity. *Brain Res.,* 86:150–154.
91. Renaud, L. P., and Martin, J. B. (1975): Electrophysiological studies of connections of hypothalamic ventromedial nucleus neurons in the rat: Evidence for a role in neuroendocrine regulation. *Brain Res.,* 93:145–151.
92. Renaud, L. P., Martin, J. B., and Brazeau, P. (1975): Depressant action of TRH, LH-RH and somatostatin on activity of central neurons. *Nature,* 255:233–235.
93. Renaud, L. P., Martin, J. B., and Brazeau, P. (1976): Hypothalamic releasing factors: Physiological evidence for a regulatory action on central neurons and pathways for their distribution in brain. *Pharmacol. Biochem. Behav.,* 5(1):171–178.
94. Riskind, P., and Moss, R. L. (1977): Midbrain central grey: An extrahypothalamic site for LRH potentiation of lordosis behavior in female rat. *Soc. Neurosci. Abstr.,* 3:356.
95. Rodriguez-Sierra, J. F., Crowley, W. R., and Komisaruk, B. R. (1977): Induction

of lordosis responsiveness by vaginal stimulation in rats is independent of anterior or posterior pituitary hormones. *Horm. Behav.* 8(3):348–355.

96. Rodriguez-Sierra, J. F., and Komisaruk, B. R. (1977): Effects of prostaglandin E_2 and indomethacin on sexual behavior in the female rat. *Horm. Behav.*, 9:281–289.

97. Rodriguez-Sierra, J. F., and Komisaruk, B. R. (1978): Lordosis induction in the rat by prostaglandin E_2 systematically or intracranially in the absence of ovarian hormones. *Prostaglandins (in press).*

98. Sanghera, M., Harris, M. C., and Morgan, R. A. (1978): Effects of microiontophoretic and intravenous application of gonadotrophic hormones on the discharge of medial basal hypothalamic neurones in the rat. *Brain Res.*, 140:63–74.

99. Schwartz, N. B. (1969): A model for the regulation of ovulation in the rat. *Recent Prog. Horm. Res.*, 25:1–55.

100. Schwarzstein, L., Aparicio, N. J., Turner, D., Calamera, J. C., Mancini, J. F., and Schally, A. V. (1975): Use of synthetic luteinizing hormone-releasing hormone in treatment of oligospermia men: A preliminary report. *Fertil. Steril.*, 25:331–336.

101. Silverman, A. J., and Zimmerman, E. A. (1978): Pathways containing luteinizing hormone-releasing hormone (LHRH) in the mammalian brain. Brain endocrine interaction III. *Neural Hormones and Reproduction*, pp. 83–96. 3rd International Symposium, Wurzburg.

102. Singer, J. J. (1968): Hypothalamic control of male and female sexual behavior in female rats. *J. Comp. Physiol. Psychol.*, 69:738–742.

103. Steiner, F. A. (1972): Effects of locally applied hormones and neurotransmitters on hypothalamic neurons. In: *Proceedings of the IV International Congress of Endocrinology*, pp. 202–204. Excerpta Medica, Amsterdam.

104. Terasawa, E. I., Whitmoyer, D. I., and Sawyer, C. H. (1969): Effects of luteinizing hormone on multiple-unit activity in the rat hypothalamus. *Am. J. Physiol.*, 217:1119–1126.

105. Turgeon, J. L., and Barraclough, C. A. (1976): The existence of a possible short-loop negative feedback action of LH in proestrous rat. *Endocrinology*, 98:639–644.

106. Vale, W., Rivier, C., and Brown, M. (1977): Regulatory peptides of the hypothalamus. *Annu. Rev. Physiol.*, 39:473–527.

107. Wheaton, J. E., Krulich, L., and McCann, S. M. (1975): Localization of luteinizing hormone-releasing hormone in the preoptic area and hypothalamus of the rat using radioimmunoassay. *Endocrinology*, 97:30–38.

108. Yagi, R., and Sawaki, Y. (1975): Recurrent inhibition and facilitation: Demonstration in the tuberoinfundibular system and effects of strychnine and picrotoxin. *Brain Res.*, 84:155–159.

109. Yagi, K., and Sawaki, Y. (1978): Neuroendocrinology electrophysiological characteristics of identified tubero-infundibular neurons. *Brain Res. (in press).*

110. Zimmerman, E. A., Hsu, K. C., Ferin, M., and Kozlowski, G. P. (1974): Localization of gonadotropin-releasing hormone (GN-RH) in hypothalamus of mouse by immunoperoxidase technique. *Endocrinology*, 95:1–11.

Central Nervous System Effects of Hypothalamic Hormones and Other Peptides, edited by Collu et al. Raven Press, New York © 1979.

Somatostatin: Physiological Studies and Blood Determinations

P. Brazeau, J. Epelbaum, and R. Benoit

Division of Neurology, McGill University, Montreal, Canada

In late November 1971, while investigating crude hypothalamic extracts for a still hypothetical growth hormone (GH) releasing factor, we found an active principle which was a potent inhibitor of GH release. This unexpected activity, first observed by Krulich and McCann in 1968 and still uncharacterized, was originally detected in a crude side fraction (alcohol-chloroform extract) that had been used in the luteinizing hormone-releasing factor (LH-RF) characterization program. It was then isolated and characterized. The amino acid sequence found was:

H-Ala-Gly-Cys-Lys-Asn-Phe-Phe-Trp-Lys-Thr-Phe-Thr-Ser-Cys-OH

S ———————————————————————— S

TABLE 1. *Growth hormone release-inhibiting effect of somatostatin*

Stimuli	Species studied	Year of study
None (normal and sleep pulses)	Rat, monkey, man	1973–1977
Exercise	Man	1973
Meal	Man	1974–1975
Insulin (hypoglycemia)	Dog, man	1973–1974
Arginine	Dog, monkey, man	1973–1974
L-DOPA	Dog, monkey, man	1973–1974
Barbiturates	Rat	1973
Morphine	Rat	1974
NE (third ventricle)	Monkey	1973–1974
Electrical (VM nucleus,	Rat	1973–1974
amygdala)	Rat	1973–1974
Pathological conditions		
Acromegaly	Man	1973
Diabetes ("juvenile")	Man	1974
Malnutrition	Man	1975

The synthetic replicates of both forms (dihydrosomatostatin and somatostatin) synthesized by the solid-phase technique (Merryfield technique) were found to have the same net bioactivity as native somatostatin (4).

The elucidation of the structure of somatostatin and the development of techniques for radioimmunoassay and immunocytochemistry have led to a rapid expansion of knowledge about the effects, distribution, and function of the tetradecapeptide (8). Somatostatin has well-documented inhibitory effects on GH secretion. It inhibits GH secretion in the rat induced by electrical stimulation, pentobarbital, morphine, and chlorpromazine. It prevents GH release in response to L-DOPA in man, baboon, and dog and GH secretion stimulated by insulin hypoglycemia and arginine in man. Sleep-associated GH secretion is also prevented by somatostatin (Table 1).

Somatostatin has no effect on basal physiological prolactin, FSH, LH, or ACTH secretion. It prevents basal TSH release and TRH-induced TSH secretion without affecting TRH-mediated prolactin release. It does not block LH-RH-induced LH or FSH release.

Somatostatin has a broad range of inhibitory activities in addition to its pituitary effects. It has been reported that the peptide inhibits the secretion of insulin, glucagon, gastrin, secretin, vaso-active intestinal peptide, renin, motilin, cholecystokinin, and even PTH and calcitonin. Whether or not these

TABLE 2. *Release-inhibiting effects of somatostatin*

Effect	Hormone		Year of Publication
On pituitary hormones			
Inhibit	TSH (TRF stim)	Rat, monkey, man	1973–1975
None	Prolactin	Rat, monkey, man	1973–1974
None	FSH	Rat, dog, man	1973–1974
None	LH	Rat, dog, man	1973–1974
On extrapituitary peptides			
Inhibit	Insulin	Dog, monkey, man	1973–1975
Inhibit	Glucagon	Dog, monkey, man	1973–1975
Inhibit	Gastrin	Rat, dog, man	1974–1977
Inhibit	Secretin	Dog	1975
Inhibit	Renin	Dog	1976
Inhibit	Vasoactive intestinal polypeptide	Dog	1975–1976
Inhibit	Motilin	Dog	1975–1976
Inhibit	Cholecystokinin	Man, rat	1977
Inhibit	Parathyroid hormone	Rat, monkey	1977
Inhibit	Calcitonin	Rat, monkey	1977
On neurotransmitters			
Inhibit	Acetylcholine	Guinea pig	1976

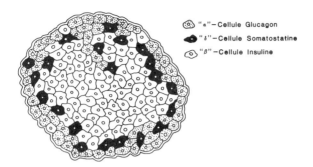

FIG. 1. Cell distribution in Langerhans' islet.

are physiological effects is still debatable for many of these hormones (Table 2).

In view of such a diversity of release-inhibiting properties, one might question the physiological significance and validity of some of them. In fact, in most *"in vivo"* studies from which these data were obtained, massive intravenous doses (bolus and/or infusion) of somatostatin were given; i.e., doses often thousands of times higher than the content of the target gland studied. One can therefore legitimately question whether the observed activities could result from nonspecific and/or indirect effects.

Somatostatin is known to be a natural substance found in specific cells (1) in the central nervous system (CNS) and upper gut organs which can be stimulated to secrete by either physiological or pharmacological means. The lack of appropriate technology for measuring endogenous somatostatin in body fluids (3) has made direct study of somatostatin physiology difficult. In addition, it is interesting that in the pancreatic islets, the anatomical position of the "δ" cells between the α and β cells suggests a possible paracrine role (Fig. 1). Therefore, one should question first the physiology of endogenous secretion of somatostatin since it is known that glucagon and insulin secretions can be strongly inhibited by somatostatin. In view of all these accumulated findings, we have initiated studies *in vitro* and *in vivo* on the physiology of somatostatin secretion from the brain (6,7) and from the pancreas (2). Such an orientation has required the development of a specific radioimmunoassay, tissue extraction methodology, and an affinity chromatography system. In this chapter we shall briefly describe the following aspects:

1. Subcellular localization of somatostatin in the CNS.
2. Somatostatinergic pathways and their interrelations in the CNS.
3. Modulation of somatostatin secretion from cultured islets of the pancreas.
4. Blood measurement of somatostatin.
5. Modulation of somatostatin secretion in the portal vein.

RADIOIMMUNOASSAY OF SOMATOSTATIN

In order to measure somatostatin in tissues and plasma we have developed a specific radioimmunoassay (RIA) using antisera to somatostatin raised in rabbits and adult sheep. The sheep antiserum in a 1:25,000 to 1:50,000 dilution binds approximately 30 to 40% of ^{125}I Tyr^1-somatostatin and the sensitivity of the RIA is 10 pg somatostatin per tube. No cross-reactivity was detected to 23 peptides and biogenic amines tested.

A rabbit anti-sheep γ-globulin is used as second antibody with a supplement of normal sheep serum. The labeling technique of Tyr^1-somatostatin is the Chloramine T technique at a dilution of 1/10. This labeled antigen was purified at 4°C on a CM-52 column (0.5 × 15 cm) for the first 5 ml with 0.002 N NH$_4$OAc, then secondly for the remaining 50 ml with 0.2 N of NH$_4$OAc at a pH 4.6.

Bioassay and radioimmunoassay studies have shown that somatostatin is localized in a number of brain regions outside the hypothalamus (Table 3).

TABLE 3. *Regional distribution of SRIF in brain*

Brain region	No. of experiments	Wet weight (mg)	PG SRIF/ fragment	PG SRIF (mg wet weight)
Total MBH[a]	7	16.7 ± 0.8	22,239 ± 2,160	1,397 ± 208
Median eminence	7	1.45 ± 0.2	17,656 ± 1,036	15,470 ± 2,421
Remaining[b]				
HPT	7	13.9 ± 1.4	3,837 ± 604	266 ± 45
Anterior preoptic area	7	13.3 ± 0.5	4,414 ± 387	338 ± 37
CMA	7	30.5 ± 1.2	8,212 ± 574	272 ± 23
BLA	7	34.1 ± 1.9	12,214 ± 1,472	351 ± 23
Cortex	7	42.0 ± 4.4	3,750 ± 404	92 ± 16
Spinal cord	7	34.0 ± 3.2	3,696 ± 508	114 ± 18
Pineal gland	7	2.3 ± 0.3	350	—

[a] MBH, medial basal hypothalamus; mean ± SE.
[b] Hypothalamus excluding medial basal hypothalamus.

Highest concentrations of extrahypothalamic somatostatin have been reported in the preoptic area, amygdala, brainstem, and spinal cord, but it is also present in the cerebral cortex, thalamus, cerebellum, pineal gland, and peripheral nerve (5).

Subcellular Localization of Somatostatin in the CNS

Tissues for subcellular fractionation were processed according to the technique of Whittaker (9). The B zone represents the synaptosomal band (Fig. 2).

Subcellular distribution studies indicate that somatostatin in the hypothala-

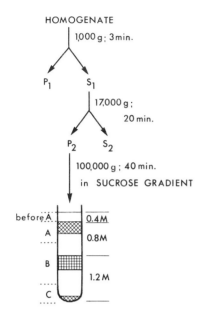

FIG. 2. Organelles extraction procedure from nervous tissue.

mus, preoptic area, and amygdala is localized predominantly in synaptosomes or nerve terminals. This localization is consistent with a function of the peptide as a synaptic neurotransmitter and/or modulator. Presumably somatostatin is released both from nerve terminals in the median eminence and from synaptic terminals that end in other brain areas.

Somatostatinergic Pathways and Their Interrelations in the CNS

To investigate somatostatinergic pathways in the medial basal hypothalamus or preoptic area, we made selective lesions in these regions and measured

TABLE 4. *Effect of CNS lesions on somatostatin[a]*

Site of lesion	ME	POA	CX	AMYGD
Ventromedial nucleus	—	↓[b]	—	—
Anterior hypothalamic area	↓[c]	—	—	—
Ventromedial preoptic area	↓[c]	N.M.	—	—
Dorsomedial preoptic area	—	N.M.	—	—
	MBH	POA	CX	AMYGD
Amygdala	—	—	—	N.M.
Deafferentation	↓[c]	↓[b]	—	—

[a] ME, median eminence; MBH, mediobasal hypothalamus; POA, preoptic area; CX, cortex; AMYGD, amygdala; N.M., not measured; ↓, decrease; —, no change.
[b] $p < 0.05$.
[c] $p < 0.005$.

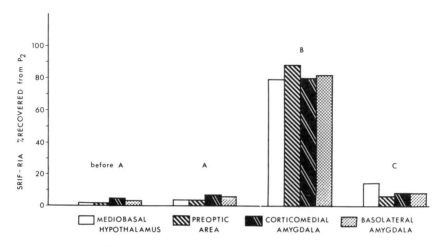

FIG. 3. Percent of somatostatin recovered from organelles.

the content of somatostatin by radioimmunoassay in the amygdala and cortex (Fig. 3).

All lesions were carried out under pentobarbital anesthesia (50 mg/kg i.p.) following De Groot coordinates with bilateral anodal platinum wire with 0.5-mm exposed tips. Lesion sizes were 30 to 90 mc depending on the nucleus size. Hypothalamic deafferentation was performed according to the Halasz and Pupp technique (10), the depth of the knife reference being the anterior skull base. Four days after lesions or 3 weeks after deafferentation, these animals were killed by decapitation and the dissected tissues were homogenized in 0.2 N acetic acid and kept frozen until assayed. Prior to assay the homogenate fragments were centrifuged (1,000 g) for 10 min. The supernatants were neutralized to pH 7.2 with 4 N NaOH, and somatostatin concentration was determined using our RIA.

The inter- and intra-assay variations using this extraction method were 3 and 4%, respectively.

Bilateral anterior hypothalamic or ventromedial preoptic lesions reduced somatostatin content in the median eminence to less than 10% of control levels (Table 4). However, such lesions had no effect on somatostatin concentration in the amygdala or cortex. Combined preoptic and VMN lesions also had no effect on amygdaloid or cortex somatostatin content. Hypothalamic islands that preserved the ventromedial-arcuate region attached to the pituitary stalk resulted in the reduction in somatostatin content in the ME and the preoptic area, but had no effect on levels in the amygdala and cortex (6).

Conclusion

These findings argue in favor of an anterior-hypothalamic-preoptic somatostatinergic pathway to the median eminence but indicate that extrahypothalamic somatostatin is not derived from hypothalamic regions. These results are in agreement with immunohistochemical studies which indicate that the primary localization of cell perikarya is the anterior hypothalamic region (9), but that other brain areas also contain cells that react with somatostatin antisera.

Somatostatin Secretion from Cultured Islets

We have studied the physiology of somatostatin secretion on enzymatically dispersed newborn rat islets. This investigation was planned to identify the biochemical and/or hormonal parameters that trigger secretion of somatostatin by "δ" cells. This was done using delicately digested islets in order to preserve their fragile anatomy and prevent damage to intercellular gap junctions.

Islet Preparation

Pancreata were dissected from 1-day-old decapitated rats and pooled on ice cold PBS buffer solution at pH 7.4 (prepared as follows: to 1 liter of distilled water were added 8 g NaCl, 0.2 g KCl, 1.15 g Na_2HPO_4, 0.2 g KH_2PO_4, 0.1 g $CaCl_2$, and 0.1 g $MgCl_2$–6 H_2O; this solution was buffered and filter sterilized).

After they were cut in a few pieces, the pancreata were washed twice with a second PBS buffer without calcium and magnesium, and digested in 25 ml of the same buffer containing 30 mg of collagenase (Worthington CLS IV) for 26 to 28 min. This timing of digestion was chosen because it was found (empirically) to be critical in dispersing the islets from connective tissue without altering the integrity of cell layers and the islet capsule. After the digestion broth was sedimented in a sterile 50-ml tube (Falcon No. 2070) for 40 to 50 sec, the supernatant was gently removed and the precipitate discarded. This supernatant, containing more than 90% of the well-dispersed islets, was centrifuged 3 min at 40 to 50 g. The islets obtained in the precipitate were then washed twice with culture medium "199" (Gibco: 115E) supplemented with 10% fetal calf serum (Gibco: 614H) and penicillin G (400 μm/ml; Gibco 180030). The islets were plated (35-mm culture dishes, Corning; No. 25,000) in this same medium, 2 pancreata equivalent per 2 ml of medium, and cultured at 37°C under 5% CO_2 for 2 days, until stabilized and fixed for the assay.

Assay Procedure

The day of the assay, the fixed islets were washed twice with Kreb's-Ringer bicarbonate buffer, and 0.450 ml of buffer was immediately added for the assay (112 mM NaCl, 5.6 mM KCl, 30 mM $CaCl_2$, 1.4 mM KH_2PO_4, 1.5 mM $MgSO_4$, 29.4 mM $NaHCO_3$, 10 mg/liter of phenol red, pH 7.2, supplemented with α-D $(+)$ glucose). It should be understood that in these experiments where the effect of variable concentration of the sugar was studied, no adjustment of the ionic strength of the medium was made, but when the concentrations of Ca^{2+} and K^+ were studied, the concentration of NaCl was appropriately adjusted. $NaHCO_3$ was added to the Kreb's solution just before use and was equilibrated under the same incubation conditions as previously described.

In some experiments insulin (Insulin-Toronto; Pork Insulin, Connaught La.) and glucagon (Sigma A-4250) were added to the cultured islets diluted in Kreb's Ringer solution. The Kreb's solution was preheated and gassed 30 min before to the incubation conditions. After 2 hr of incubation, a 400- to 500-μl aliquot from each dish was collected and mixed with an equal volume of 2 N acetic acid. The samples were kept at $-20°C$ until the following day when they were assayed in our RIA for somatostatin, after being centrifuged and the supernatant buffered with 5 N NaOH to pH 7.2 to 7.4.

The data clearly show that both hypoglycemia and hyperglycemia have a significant stimulating effect on somatostatin secretion. However, compared to the stimulatory releasing effect seen with insulin and glucagon, it is marginal. This can best be explained by the fact that the stimulatory effect of both hyper- and hypoglycemia is indirect and slower. Therefore the response is less prominent than the direct effects of insulin and glucagon (Table 5).

In this assaying model a treatment with 10-fold the control concentration of K^+ causes a significant rise in RIA somatostatin secreted ($p < 0.01$) up to three times the control level, whereas two times the concentration of Ca^{2+} had no effect on RIA somatostatin secretion.

It is also interesting to note that the treatment of the cultured islets with

TABLE 5. Somatostatin secretion from pancreatic islets

	Somatostatin (pg/ml)	
Glucose	Control period	Assay period
1.4 mM	210 $\pm$ 35 (6)[a]	590 $\pm$ 65[b]
2.8 mM	180 $\pm$ 65 (6)[a]	340 $\pm$ 55
5.6 mM	380 $\pm$ 90 (6)[a]	365 $\pm$ 60
11.0 mM	200 $\pm$ 50 (6)[a]	165 $\pm$ 65
16.5 mM	240 $\pm$ 50 (6)[a]	700 $\pm$ 85[b]
22.0 mM	175 $\pm$ 30 (6)[a]	910 $\pm$ 50[b]
Glucagon		
0.5 μg/ml	135 $\pm$ 15 (4)	2,800 $\pm$ 250[b]
5.0 μg/ml	430 $\pm$ 35 (4)	3,500 $\pm$ 230[b]
Insulin		
1 mU/ml	405 $\pm$ 50 (4)	4,350 $\pm$ 195[b]
100 mU/ml	415 $\pm$ 115 (4)	3,165 $\pm$ 675[b]

[a] Mean $\pm$ SE (number of plates).
[b] $p < 0.01$ as compared to control period.

high concentrations of insulin and glucagon has augmented significantly ($p < 0.02$) the content of RIA somatostatin in the "δ" cells (from 45 to 75%) after a pulse incubation of only 2 hr.

Blood Measurement of Somatostatin

We found that unextracted plasma completely destroyed Tyr_1-somatostatin (Table 6) even with high concentrations of EDTA added to the plasma samples. Therefore our problem in measuring somatostatin in blood was to find a technique to extract the peptide before degradation and/or protein adsorption. Two methods of extraction were studied extensively. Acetic acid (2 N,1:1) and acetone (2:1) were compared on the basis of percentage of recovery of added synthetic somatostatin. Plasma or serum, deactivated by incubation at room temperature for 48 hr, was used as a substrate to which variable known amounts of synthetic somatostatin were added. The acetic acid extracts were buffered and the acetone extracts were evaporated. The percentage of recovery after extraction was evaluated by radioimmunoassay. Trasylol (1,000 KIU/ml) was added to some samples to evaluate its ability to inhibit peptic degradation of somatostatin.

The data suggest (Table 7) that both acetic acid and acetone are reliable for extraction of somatostatin from rat and human plasma or serum. Trasylol did not improve recovery. We did not evaluate benzamidine's effect on recovery of somatostatin, since it was found to decrease the binding of our sheep antibody to somatostatin by 12% at a final concentration of 5 mM per assay tube.

We have also studied the effect of anesthetic on levels of RIA-somatostatin in plasma (Table 8). Two groups of 14 rats were studied: the first group received Na-pentobarbital anesthesia (50 mg/kg, i.p.) and the second group received urethane (150 mg/100 g body weight). In the Na-pentobarbital group, mean immunoreactive somatostatin was 182 ± 15.7 pg/ml plasma in the jugular vein and 432 ± 48 pg/ml plasma in the portal vein. In the

TABLE 6. *Effect of acetic acid extraction on binding of* [125]*I-Tyr-*[1]*SRIF*

	% B/Bo (Buffer I)	% B/Bo (Buffer II)
Extracted plasma (100 μl)	87.7	81.8
Unextracted plasma (100 μl)	7.9	8.4

Buffer I: 25 mM EDTA, 4 mM PO_4, 150 mM NaCl, 1 g/liter Na azide and 1 g/liter human serum albumin (fraction V) at pH 7.2.

Buffer II: 50 mM EDTA, 10 mM PO_4, 150 mM NaCl, 1 g/liter Na azide and 4 g/liter human serum albumin (fraction V) at pH 7.8.

TABLE 7. *Recovery of synthetic somatostatin (SS) from deactivated plasma or serum*

Sub-strate[a]	No. of samples	Extraction	% Recovery RIA-SS
D.H.S.	6	2 N Acetic acid	93.3 ± 3.3
D.H.P.	8	"	93.6 ± 4.4
D.H.S.+T	6	"	107.8 ± 7.4
D.H.P.+T	8	"	79.1 ± 5.7
D.R.P.	7	"	76.4 ± 7.0
D.R.P.+T	7	"	71.3 ± 4.3
D.H.P.+T	4	Acetone	85.5 ± 11.0
D.R.P.+T	4	Acetone	77.3 ± 4.5

D, deactivated 48 hr; H, human; R, rat; S, serum; P, plasma; T, trasylol; +, 5 days freezing.

[a] SS added 62.5 to 4,000 pg/ml.

TABLE 8. *Effect of anesthesia on immunoreactive SS in plasma (acetic acid extracted)*

	Jugular vein	Portal vein
Na pentobarbital 50 mg/kg B.W. (i.v.)	182.7 ± 15.7 (14)	432 ± 48 (17)[b]
Urethane 150 mg/100 B.W. (i.p.)	343.9 ± 31 (14)[b]	678 ± 94 (21)[a]

[a] $p < 0.05$.
[b] $p < 0.001$ as compared to Na pentobarbital.

urethane group, mean immunoreactive somatostatin was 343.9 ± 31 pg/ml plasma ($p < 0.001$) in the jugular vein and 678 ± 94 pg/ml ($p < 0.05$) in the portal vein. This increased level of RIA-somatostatin in the urethane-anesthetized rat can best be explained by the toxicity of the chemical at the upper gut level.

Modulation of Somatostatin Secretion in the Portal Vein

In vivo *Physiological Preliminary Studies*

Male rats weighing 350 to 500 g were anesthetized with pentobarbital (50 mg/kg i.p.). Three groups of rats were studied using a jugular catheter ending in the right atrium. Via this catheter, a first group of 11 rats received 2 g/kg of glucose 50%. A second group of 8 rats received 10 μg of glucagon, and a third group of 11 rats, 1 cc of normal saline. Portal blood was rapidly collected, the plasma extracted with 2 N acetic acid (1:1) and stored at −20°C.

The effect of glucose administration on RIA somatostatin levels in the

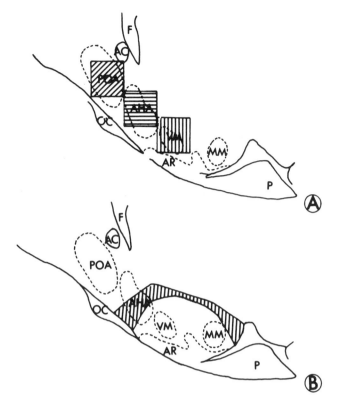

FIG. 4. (A): Diagrammatic representation of histologically determined hypothalamic lesions to indicate size and location as projected on a parasagittal (L 0.2) plane of De Groot's stereotaxic atlas. (B): Diagrammatic representation of location of lesion in hypothalamic island preparations. Abbreviations: AC, anterior commissure; AHA, anterior hypothalamic area; AR, arcuate nucleus; F, fornix; MM, mammillary bodies; OC, optic chiasm; P, pituitary; POA, preoptic area; VM, ventromedial nucleus.

portal blood was not significant: this is in agreement with our results obtained *in vitro* when the glucose concentration was twice the physiological level (i.e., 11 mM). On the other hand, glucagon caused a significant increase in the RIA somatostatin of the portal vein (Fig. 4).

CONCLUSION

In Vitro (Islets of Langerhans)

1. Marked hyperglycemia or hypoglycemia is a potent stimulator of somatostatin from the islets.
2. High insulin levels or high glucagon levels are more potent inducers of somatostatin synthesis and release.

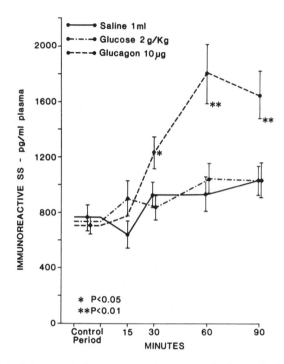

FIG. 5. Effect of glucose and glucagon on somatostatin secretion in portal vein of the rat.

In Vivo (Blood Measurements)

1. Somatostatin immunoreactivity is 2 to 2.4 times higher in portal blood than in systemic venous blood.
2. Urethane appears to increase RIA somatostatin concentration in both jugular and portal blood.
3. Hyperglycemia *per se,* as long as it does not exceed the physiological range, does not stimulate somatostatin release from the pancreas from 15 to 90 min after glucose administration.
4. Hyperglucagonemia increases RIA somatostatin levels in the portal vein.

These findings suggest that in pathological situations with marked hyperglycemia, hyperinsulinemia, or hyperglucagonemia, hypersomatostatinemia does occur.

ACKNOWLEDGMENTS

The authors wish to express their gratitude to Tina Crossfield, Wendy Gurd, and Darlene Martineau for their technical assistance and to Dr. J. B. Martin for his continuing encouragement. This research was funded by the

Medical Research Council of Canada (Grant No. MA-5298) and by a grant from the Canadian Diabetes Association to Dr. P. Brazeau.

REFERENCES

1. Alpert, L. C., Brawer, J. R., Patel, Y. C., and Reichlin, S. (1976): Somatostatinergic neurons in anterior hypothalamus: Immunohistochemical localization. *Endocrinology*, 98:255–256.
2. Brazeau, P., and Epelbaum, J. (1977): Physiology of somatostatin secretion of rat cultured islets: Preliminary studies on the effects of glucose concentration, glucagon and insulin. International Symposium on Somatostatin, Freiburg, Germany, September 25–27, 1977.
3. Brazeau, P., Epelbaum, J., Tannenbaum, G. S., Rorstad, O., and Martin, J. B. (1978): Somatostatin: Isolation, characterization, distribution and blood determination. *Proceedings of the 1st International Congress on Somatostatin*, Raven Press, New York (*in press*).
4. Brazeau, P., Vale, W., Burgus, R., Ling, N., Butcher, M., Rivier, J., and Guillemin, R. (1973): Hypothalamic polypeptide that inhibits the secretion of immunoreactive pituitary growth hormone. *Science*, 197:77–79.
5. Brownstein, M. J., Arimura, A., Sato, M., Schally, A. V., and Kizer, J. (1975): The regional distribution of somatostatin in the rat brain. *Endocrinology*. 96: 1456–1459.
6. Epelbaum, J., Brazeau, P., Tsang, D., Braver, J., and Martin, J. B. (1977): Subcellular distribution of radioimmunoassayable somatostatin in rat brain. *Brain Res.*, 126:309–323.
7. Epelbaum, J., Willoughby, J. O., Brazeau, P., and Martin, J. B. (1977): Effects of brain lesions and hypothalamic deafferentation on somatostatin distribution in the rat brain. *Endocrinology*, 101:1495–1502.
8. Guillemin, R., and Gerich, J. E. (1976): Somatostatin: Physiological and clinical significance. *Annu. Rev. Med.*, 379–388.
9. Whittaker, V. P., Michaelson, I. A., and Kirkland, R. S. A. (1964): The separation of synaptic vesicles from nerve ending particles (synaptosomes). *Biochem. J.*, 90:293–303.
10. Willoughby, J. O., Terry, L. C., Brazeau, P., and Martin, J. B. (1977): Pulsatile growth hormone, prolactin and thyrotropin secretion in rats with hypothalamic deafferentation. *Brain Res.*, 127:137–152.

Central Nervous System Effects of Hypothalamic Hormones and Other Peptides, edited by Collu et al.
Raven Press, New York © 1979.

Comparison of Behavioral Effects of Somatostatin and β-Endorphin in Animals

Viktor Havlicek and Henry G. Friesen

Department of Physiology, Faculty of Medicine, University of Manitoba, Winnipeg, Canada

It has become increasingly apparent that some hormonal peptides play physiological roles in neuronal and behavioral functions of the central nervous system (CNS). The search for hypothalamic factors controlling the function of the adenohypophysis and for endogenous opioid peptides has led to the isolation of several polypeptides whose chemical structure has been established (5,8,10,34,44,47,65). By using sensitive immunoassays for the detection of peptides it has been established that many of them, although present in the highest concentration in the hypothalamus, are distributed widely in the brain and extraneuronal sites (3,7,32,37,74). In addition to their influence on pituitary function, neuronal and behavioral effects have been documented (49). For example, systemic and intrahypothalamic injection of luteinizing hormone-releasing hormone (LH-RH) in ovariectomized, estrogen-pretreated female rats induces lordosis reflex (17,50); intracranial injections of renin, angiotensin I, or angiotensin II cause drinking behavior in rats (15,16,67); intracerebroventricular injection of somatostatin and beta-endorphin in rats, in addition to having analgesic properties (4,30), leads to disorganization of normal behavior inducing, in lower doses, an opiate-withdrawal syndrome (such as stiffly arching tail or Straube sign, wet dog shakes, excessive grooming, etc.), whereas higher doses result in akinesia, which was described as a catatonia-like state (4,27,28). These examples indicate the importance of some brain peptides in specific neuronal integration of complicated behaviors such as mating or drinking, whereas some other peptides alter normal behavior more generally. Induction of both normal and abnormal behavior patterns makes these peptides potential etiologic factors in certain disease states. This was suggested for beta-endorphin and schizophrenia by Guillemin and associates (4). Findings from our laboratory indicate that several peptides, such as somatostatin (27,28) alpha-endorphin (29), and beta-endorphin (26), when injected intracerebrally to rats cause insomnia and in many instances have powerful epileptogenic effects. Epileptogenic properties of enkephalins and endorphins have been recently confirmed in other laboratories (3,71). Although intracerebroventricular application of beta-endorphin precipitates epileptiform

EEG activity which never develops into generalized motor convulsions (3, 31), somatostatin is able to induce violent tonic-clonic seizures and animals may even die in status epilepticus (27,28). These findings indicate the possible pathogenic role of somatostatin in two pathological states of the brain: epilepsy and insomnia. The purpose of this chapter is to describe somatostatin-induced behavioral syndrome and to review our recent investigations into the mechanisms by which somatostatin produces these complex behavioral effects and into differentiation between this syndrome and that which was induced by beta-endorphin.

IMMUNOCHEMICAL STUDIES

Distribution of Somatostatin

The radioimmunoassay method (RIA) using specific antiserum to somatostatin was originally reported by Brownstein et al. (7). Later several other research groups developed their own antisera and reported data on the distribution of somatostatin in brain and other tissues (14,40,52). In our laboratory antisomatostatin-specific antibody was generated in rabbits by using conventional immunological procedures. The rabbits were immunized

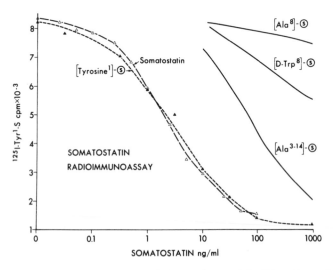

FIG. 1. Tyr¹-somatostatin was iodinated and purified on carboxymethyl cellulose. Tracer that was more than 80% precipitable with excess antibody was used in the radioimmunoassay. A dilution of 1/10,000 of the rabbit antibody was incubated along with tracer, standards, or unknowns for 20 hr, at which time antibody-bound somatostatin was separated from free by dextran-coated charcoal or by a second antibody addition (after incubation for 2 days). No cross-reactivity was noted at 1 μg/ml for a large number of peptides including: TRH, LHRH, enkephalin, alpha-endorphin, beta-endorphin, β-LPH, ACTH, porcine glucagon, vasopressin, oxytocin, secretin, prolactin growth hormone, luteinizing hormone, and follicle-stimulating hormone.

TABLE 1. *Distribution of immunoreactive somatostatin in the rat brain*

Region	N	Weight (mg) ± SEM	Somatostatin		
			ng/mg wet weight ± SEM	ng/region ± SEM	ng/mg protein[b]
Cerebral cortex	8	1,000[a]	0.03 ± 0.002	30.0	0.26
Cerebellum	9	228.9 ± 3.5	0.02 ± 0.005	4.8 ± 1.3	0.18
Hindbrain	7	206.3 ± 11.6	0.02 ± 0.002	4.9 ± 0.56	0.18
Midbrain	8	120.3 ± 9.7	0.04 ± 0.01	4.5 ± 1.06	0.35
Hippocampus	10	83.1 ± 5.0	0.06 ± 0.004	5.3 ± 0.35	0.53
Striatum	7	60.8 ± 6.0	0.08 ± 0.008	4.5 ± 0.29	0.70
Hypothalamus	8	32.9 ± 1.5	1.11 ± 0.27	36.3 ± 8.2	9.77

Animals were killed by microwave irradiation and the brain was dissected as described by Glowinsk and Iversen (21). The somatostatin content of each region was determined. The means and SEM of 7–10 separate determinations are given.

[a] Only partial samples of cerebral cortex were used. Weight of the entire region was taken from Brownstein et al. (7).

[b] Protein content was determined by method of Lowry et al. (48) and has been found to be 11.4% of the wet weight (average from different regions).

with somatostatin conjugated with bovine albumin. The antisera obtained were tested using a double-antibody method or dextran-coated charcoal. As tracer ^{125}I-Tyr^1-somatostatin was used and the assay procedure outlined in the legend of Fig. 1 was employed. Figure 1 indicates the sensitivity and specificity of the assay. As can be seen, the assay sensitivity was 0.1 ng/ml

TABLE 2. *Immunoreactive somatostatin in cerebral cortex of the rat brain (values obtained in this study compared with other reports)*

	This study A	Brownstein et al. (7) B	Patel and Reichlin (52) C	Kronheim et al. (40) D
ng/mg wet wt. ± SEM	0.03 ± 0.002	0.03 ± 0.002	0.03	98.3 ± 23.7 (0.098)[a]
ng/region	30.0	30.0	516.0 ± 34.0	
ng/mg protein	0.26	2.4 ± 0.03[b]	6.7 ± 1.7	35.79 ± 7.54

Comment: According to our measurements using the Lowry method, the protein content of the cerebral cortex is approximately 11% of the wet weight. Thus values expressed as ng/mg protein should be about nine times higher in comparison with values expressed as ng/mg wet weight. Such a comparison for data B gives 80 × higher values; for C, 223 × higher values; whereas D gives approximately 3 × lower, or after correction (52) 365 × higher, values. This would correspond to protein content ranging from 1.25 to 0.27% of the wet weight.

Weight of the rat's cerebral cortex in data C must be 17,200 mg in order to obtain 516 mg/region (based on 0.03 ng/mg wet weight).

[a] As corrected from the original report; see Patel and Reichlin (52).

[b] Data for parietal cortex only in Table 2 (7).

TABLE 3. *Immunoreactive somatostatin content of the whole cerebral cortex and two ultracentrifugal fractions in the rat brain*

Tissue treatment	Somatostatin ng/mg protein ± SEM (N)
Whole cerebral cortex	0.33 ± 0.01 (8)
Crude mitochondrial pellet	1.5 ± 0.15 (3)
Synaptosomal pellet	13.2 ± 3.1 (4)

Animals were killed by decapitation, the cerebral cortex rapidly removed, chilled in ice-cold sucrose, and processed according to the method of Whittaker et al. (73).

and only minimal cross-reaction was noted with several analogs, whereas all other unrelated peptides failed to cross-react.

The regional distribution of somatostatin in the rat brain is presented in Table 1. Our data show that the highest concentration of somatostatin is in the hypothalamus. However, other areas of the brain also contain considerable amounts of somatostatin. Nevertheless, due to the large size of the cerebral cortex the total amount of somatostatin in this structure is similar to that in the hypothalamus. In the cerebral cortex the concentration of somatostatin is relatively low. Our data for the regional distribution of somatostatin in brain are very close to those reported by Brownstein et al. (7); however, they differ from values reported by some other authors (40, 53) (Table 2). Using Whittaker's method (73) of preparing synaptosomal fraction, Lee et al. (46) were able to show that synaptosomal pellet of the cerebral cortex has 40 times higher concentrations of somatostatin than the whole cerebral cortex (Table 3). These findings, which are in good agreement with data of Epelbaum et al. (14), indicate that somatostatin is present intraneuronally in highest concentrations in nerve endings. Recent immunohistochemical findings in the human cerebral cortex support this notion (33).

Release of Somatostatin

The next question to be answered was whether immunoreactive somatostatin in the cerebral cortex could be released by tissue depolarization and whether such a release, if present, was calcium dependent (13).

Experiments were performed *in vitro* on cortical slices (45) since very high basal release from cortical synaptosomes indicated that unstable membranes in this preparation were most likely due to tissue damage (46). Results of these experiments are presented in Table 4. Membrane depolarization by high extracellular potassium concentration caused approximately four-fold increase in release of somatostatin. This significant increase in release of somatostatin was suppressed when extracellular Ca^{2+} was replaced by Mn^{2+}. Thus our immunochemical studies have shown that: (a) Immuno-

TABLE 4. Effect of high K^+ and low Ca^{2+} on the release of immunoreactive somatostatin from cortical slices

Krebs solution	Somatostatin release[a]	Statistical significance
1. 5 mM K^+ 1.5 mM Ca^{2+}	1.24 ± 0.3 (N = 8)	
2. 56 mM K^{+b} 1.5 mM Ca^{2+}	4.87 ± 1.0 (N = 6)	$p \leq 0.01$
3. 5 mM K^+ 1.5 mM Mn^{2+}	0.53 ± 0.1 (N = 8)	
4. 56 mM K^{+b} 1.5 mM Mn^{2+}	0.9 ± 0.26 (N = 8)	

[a] ng/ml/100 mg dry wt. during 15 min incubation.
[b] Iso-osmolality was maintained by decreasing Na^+ concentration from 150 to 100 mM in oxygenated Krebs solution. The basal release of somatostatin was not affected by lowering Na^+ concentration: when iso-osmolality in 100 mM Na^+ Krebs solution was maintained by equimolar choline-Cl, the release of somatostatin was not significantly different from control values $(1.34 \pm 0.33$ ng/ml/100 mg dry wt.).

reactive somatostatin is present in the brain not only in the hypothalamus, but also in other CNS structures. Regional distribution shows that cerebral cortex contains large amounts of somatostatin (30 ng/region). (b) In the cerebral cortex somatostatin is highly concentrated in synaptosomes (13.2 ng/mg protein versus 0.33 ng/mg protein in the whole cortex). (c) Upon cell depolarization with high extracellular potassium ions, tissue slices of the cerebral cortex significantly increase release of somatostatin (fourfold increase). Such increased release is calcium dependent, since it is suppressed in calcium-free medium. All these findings allow us to speculate that somatostatin has some physiological role in the CNS; it could be a neurotransmitter or a neuromodulator-neurohormone.

BEHAVIORAL AND ELECTROPHYSIOLOGICAL STUDIES

Systemic and Intracerebral Applications

In the first reports on behavioral effects of somatostatin systemic applications of this peptide were employed (6,54). The results were difficult to assess and interpret. One laboratory described significant potentiation by somatostatin of the excitatory behavioral effects of DOPA. This result was interpreted to mean that somatostatin had psychogenic effects (54). Others observed reduction of strychnine-induced seizures and a potentiation of pentobarbital depression and concluded that somatostatin caused central depression (6). Experiments of this nature must be interpreted with extreme caution for at least two reasons: first, it is difficult to differentiate between the direct central effects and the multiple peripheral actions of this peptide which can secondarily affect brain function by stimulation of peripheral receptors and/or metabolic peripheral changes. Secondly, the free passage of somatostatin across the blood-brain barrier has not as yet been demonstrated conclusively.

Central application avoids some of these problems. In our experiments, when somatostatin was applied intracerebroventricularly (i.c.v.) (27,28), supracortically (58), into the amygdala (60), into the hippocampus (59), and into the striatum (63), no sedative effects were noted. In all doses tested (100 pg to 50 μg) somatostatin exerted a remarkable effect on the spontaneous sleep and on the motor activity in the freely moving rat. A significant reduction of both the slow-wave sleep and particularly the paradoxical sleep can be detected after infusion of somatostatin into any brain structure tested (see above). This effect was dose dependent and after i.c.v. application was dependent on the speed of infusion. This effect is reproducible in hypophysectomized rats (28). Analogs of somatostatin (both those that suppress GH secretion, e.g., Ala^2-somatostatin, and those that do not, e.g., Ala^8-somatostatin) have little or no effect on the sleep-waking cycle or EEG.

Dramatic changes in motor activity and in the EEG were detected after i.c.v. administration of somatostatin. On the basis of this action we were able to distinguish several stages of the central somatostatin effects starting with excessive grooming and exploring and ending with violent tonic-clonic seizures and ultimately stuporous immobility which we erroneously described as a catatonic state (28).

Stuporous immobility or "frozen stares" and aphagia with flattening of the EEG and eventually with epileptic-like EEG activity could also be induced by systemic (i.p.) application of somatostatin. However, this effect seems to be mediated by peripheral glucoprivic action of somatostatin because it was instantaneously reversed by systemic application of glucose (57,61). On the other hand, i.c.v. somatostatin-induced syndrome was glucose insensitive (61).

Motor Incoordination

After somatostatin was administered into any brain structure, signs of motor incoordination developed (Table 5). The lowest threshold doses for induction of motor incoordination were detected after infusions into striatum and amygdala. In these structures as little as 0.1 ng of somatostatin induced clear signs of motor coordination difficulties. It is necessary to describe certain details of the experimental conditions.

Rats were placed in a cage (20 × 21 × 25 cm) that was isolated from the experimentor in a soundproof and electrically shielded room. The cage was equipped with a grid floor to permit detection of changes in the fine motor

TABLE 5. *Motor incoordination in rats after administration of somatostatin into different brain regions*

Dose of somatostatin (μg)	Motor incoordination infusion site					
	Striatum[a]	Hippocampus[b]	Dentate[b] gyrus	Amygdala[c]	Cortex[d]	i.c.v.[e]
0.01	—	—	—	—	*	*
0.1	+	—	—	+	*	*
1.0	++	+	+	++	*	*
5.0	*	++	++	*	*	*
10.0	+++	+++	+++	+++	+++	+++

Motor incoordination was assessed in a chamber with a grid floor: (+), legs occasionally slip between bars of the grid floor during exploration and grooming activity without loss of balance; (++), legs slip between bars in moving or sitting animals with short-lasting (2–3 sec) loss of balance; (+++), legs slip between bars with lengthy (> 10 sec) loss of balance; (*), not tested.
[a] Rezek et al. (63).
[b] Rezek et al. (59).
[c] Rezek et al. (60).
[d] Rezek et al. (58).
[e] Havlicek et al. (28).

coordination necessary for a proper grip, movement, and maintenance of balance on the bars of the grid floor. In this way the motor coordination of a rat was continuously tested even when the rat was motionless in a sitting position. Even minor coordination difficulties could be detected because the legs might slip between the bars with or without a loss of balance. Coordination difficulties often cause animals to remain motionless in order to avoid loss of balance (Fig. 2A). On an ordinary flat floor of the "motility box," such changes will not be detected. Moreover, minor incoordination will cause a decrease in motor activity counts which can easily be misinterpreted as sedation or the "calming effect" (66).

Akinesia and Muscle Rigidity

After higher doses of somatostatin (5 to 10 μg i.c.v.), motor incoordination can evolve into a hemiplegia-in-extension, due to spastic rigidity which predominates in the extensors in legs contralateral to the side of infusion (Fig. 2C), or into a generalized rigidity of all body muscles—a state we have described as catatonia (28). Since immobility and muscle rigidity also develop after i.c.v. infusion of another brain peptide—beta-endorphin (9)— we have compared this aspect of central action of somatostatin with that of beta-endorphin (31). The most obvious differences were noted in the EEG patterns. When compared with the cortical EEG during the normal wakeful state, somatostatin-induced akinesia (10 μg i.c.v.) was associated with depression of the EEG (Fig. 3). Frequency analysis of the EEG (fast Fourier transform) showed significant decrease of the power in all frequencies from

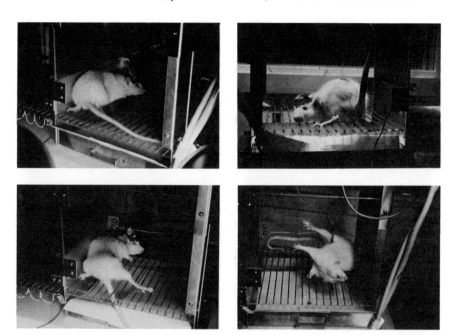

FIG. 2. Effect of somatostatin on motor behavior. Top left: incoordination (note from left leg with extended digits hanging between bars of the floor). Top right: stiffly arched tail (Straube sign). Bottom left: hemiplegia-in-extension of the limbs on the right side. Bottom right: tonic-clonic seizures with opisthotonus and extension prevailing on the right side of the body.

1.5 to 25 Hz (Fig. 4). At the same time beta-endorphin-induced akinesia (50 μg i.c.v.) was associated with a significant increase in power in all frequencies tested (Fig. 4). Initially, during the first 20 to 25 min after infusion this hypersynchrony can be interrupted by an EEG arousal response to any external stimulus, such as acoustic, somesthetic, or nociceptive stimulation, particularly when applied to the head area (ear pinprick, corneal stimulation). Approximately 30 min after application of beta-endorphin,

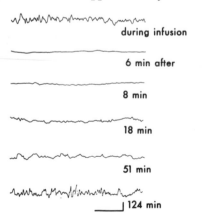

during infusion

6 min after

8 min

18 min

51 min

124 min

FIG. 3. Depression of the EEG of the sensorimotor cortex in the rat after i.c.v. infusion of somatostatin (10 μg of somatostatin μg/μl/min). From top to bottom: EEG during infusion, 6 min after infusion, 8 min after infusion, 18 min after infusion, 51 min after infusion, and 124 min after infusion. Bottom right calibration: horizontal line 1 sec, vertical line 100 μV.

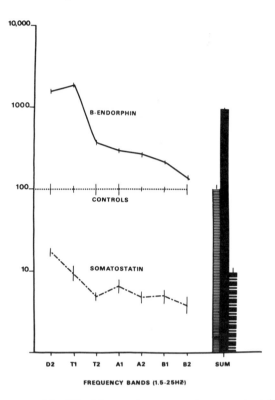

FIG. 4. The power spectrum of the EEG of the sensorimotor cortex in groups of rats (6–8 animals in each group) treated with either somatostatin (10 μg i.c.v.) or beta-endorphin (50 μg i.c.v.). Control values were taken in animals during wakeful state as 100%. Spectral analysis was performed on PDP8/E minicomputer using fast Fourier transform. EEG spectrum was integrated into the following frequency bands: D2 (1.56–3.51 Hz); T1 (3.61–5.57 Hz); T2 (5.66–7.52 Hz); A1 (7.62–9.47 Hz); A2 (9.57–12.50 Hz); B1 (12.60–17.48 Hz); B2 (17.58–25.00 Hz); SUM (1.56–25.00 Hz). Vertical bars indicate from left to right controls (*horizontal batch*), beta-endorphin (*solid bars*), and somatostatin (*solid and horizontal batch*).

animals became behaviorally and electroencephalographically unresponsive to any stimulation (Fig. 5). During this time we were able to perform even minor surgery without any EEG or behavioral response, therefore we have defined this state as general anesthesia with muscle rigidity (25). The initial stage of beta-endorphin akinesia in several respects corresponds to a pre-anesthetic stuporous state.

These findings underline the inappropriateness of the term "catatonia" for a state induced by beta-endorphin: catatonia is a well-recognized psychiatric condition that includes additional symptoms such as willful resistance and negativism, and most importantly consciousness is not affected. Thus the EEG of catatonic patients has a normal wakeful pattern (55).

Somatostatin-induced akinesia in rats also does not correspond to human catatonic syndrome. This type of akinesia has more similarities with epileptic stupor in which consciousness is also affected. Stimulation of animals

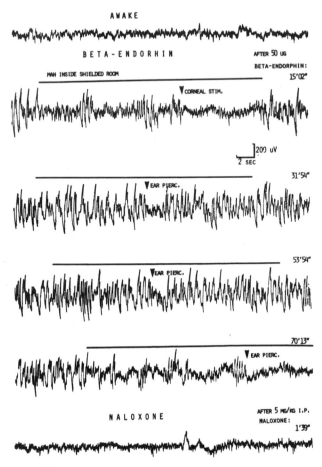

FIG. 5. EEG hypersynchrony after i.c.v. infusion of the high dose of beta-endorphin (50 μg). From top to bottom: (1) EEG in the wakeful rat before the infusion; (2) EEG 15 min after infusion. Horizontal bar marks the presence of a man close to the rat (inside the sound-shielded room), arrow marks corneal stimulation. There is a marked EEG arousal response to the presence of the man and even larger arousal to the corneal stimulation; all the time animal remains akinetic and rigid, corneal reflex is partially suppressed. (3) 31 min after infusion animal is akinetic, corneal reflex is absent. There is no arousal response to presence of the man, and even minor surgery on the ear (arrow) produced only short-lasting EEG arousal without any behavioral response; (4) 53 min after infusion animal is akinetic and rigid, corneal reflex is absent. Presence of the man and surgery on the ear remain without EEG and/or behavioral response; (5) 70 min after infusion animal is still akinetic; however, corneal reflex is present, there is EEG arousal in response to the mere presence of man, and noncicetive stimulation (ear piercing) produces strong EEG arousal and behavioral response. (6) Systemic naloxone treatment (5 mg/kg i.p.) instantaneously removes the EEG hypersynchrony and animal shows normal wakeful behavior with no incoordination or muscle rigidity. Calibration between the second and third EEG sample applies to all samples. EEG recordings are bipolar from the sensory motor cortex.

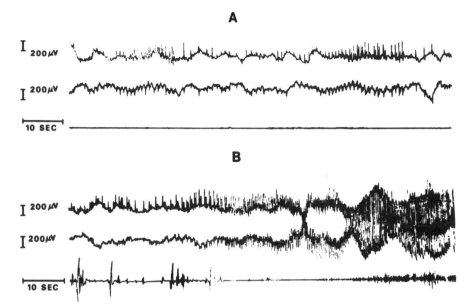

FIG. 6. EEG and behavioral seizures after i.c.v. administration of somatostatin (10 μg). A: Two clusters of EEG spikes and singular spike in between. No motor seizures are present, only akinesia or "frozen stares." B: Epileptic-like EEG activity becomes more regular, frequency and amplitude of spikes gradually increase until it evolves into generalized EEG and motor epileptic fit. A and B from top to bottom: (1) EEG of the left sensorimotor cortex; (2) EEG of the right sensorimotor cortex (both are bipolar recordings); (3) actogram. Calibration on the left side.

in this state produced two types of responses: in some rigid and akinetic animals sound or soft touch provoked violent tonic-clonic seizures (Fig. 6), whereas other animals remained behaviorally and EEG (flat, depressed pattern) unresponsive even to lifting and handling. The latter state typically occurred during postictal periods (post-seizure stupor); however, it was also observed in animals that never developed any motor seizure activity.

Systemic administration of naloxone (5 mg/kg i.p.) completely abolished endorphin-induced EEG hypersynchrony (Fig. 5) within 2 to 3 min after infusion and replaced it with normal wakeful EEG patterns which were, after an additional 30 to 60 sec delay, followed by behavioral arousal. Muscle rigidity also dissipated after naloxone administration. By contrast, somatostatin-induced akinesia remained unaffected by naloxone treatment.

Behavioral Seizures and Epileptic-like EEG

After i.c.v. infusion of somatostatin, 33% of animals developed violent tonic-clonic seizures (Fig. 6). In some instances seizures developed "spontaneously" (without any additional stimulation) during the infusion of the peptide (10 μg at the rate of 1 μg/μl/min), whereas in other cases the first grand mal type fit was seen 5 to 15 min after the end of the infusion. Behavioral seizures lasted from 1 to 5 min and occurred in cycles every 10 to 20 min during the first hour postinfusion. During the first seizures, particularly those which developed with a short latency, more violent contractions of limbs contralateral to the side of infusion often caused animals to rotate unidirectionally along the body axis (Fig. 2D). This condition, designated "barrel rotation," differs from "close head-to-tail" rotations induced by TRH (9). We feel that such description conceals the epileptic-nature of this state.

Electrocorticogram in most instances showed generalized epileptic-like activity; however, occasionally there was a depression of the EEG which was most often seen during akinetic spells. Topical microinfusion of somatostatin to hippocampus, amygdala, dentate gyrus, or sensorimotor cortex caused local depression of the electrical activity and/or epileptic-like spiking, but generalized motor seizures were not detected. Thus our experiments indicate that only i.c.v. infusion of somatostatin is able to elicit grand mal-type epileptic fits. Indeed, in some instances we have seen generalized motor seizures even after 100 pg of peptide (Tyr^1-somatostatin) was applied rapidly (1 to 2 sec) i.c.v. On the other hand, our experiments have shown that epileptogenic effects seen after 10 μg of somatostatin can be completely avoided if the rate of intraventricular infusion is reduced from 1 to 0.5 μg/min.

All these findings indicate that in order to produce generalized motor seizures somatostatin must reach a critical concentration in certain large periventricular (hippocampal?) areas of the brain. During a slow infusion this concentration was not reached due to several possible mechanisms such as passive removal with the flow of the cerebrospinal fluid, metabolic deactivation, or uptake mechanisms. Similarly, topical microinjection of somatostatin did not affect large enough neuronal populations to initiate spread of the epileptic activity into the CNS motor system.

Intracerebroventricular infusion of beta-endorphin in doses ranging from 2 to 50 μg caused a variety of epileptiform EEG changes; however, none of the animals tested developed generalized tonic-clonic seizures (26). This is in good agreement with recently published findings (3). Electrical epileptic-like activity usually preceded "frozen stares," and some other opiate withdrawal symptoms (see below). Therefore we have compared this syndrome with petit mal epilepsy in humans (31).

Again, as with akinetic state, naloxone completely abolished the electrophysiological and behavioral changes induced by beta-endorphin but did not alter somatostatin effects.

Opiate Withdrawal Symptoms and Analgesic Properties of Somatostatin

Central infusion of somatostatin promotes behavioral responses that generally are associated with opiate withdrawal syndrome (18). Thus wet

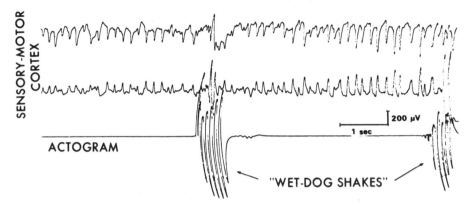

FIG. 7. Wet dog shakes in the rat after i.c.v. infusion of beta-endorphin (2 µg) are preceded by multiple spikes in the EEG of the sensorimotor cortex. From top to bottom: (1) left sensorimotor cortex; (2) right sensorimotor cortex; (3) actogram. Calibration bottom right.

dog shakes, stiffly arching tail or Straube's sign (Fig. 2B), excessive exploring and grooming, hyperreactivity to stimuli, seizures, salivation, urination, and defecation may be seen after infusion of somatostatin. Similar activities have been reported for central administration of morphine (11), enkephalin (71), alpha-endorphin (29), and beta-endorphin (4,26).

Among these opiate withdrawal signs of particular interest are wet dog shakes, which are not present in the rat under ordinary circumstances but are provoked in a dose-related manner by central administration of opiates (11). We have shown that the initial occurrence of this symptom is always preceded by clusters of EEG spikes (Fig. 7). Maximal number of wet dog shakes is seen after low doses of beta-endorphin (2 µg i.c.v.), whereas higher doses cause akinesia when any excitatory opiate withdrawal symptoms including wet dog shakes are suppressed. Central administration of somatostatin also generates wet dog shakes, but in lesser number than beta-endorphin. The main difference, however, between somatostatin-induced "opiate withdrawal signs" including wet dog shakes and similar signs induced by beta-endorphin is that naloxone very efficiently removes or prevents endorphin-induced signs, although somatostatin's effect remains unaffected.

In a collaborative study with Dr. Frank LaBella (41), we have observed that central application of calcium chelators (EGTA, 25 µg ICV) promotes an excitatory syndrome which is naloxone insensitive and is similar to that of opiate withdrawal including wet dog shakes and EEG and behavioral seizures. These signs, which were caused by depletion of extracellular calcium primarily within periventricular and periaqueductal structures, were also insensitive to naloxone treatment.

Similarities between central effects of somatostatin and beta-endorphin promoted experiments in which we have tested analgesic properties of

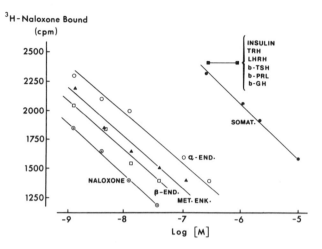

FIG. 8. Relative potencies of naloxone, alpha-endorphin, beta-endorphin, methionine-enkephalin, somatostatin, and other peptides and bovine protein hormones in the opiate radioreceptor assay, at 0°C and no sodium. Diminished radioactivity (cpm) reflects displacement of ³H-naloxone from rat brain membranes.

somatostatin. Central administration of somatostatin (1 to 10 μg i.c.v.) significantly prolonged the latency of the tail flick response, and this analgesic effect of somatostatin was naloxone reversible (30,62). In the opiate radioreceptor assay somatostatin showed relatively weak activity: IC_{50} about 8 μM as compared to IC_{50} about 10 nM for beta-endorphin (Fig. 8). Such relatively weak activity of somatostatin in the opiate radioreceptor assay makes the specific interaction of this peptide with opiate receptors questionable. However, LaBella et al. (42,43) have shown that androsterone sulfate also competes weakly in the receptor assay, but is a potent, naloxone-reversible analgesic when administered i.c.v. Similarly, ACTH also shows weak *in vitro* binding (69), although *in vivo* it has a potent naloxone-reversible action (20). All these observations indicate that opiate potency as determined by the radioreceptor assay does not always parallel *in vivo* potency.

Microelectrode Application

The above-described behavioral and gross electrophysiological studies indicate predominantly a CNS stimulatory effect of somatostatin. In contrast to these findings, iontophoretic application of this peptide to individual CNS neurons has been exclusively associated with a decrease in excitability (56). These experiments have been performed on anesthetized rats. In order to avoid all possible anesthetic effects on the results, in our laboratory we have performed microelectrophoresis in unanesthetized rabbits (35).

Using this technique the effect of iontophoretically administered somato-

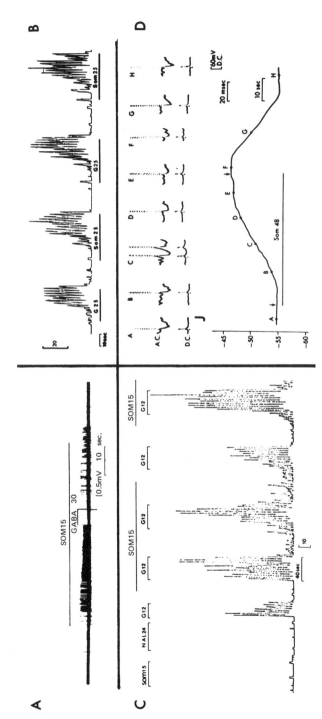

FIG. 9. A: Excitatory effect of somatostatin on cortical neuron in the unanesthetized restrained rabbit is inhibited by superimposed application of GABA. Top horizontal bar indicates iontophoretic administration of somatostatin as cation (Som, 15 nA), shorter horizontal bar indicates application of GABA (30 nA). Calibration: 0.5 mV and 10 sec. B: Effect of successive iontophoretic administrations of glutamate (G, 25 nA) and somatostatin (Som, 25 nA) on the discharge rate of the cortical neuron in the unanesthetized rabbit. Ratemeter record. Calibration: 10 sec and 20 Hz. C: Subthreshold dose of somatostatin potentiates excitatory effect of glutamate on cortical neuron. Simultaneous iontophoretic administration of glutamate (G, 12 nA) and somatostatin (Som, 15 nA) is marked by horizontal bars. D: Effect of the extracellular applied somatostatin on the membrane potential of the cortical neuron in the sensorimotor cortex of the unanesthetized rabbit. From top to bottom: (1) AC recordings of action potentials at points from A to H in bottom trace; (2) DC recordings of action potentials from the same points; (3) Penwriter trace of the membrane potential recorded intracellularly before, during, and after extracellularly applied somatostatin. The bar indicates iontophoretic administration of somatostatin (Som, 48 nA).

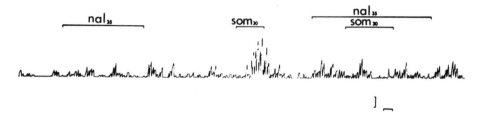

FIG. 10. Naloxone suppresses excitatory effect of somatostatin on neuronal activity in the sensorimotor cortex of the unanesthetized rabbit. Horizontal bars indicate iontophoretic administration of naloxone (nal, 35 nA) or somatostatin (Som, 30 nA). Delayed excitatory effect of somatostatin is abolished by simultaneous administration of naloxone. Ratemeter tracing. Calibration in the bottom right corner: horizontal bar, 5 sec; vertical bar, 20 Hz.

statin has been tested on 60 neurons in the somatosensory cortex. In our experiments none of the cells responded with a decrease in firing rate, but 35 neurons (58% of the neuronal population) showed significant increase in firing (Fig. 9A and B). Subthreshold stimulation by somatostatin showed a significant potentiation of the excitatory action of glutamic acid (Fig. 9C). In 81% of neurons responsive to somatostatin, GABA suppressed the somatostatin-induced excitation whereas naloxone inhibited only 32% of these cells (Fig. 10). Extracellular effect of somatostatin has been also tested on 17 neurons recorded intracellularly (36). In these experiments seven cells responded to somatostatin with prolonged depolarization (6 to 12 mV) (Fig. 9D), whereas none of the cells showed hyperpolarization.

MOLECULAR MECHANISMS—DISCUSSION

Role of Calcium Ions

Free calcium ions outside and within neurons are essential for normal functioning of the nervous system. Thus the action potential is associated with an influx of calcium ions (1), the release of neurotransmitters is calcium dependent (2,38), whereas depletion of extracellular calcium from postsynaptic sites causes a diminution and instability of the membrane potential, increasing membrane excitability and facilitating spontaneous firing (19,39).

In the mechanism of the central action of somatostatin, the role of calcium ions occurs at several critical points. First of all, we have found that the release of somatostatin from the cerebral cortex upon membrane depolarization by high extracellular potassium is calcium dependent (45,46). Similar results were described for the hypothalamus (70,72) and spinal cord primary afferents (51). Secondly, it has been established that membrane depolarization caused by glutamate or high extracellular potassium is associated with calcium uptake into cerebral synaptosomes (23). Such glutamate action in the cerebral cortex was potentiated by somatostatin (68). These findings are in good agreement with our data in which iontophoretic application of somatostatin to cortical neurons in an unanesthetized animal potentiated the excitatory effect of glutamate (35,36). This picture, however, is complicated by findings that somatostatin inhibits the release of calcium ions from synaptosomes previously loaded with $^{45}Ca^{2+}$. These data have been interpreted as a possible mechanism underlying the depressant action of somatostatin on neuronal activity (56,68). Nevertheless, such a conclusion seems premature, since strong depolarizing agents such as KCl (50 mM) were also associated with significant retention of calcium in ^{45}Ca-preloaded synaptosomes, whereas glutamate exerted no significant effect in $^{45}Ca^{2+}$-preloaded synaptosomes—in fact, there was 14% increase of retention [see Table 6, p. 344, in Goddard and Robinson (23)]. Thus it is tempting to speculate that synaptosomal uptake and retention of calcium ions which is induced by somatostatin may lead to a decrease in concentration of extracellular calcium which, in turn, will cause instability and depolarization of membranes. In this regard our observations that calcium chelators applied i.c.v. promote an excitatory syndrome very similar to that induced by somatostatin and/or opiates (41) indicate that calcium translocation may in some way be responsible for behavioral changes described as opiate withdrawal (wet dog shakes, excessive grooming and exploring, frozen stares, stiffly arching tail and seizures, salivation, defecation, and urination). Brain calcium is significantly depleted by an acute adminstration of opiate (64) and during the withdrawal syndrome resulting from abrupt discontinuation of opiates (24).

Calcium complexing agents applied i.c.v. deplete extracellular calcium primarily within periventricular and periaqueductal structures (41). The hippocampus and amygdala are situated periventricularly and are known to be readily driven into epileptic activity (12,22). This would be accomplished by calcium depletion in these structures, which would cause direct postsynaptic activation. Also, suppression of transmitter release would remove all synaptically mediated inhibitory mechanisms, thus causing unrestrained excitation in these structures. Whether similar mechanisms are involved in somatostatin-induced "opiate withdrawal" signs has yet to be elucidated. Of particular interest are our findings that wet dog shakes caused by somatostatin, beta-endorphin, or calcium chelating agents are usually preceded by EEG epileptic activity. The degree of central excitation associated with acute infusion of somatostatin opiates or calcium chelators may represent a graded response pattern, with wet dog shakes and frozen stares at one end of the spectrum and motor seizures including status epilepticus at the other end.

Central Somatostatin Action and Opiate Receptors

As has already been mentioned central application of somatostatin induces a pattern of behavioral responses generally associated with opiate withdrawal syndrome. Acute administration of opioids, enkephalins, and endorphins shows similar behavioral effects. Nevertheless, in the opiate radioreceptor assay somatostatin shows relatively weak activity—IC_{50} about 8 μM compared with IC_{50} of about 5 nM for beta-endorphin (Fig. 8) (62). These data argue against a specific interaction of somatostatin at the opiate receptor sites. There are at least four dissimilarities between behavioral syndrome of somatostatin and that of beta-endorphin:

1.   Although somatostatin produced flattening of the EEG, or EEG depression with significant decrease in power in all frequencies tested, beta-endorphin in high doses induced EEG hypersynchrony with significant increase in power in all frequencies.

2.   Both peptides induced epileptic-like EEG activity. However, whereas somatostatin caused grand mal type seizures in 33% of animals, beta-endorphin-induced behavioral syndrome never progressed to generalized motor seizures.

3.   Somatostatin-induced akinesia resembles postictal stupor, whereas beta-endorphin causes immobility which after high doses evolves into a state of general anesthesia.

4.   Naloxone had no effect on the EEG and/or motor seizures caused by somatostatin, whereas beta-endorphin-induced behavioral and/or EEG changes were completely prevented or abolished by naloxone.

However, one action of both peptides was in both instances completely abolished by naloxone: analgesic effect of somatostatin was naloxone-reversible identically to that of beta-endorphin. The relatively weak activity of somatostatin in the opiate radioreceptor assay contrasts with potent, naloxone-reversible analgesic properties of this peptide. However, such dissociation between *in vitro* and *in vivo* actions is not unique for somatostatin. Similar dissociation has been described for aldosterone (42,43), and ACTH also shows weak *in vitro* binding (69), apparently inconsistent with its potent *in vivo* actions that are antagonized by naloxone (20).

These data suggest that somatostatin in the CNS influences at least two types of receptors: (a) receptors responsible for analgesic properties of this peptide and (b) some other receptor (yet to be identified) responsible for epileptogenic properties of somatostatin.

ACKNOWLEDGMENTS

This research was supported by MRC of Canada. We are indebted to Dr. M. Goetz, Ayerst Research Laboratories, Montreal, for the generous supply of cyclic form of somatostatin (AY-24,910), and to Dr. R. Guillemin of Salk Institute for generous supply of cyclic somatostatin and somatostatin analogs.

REFERENCES

1. Baker, P. F., Hodkin, A. L., and Ridgeway, E. B. (1971): Depolarization and calcium entry in squid axons. *J. Physiol. (Lond.)*, 218:709–755.

2. Blaustein, M. P., Kendrick, N. C., Fried, R. C., and Ratzlaff, R. W. (1977): Calcium metabolism at the mammalian presynaptic nerve terminal: Lessons from the synaptosome. *Soc. Neurosci. Symp.*, 2:172–194.
3. Bloom, F. E., Rossier, J., Battenberg, E. L. F., Bayon, A., French, E., Henriksen, S. J., Siggins, G. R., Segal, D., Browne, R., Ling, N., and Guillemin, R. (1978): β-Endorphin: Cellular localization, electrophysiological and behavioral effects. In: *Advances in Biochemical Psychopharmacology*, Vol. 18, edited by E. Costa and M. Trabucchi, pp. 89–109. Raven Press, New York.
4. Bloom, F., Segal, D., Ling, N., and Guillemin, R. (1976): Endorphins: Profound behavioral effects in rats suggest new etiological factors in mental illness. *Science*, 194:630–632.
5. Brazeau, P., Vale, W., Burgus, R., Ling, N., Butcher, M., Rivier, J., and Guillemin, R. (1973): Hypothalamic polypeptide that inhibits the secretion of immunoreactive pituitary growth hormone. *Science*, 179:77–79.
6. Brown, M., and Vale, M. (1975): Central nervous system effects of hypothalamic peptides. *Endocrinology*, 96:1333–1336.
7. Brownstein, M., Arimura, A., Sato, H., Schally, A. V., and Kizer, J. S. (1975): The regional distribution of somatostatin in the rat brain. *Endocrinology*, 96:1456–1461.
8. Burgus, R., Dunn, T. F., Desiderio, D., Ward, D. N., Vale, W., and Guillemin, R. (1970): Characterization of ovine hypothalamic hypophysiotropic TSH-releasing factor. *Nature*. 226:321–325.
9. Cohn, M. L., and Cohn, M. (1975): "Barrel rotation" induced by somatostatin in the non-lesioned rat. *Brain Res.*, 96:138–141.
10. Cox, B. M., Goldstein, A., and Li, C. H. (1976): Opioid activity of a peptide, β-lipotropin-(61–91), derived from β-lipotropin. *Proc. Natl. Acad. Sci. USA*, 73:1821–1823.
11. Criswell, H. E. (1976): Analgesia and hyperreactivity following morphine microinjection into mouse brain. *Pharmacol. Biochem. Behav.*, 4:23–26.
12. Dichter, M., and Spencer, W. A. (1969): Penicillin-induced interictal discharges from the cat hippocampus. I. Characteristics and topographic features. *J. Neurophysiol.*, 32:649–662.
13. Douglas, W. W. (1976): The role of calcium in stimulus-secretion coupling, In: *Stimulus-Secretion Coupling in the Gastrointestinal Tract*, edited by R. M. Case and H. Goebell, pp. 17–48. University Park Press, Baltimore, Maryland.
14. Epelbaum, J., Brazeau, P., Tsang, D., Brawer, J., and Martin, J. B. (1977): Subcellular distribution of radioimmunoassayable somatostatin in rat brain. *Brain Res.*, 126:309–323.
15. Epstein, A. N., Fitzsimons, J. T., and Rolls, B. J. (1970): Drinking induced by injection of angiotensin into the brain of the rat. *J. Physiol. (Lond.)*, 210:457–474.
16. Fitzsimons, J. T. (1971): The effect on drinking of peptide precursors and of shorter chain peptide fragments of angiotensin II injected into the rat's diencephalon. *J. Physiol. (Lond.)*, 214:295–303.
17. Foreman, M., and Moss, R. L. (1975): Enhancement of lordotic behavior by intrahypothalamic infusion of luteinizing hormone-releasing hormone. *Neurosci. Abstr.*, 1:435.
18. Francis, D. L., Roy, A. C., and Collier, H. O. J. (1975): Morphine abstinence and quasi-abstinence effects after phosphodiesterase inhibitors and naloxone. *Life Sci.*, 16:1901–1906.
19. Frankenhauser, B., and Hodkin, A. L. (1957): The action of calcium on the electrical properties of squid axons. *J. Physiol. (Lond.)*, 137:218–244.
20. Gispen, W. H., and Wiegant, V. M., (1976): Opiate antagonists suppress ACTH induced excessive grooming in the rat. *Neurosci. Lett.*, 2:159–164.
21. Glowinski, J., and Iversen, L. L. (1966): Regional studies of catecholamines in the rat brain. I. The disposition of [³H]norepinephrine, [³H]dopamine and [³H] dopa in various regions of the brain. *J. Neurochem.*, 13;655–659.
22. Goddard, G. V., McIntyre, D. C., and Leech, C. K. (1969): A permanent change

in brain function resulting from daily electrical stimulation. *Exp. Neurol.,* 25:295–330.

23. Goddard, G. A., and Robinson, J. D. (1976): Uptake and release of calcium by rat synaptosomes. *Brain Res.,* 110:331–350.
24. Harris, R. A., Yamamoto, H., Loh, H. H., and Way, E. L. (1977): Discrete changes in brain calcium with morphine analgesia. *Life Sci.,* 20:501–506.
25. Havlicek, V., LaBella, F., Rezek, M., and Friesen, H. G. (1977): General anaesthesia induced by intracerebroventricular (ICV) beta-endorphin. *Physiologist,* 20(4): 41 (abstr.).
26. Havlicek, V., Leybin, L., Rezek, M., and Pinsky, C. (1977): Two opposite behavioral and EEG effects of low and high doses of beta-endorphin. *Endocrinology Society 59th Annual Meeting,* p. 178.
27. Havlicek, V., Rezek, M., and Friesen, H. (1975): Sleep-disturbing action of somatostatin release inhibiting factor (SRIF or somatostatin) and thyrotropin releasing hormone (TRH), Sixth International Congress of Pharmacology, Helsinki, p. 523 (abstr.).
28. Havlicek, V., Rezek, M., and Friesen, H. (1976): Somatostatin and thyrotropin releasing hormone: Central effect on sleep and motor system. *Pharmacol. Biochem. Behav.,* 4:455–459.
29. Havlicek, V., Rezek, M., and Friesen, H. (1976): Hexadecapeptide alpha-endorphin: Central effects on motor function, EEG and sleep-waking cycle. *Neurosci. Abstr.,* 2:568.
30. Havlicek, V., Rezek, M., Leybin, L., and Friesen, H. (1977): Analgesic effect of cerebroventricular administration of somatostatin (SRIF). *Fed. Proc.,* 36:363.
31. Havlicek, V., Rezek, M., Leybin, L., Pinsky, C., and Friesen, H. (1977): Central effect of two brain peptides, somatostatin and beta-endorphin (fragment C of beta-lipotropin). *Proc. Int. Union Physiol. Sci.,* 13:312.
32. Hökfelt, T., Efendic, C., Johansson, O., Luft, R., and Arimura, A. (1974): Immunohistochemical localization of somatostatin (growth hormone release inhibiting factor) in the guinea pig brain. *Brain Res.,* 80:165–169.
33. Hökfelt, T., Sachs, C., Meyerson, B., Elde, R., and Rehfelt, G. (1976): Peptide neurons in human cerebral cortex. 11th World Congress of Neurology, Amsterdam, pp. 220–221 (abstr.).
34. Hughes, J., Smith, T. W., Kosterlitz, H. W., Fothergill, L. A., Morgan, B. A., and Morris, H. R. (1975): Identification of two related pentapeptides from the brain with potent opiate agonist activity. *Nature,* 258:577–580.
35. Ioffe, S., Havlicek, V., Friesen, H., and Chernick. V. (1977): The excitatory effect of iontophoretically applied somatostatin (SRIF) on cortical neurons in awake unanesthetized animals. *Fed. Proc.,* 36:364.
36. Ioffe, S., Havlicek, V., Friesen, H., and Chernick, V. (1978): The postsynaptic changes and effect of L-glutamate, GABA and naloxone on somatostatin (SRIF) sensitive cells in cerebral cortex of awake nonparalyzed rabbits. *Fed. Proc.,* 37:523.
37. Jackson, I. M. D., and Reichlin, S. (1974): Thyrotropin-releasing hormone (TRH): Distribution in hypothalamic and extrahypothalamic brain tissues of mammalian and submammalian chordates. *Endocrinology,* 95:854–862.
38. Katz, B., and Miledi, R. (1968): The role of calcium in neuromuscular facilitation. *J. Physiol.,* 195:481–492.
39. Koketsu, K. (1969): Calcium and the excitable cell membrane. *Neurosci. Res.,* 2:1–39.
40. Kronhein, S., Berelowitz, M., and Pimstone, B. L. (1976): A radioimmunoassay for growth hormone release-inhibiting hormone: Method and quantitative tissue distribution. *Clin. Endocrinol.,* 5:619–630.
41. LaBella, F., Havlicek, V., and Pinsky, C. (1978): Opiate action: Evidence for the role of steroid sulfates and calcium in acute and withdrawal responses. *Brain Res. (in press).*
42. LaBella, F., Havlicek, V., Pinsky, C., and Leybin, L. (1977): Opiate-like, naloxone-reversible effects of androsterone sulfate in rats. *Soc. Neurosci. Abstr.,* 3:295.
43. LaBella, F., Havlicek, V., Pinsky, C., Vivian, S., and Leybin, L. (1978): Opiate-

like, naloxone-reversible effects of androsterone sulfate in rats. *Can. J. Physiol.,* (*in press*).

44. Lazarus, L. H., Ling, N., and Guillemin, R. (1976): β-Lipotropin as a prohormone for the morphinomimetic peptides endorphins and enkephalins. *Proc. Natl. Acad. Sci. USA,* 73:2156–2159.

45. Lee, S. L., Havlicek, V., Panerai, A. E., and Friesen, H. G. (1978): High K⁺ induced release of somatostatin (SRIF) from the cortical preparation of rat brains. *Physiol. Can.,* 9:45.

46. Lee, S. L., Havlicek, V., Panerai, A. E., and Friesen, H. G. (1978): Release of endogenous somatostatin (SRIF) from the rat cortical synaptosomes RCS. *Fed. Proc.,* 37:665.

47. Ling, N., Burgus, R., and Guillemin, R. (1976): Morphinomimetic activity of synthetic fragments of B-lipotropin and analogs. *Proc. Natl. Acad. Sci. USA,* 73:3308–3310.

48. Lowry, O. H., Rosenbrough, N. J., Farr, L. A., and Randall, R. J. (1951): Protein measurement with the folin phenol reagent. *J. Biol. Chem.,* 193:265–275.

49. Martin, J. B., Renaud, L. P., and Brazeau, P. (1975): Hypothalamic peptides: New evidence for "peptidergic" pathways in the C.N.S. *Lancet,* 2:393–395.

50. Moss, R. L., and McCann, S. M. (1973): Induction of mating behavior in rats by luteinizing hormone releasing factor. *Science,* 181:177–179.

51. Mudge, A. W., Fischbach, G. D., and Leeman, S. E. (1977): The release of immunoreactive substance P and somatostatin from sensory neurons in dissociated cell cultures. *Neurosci. Abstr.,* 1306:410.

52. Patel, Y. C., and Reichlin, S. (1978): Somatostatin in hypothalamus, extra-hypothalamic brain, and peripheral tissues of the rat. *Endocrinology,* 102:523–530.

53. Pelletier, G., Labrie, F., Arimura, A., and Schally, A. V. (1974): Electron microscopic immunohistochemical localization of growth hormone-release inhibiting hormone (somatostatin) in the rat medium eminence. *Am. J. Anat.,* 140:445–450.

54. Plotnikoff, N. P., Kastin, A. J., and Schally, A. V. (1974): Growth hormone release inhibiting hormone: Neuropharmacological studies. *Pharmacol. Biochem. Behav.,* 2:693–696.

55. Plum, F., and Posner, J. B. (1972): *The Diagnosis of Stupor and Coma,* 2nd edition. F. A. Davis Co., Philadelphia.

56. Renaud, L. P., Martin, J. B., and Brazeau, P. (1975): Depressant action of TRH, LH-RH and somatostatin on activity of central neurones. *Nature,* 255:233–235.

57. Rezek, M., Havlicek, V., and Friesen, H. (1978): The role of somatostatin (SRIF) in the control of alimentation. Part I: Differential effect on food intake as a function of the dose and infusion site. *Fed. Proc.,* 37:620.

58. Rezek, M., Havlicek, V., Hughes, K. R., and Friesen, H. (1976): Cortical administration of somatostatin (SRIF): Effect on sleep and motor behavior. *Pharmacol. Biochem. Behav.,* 5:73–77.

59. Rezek, M., Havlicek, V., Hughes, K. R., and Friesen, H. (1976): Central sites of action of somatostatin (SRIF): Role of hippocampus. *Neuropharmacology,* 15:499–504.

60. Rezek, M., Havlicek, V., Hughes, K. R., and Friesen, H. (1977): Behavioral and motor excitation and inhibition induced by the administration of small and large doses of somatostatin into the amygdala. *Neuropharmacology,* 16:157–162.

61. Rezek, M., Havlicek, V., and Friesen, H. (1977): Reversal of peripheral but not central effects of somatostatin by glucose. *Can. Fed. Biol. Soc.,* 20:67.

62. Rezek, M., Havlicek, V., Leybin, L., Labella, F. S., and Friesen, H. (1978): Opiate-like, naloxone-reversible actions of somatostatin given intracerebrally. *Can. J. Physiol. Pharmacol,* 56:227–231.

63. Rezek, M., Havlicek, V., Leybin, L., Pinsky, C., Kroeger, E. A., Hughes, K. R., and Friesen, H. (1977): Neostriatal administration of somatostatin: Differential effect of small doses on behavior and motor control. *Can. J. Physiol. Pharmacol.,* 55:234–242.

64. Ross, D. H., Lynn, S. C., and Cardenas, H. L. (1976): Cellular adaptation to opiates. *Fed. Prod.,* 35:385.

65. Schally, A. V., Arimura, A., Baba, Y., Nair, R. M. G., Matsuo, J., Redding, R. W., Debeljuk, L., and White, W. F. (1971): Isolation and properties of the FSH- and LH-releasing hormone. *Biochem. Biophys. Res. Commun.*, 43:393–399.
66. Segal, D. S., and Mandell, A. J. (1974): Differential behavioral effects of hypo-thalamic polypeptides. In: *The Thyroid Axis, Drugs, and Behavior*, edited by Arthur J. Prange, Jr., pp. 129–133. Raven Press, New York.
67. Simpson, J. B., and Routtenberg, A. (1973): Subfornical organ: Site of drinking elucidation by angiotensin II. *Science*, 181:1172–1175.
68. Tan, A. T., Tsang, D., Renaud, L. P., and Martin, J. B. (1977): Effect of soma-tostatin on calcium transport in guinea pig cortex synaptosomes. *Brain Res.*, 123:193–196.
69. Terenius, L. (1976): Somatostatin and ACTH are peptides with antagonist-like selectivity for opiate receptors. *Eur. J. Pharmacol.*, 38:211–213.
70. Terry, L. C., and Martin, J. B. (1978): Release of somatostatin (SRIF) from pre-infused rat hypothalamic fragments. *Fed. Proc.*, 37:665.
71. Urca, G., Erenk, H., Liebeskind, J. C., and Taylor, A. N. (1977): Morphine and enkephalin: Analgesic and epileptic properties. *Science*, 197:83–86.
72. Wakabayashi, I., Miyazawa, Y., Kanda, M., Miki, N., Demura, H., and Shizume, K. (1977): Stimulation of immunoreceptive somatostatin release from hypothalamic synaptosomes by high (K+) and dopamine. *Endocrinol. Jpn.*, 24:601–604.
73. Whittaker, V. P. (1965): The application of subcellular fractionation techniques to the study of brain function. *Prog. Biophys. Mol. Biol.*, 15:39–91.
74. Winokur, A., and Utiger, R. D. (1974): Thyrotropin-releasing hormone: Regional distribution in rat brain. *Science*, 185:265–267.

Central Nervous System Effects of Hypothalamic Hormones and Other Peptides, edited by Collu et al. Raven Press, New York © 1979.

Role of Peptides in the Pathogenesis and Treatment of Parkinson's Disease

André Barbeau

Department of Neurobiology, Clinical Research Institute of Montreal, Montreal, Quebec, Canada

PEPTIDES IN THE BRAIN

The last 15 years have seen the extraordinary growth of knowledge in the physiology, pharmacology, and biochemistry of monoamines, particularly spurred on by the findings of abnormal dopamine metabolism in Parkinson's disease and the encouraging success of levodopa therapy in that illness (1,2,6).

In parallel with this activity, the field of neuroendocrinology has been steadily growing, leading to exciting new findings. One of the products of these studies is undoubtedly the recognition that a number of peptide hormones act directly on the brain to affect learning and behavior. Prominent among these active hormones are substances isolated from the hypothalamus which, on the one hand, act as releasing or release-inhibiting factors and, on the other hand, possess independent behavior-modifying properties.

A number of well-known and important functions of the organism are dependent on the action of peptide hormones: sexual behaviors, including female receptivity state and mating, are influenced by gonadotropins; eating can be induced by insulin; thirst and the consequent drinking are inhibited by vasopressin, whereas motivated drinking is induced by angiotensin; parturition can be triggered or accelerated by oxytocin; it is also well known, particularly in frogs, that melanocyte-stimulating hormone (MSH) can produce skin color changes; lipolysis can be induced by both MSH and β-lipotropic hormone (β-LPH). Finally, the best studied phenomenon is neurosecretion in the hypothalamus-pituitary interphases.

Recent developments in protein and peptide biochemistry have permitted the mapping of a number of new pathways using immunohistochemical morphological explorations. Antisera have thus been raised to luteinizing hormone-releasing hormone (LH-RH), somatostatin, thyrotropin releasing hormone, oxytocin, vasopressin, neurophysin, substance P, enkephalin, endorphins, angiotensin II, vasoactive intestinal polypeptide, and many others as demonstrated in other chapters of this book. There are still problems of specificity with this technique, as well as with methods of measuring enzymes, but the future of the approach is great (27). The present chapter intends to review the possible role of peptides in the pathophysiology and treatment of Parkinson's disease.

A PEPTIDERGIC THEORY OF THE ETIOLOGY OF PARKINSON'S DISEASE

The actual cause of Parkinson's disease remains an enigma, despite the numerous studies originating from the discovery of the therapeutic activity of L-DOPA. There is still no satisfactory answer to the elementary question: what causes the deficiency in dopamine levels in the basal ganglia and elsewhere? Viruses have been implicated in the etiology of the "postencephalitic parkinsonism" which followed the epidemic of lethargic encephalitis of 1918 through 1927. However, the true nature of the actual virus involved remains unsettled, despite claims in favor of influenza A (24). In this respect it is of interest to note that Lycke and Roos (32) have indicated that such viruses induce increases in dopamine turnover in mice brain. Recent studies by Elizan and collaborators (21) failed to find an arbovirus causative factor despite an extensive survey.

In a presentation to the Association for Research in Nervous and Mental Disorders (5) we proposed a new hypothesis on the etiology of Parkinson's disease. This hypothesis envisions a primordial role for brain peptides and was thus stated: "The symptoms of Parkinson's disease are a consequence of localized amine imbalances in the brain, but the basic pathogenic mechanism is an accelerated aging phenomenon resulting from the selective atrophy of the heavily pigmented cells in the brainstem, from where originate dopaminergic and noradrenergic pathways. This aging mechanism can be accelerated by vascular, infectious, and toxic factors, but it is conditioned by a deficiency in specialized neuroendocrine (A.P.U.D.) cells in the hypothalamus. Parkinson's disease is thus a form of A.P.U.D. cell deficiency syndrome." The evidence for the first part of this proposition has been reviewed many times (1,3,5,7) and will not be repeated here. The only point to be made is the interesting similarity between the mechanisms of aging and that of parkinsonism. Thus the brainstem pigmented cells are also involved in aging as shown by a significant lowering of striatal dopamine content in both diseases (22). In such a situation, the slightest further aggression to the integrity of the nigrostriatal pathway will result in the rapid appearance of extrapyramidal signs and symptoms. In fact, various mechanisms (vascular, infectious, and toxic) are known to further worsen the concentration or turnover of brain catecholamines (11,34). The common end result is the acceleration of a random degenerative process in the basal ganglia, which eventually leads to obvious extrapyramidal signs. It is likely that these secondary factors alone could not produce the signs and symptoms of

Parkinson's disease unless they were extremely severe or accompanied by evidence of an accelerated aging process.

On the other hand, one of the main characteristics of Parkinson's disease is a deficiency in the decarboxylases necessary for synthesis of putative neurotransmitters: DOPA and 5-HTP decarboxylase, glutamic acid decarboxylase. Cells equipped with such decarboxylases are easily seen with histofluorescence and readily take up the appropriate precursors. Pearse (36) has classified such cells as belonging to the A.P.U.D. system. The term itself derives from the main characteristics of the cells: fluorogenic amine content (catecholamines, 5-HT) and/or amine precursor uptake (DOPA or 5-HTP), with presence of amino acid decarboxylases. The other main characteristic of these cells, mostly originating from the neural crest, is that they are associated with the secretion of polypeptides, some of which have hormonal actions. The A.P.U.D. cells usually manifest their presence through hypersecretion, such as in the multiple endocrine syndrome, the Zollinger-Ellison syndrome, and other secreting tumors that have received the inelegant name of "apudomas." However, in our hypothesis we propose that both aging and Parkinson's disease would be the result of specific *deficiencies* in the function of some specialized neuroendocrine (A.P.U.D.) cells.

These cells could be absent or reduced in number congenitally, or they could be damaged progressively through the cumulative effect of successive aggressions on this system (toxic, infectious, vascular, or metabolic). It is part of our proposal that the main function of peptidergic pathways is a trophic modulation of aminergic functions, pre- or post-synaptically. In a manner similar to nerve growth factor in the peripheral nervous system (33), these polypeptides could prevent cell chromatolysis and permit the growth or maintenance of neurotransmitter-producing neurons. Any decrease in this trophic action of peptidergic neurons originating from A.P.U.D. cells, through congenital absence or progressive damage, would result in eventual atrophy and death of the latter neurons (dopaminergic and noradrenergic in Parkinson's disease, GABA-ergic in Huntington's chorea). Preliminary evidence which we will now review would favor the importance of β-LPH derivatives (MSH, $ACTH_{4-10}$, β-endorphin) in this role for Parkinson's disease, with substance P and angiotensin for Huntington's chorea.

PEPTIDE SYNTHESIS IN THE BRAIN

Most of the active peptides studied are not synthesized *de novo*. Rather, they originate from the enzymatic breakdown of much larger molecules. This discovery was made simultaneously for insulin, which derives from proinsulin, by Steiner and Oyer (39) and for β-MSH, which originates from lipotropin, by Chrétien and Li (17). It has led to important advances in the chemistry of many hormones. For example, it is now known that β-LPH, a peptide with 91 amino acids, is the precursor of β-MSH (sequence 37–58),

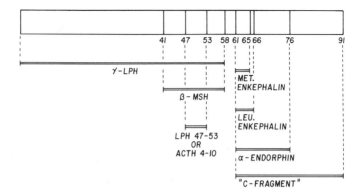

FIG. 1. Some of the breakdown products of the prohormone β-LPH.

which may not even be present as such in humans, and of γ-LPH (sequence 1–58) (Fig. 1). A recent study (28) indicates that residues 61 to 65 form the structure of methionine-enkephalin, a pentapeptide which may be the natural ligand for opiate receptors. Other fragments with biological activity are now known as α-, γ-, and β-endorphins. It now appears that both ACTH and β-LPH probably derive from a common precursor, a still larger molecule (31,000 daltons). Moreover, unpublished studies from the laboratories of Bloom and Guillemin (1978) raise doubts about the origin of the enkephalins from β-LPH. These doubts are based on the markedly different distribution in the brain of enkephalins (mainly in the basal ganglia and in local neurons) and of endorphins (intermediate lobe of the pituitary and longer fibers). Celis, Taleisnik, and Walter (15) have also demonstrated that the tripeptide proline-leucine-glycine amide resulted from the splitting of oxytocin. Such breakdown is carried out by a number of peptidases which are being isolated in the brain. It may well be that the regional concentrations of such peptidases could be the local factor responsible for specificity of peptide mapping. It is of interest that most of these peptidases are bound to a divalent metal, i.e., zinc in the hippocampus, manganese in the median eminence (8,9). In this membrane-bound form they are usually inactive until activated by hormonal or other factors, including possibly derangements in trace metal metabolism. There exists some recent evidence that manganese, probably peptide linked, is involved in the growth and maturation of dopaminergic pathways. Support for this hypothesis is obtained from recent unpublished studies from our laboratory (Barbeau, Lis, Inoue, Tsukada, and Chrétien, 1978) indicating that the intraventricular injection of manganese can cause a dose-dependent increase in serum prolactin, concomitant with a significant lowering of catecholamines in the hypothalamus.

Some of the early studies on the behavioral effects of peptide hormones were carried out in hypophysectomized animals by De Wied and his colleagues in Utrecht (20). The animals had decreased extinction of conditioned

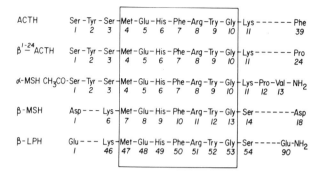

FIG. 2. Common sequence of amino acids found within behaviorly active molecules, some of which derive from β-LPH.

avoidance responses (CARs) which were corrected by the administration of ACTH, MSH, or vasopressin. These effects were not dependent on the presence of adrenals. De Wied et al. (20) are of the opinion that ACTH facilitates learning CARs by affecting motivational processes. He and his colleagues have studied many fractions of the ACTH molecules to find that the most active is composed of a 7 amino acid sequence situated between amino acids 4 and 10 (ACTH$_{4-10}$): this sequence is Met-Gly-His-Phe-Arg-Try-Gly. Modifications and substitutions of the sequence have been attempted, but most are inactive except when the methionine is oxidized to the sulfoxide, arginine is replaced by D-lysine, and tryptophan by phenylalanine. The resulting peptide is 1,000 times more active than MSH/ACTH$_{4-10}$, probably because the substitutions increase resistance to degradation by enzymes. There is evidence that MSH/ACTH$_{4-10}$ can increase visual memory on the Benton retention test in man and that the peptide prolongs the pattern of mental alertness on the EEG, by decreasing the duration of a pattern. Melanocyte-stimulating hormone possesses the same 7 amino acid sequence as MSH/ACTH$_{4-10}$, and it has essentially the same behavioral action (Fig. 2).

A very strange neurological phenomenon consisting of yawning and stretching crises of muscular hypertonus has been observed in dogs and rats after the intracerebral injection of MSH/ACTH$_{4-10}$, MSH, and β-LPH (29), all substances possessing the 7 amino acid sequence Met-Glu-His-Phe-Arg-Try-Gly.

β-LPH DERIVATIVES AND PARKINSON'S DISEASE

Cotzias, Van Woert, and Schiffer (18) had shown that the injection of MSH to parkinsonian patients rapidly exacerbated the symptoms of the illness. In subsequent studies we were able to confirm this effect, particularly on tremor. Later Shuster et al. (38) demonstrated that plasma MSH values were elevated in Parkinson's disease. However, this finding is still in doubt, mainly because the specificity of MSH determination is not as clear as previously thought. The assay may in fact be measuring β-LPH as well as MSH.

Another part of the β-LPH molecule may play an important role in Parkinson's disease. As mentioned before, the 61–65 sequence of β-lipotropin has been isolated and chemically characterized and more recently shown to possess morphine-like properties. Subsequent reports showed that these peptides administered intraventricularly in rats and mice have an analgesic action. The C-fragment (β-LPH 61–91), designated as β-endorphin, has been found to have potent and long-lasting analgesic action when administered intraventricularly in cats, rats, and mice. Recently, β-endorphin injected into the cisterna magna, in the periaqueductal gray, or in the lateral ventricle in rats has been demonstrated to produce catalepsy or catatonia in addition to analgesia. However, our own experience indicates that the phenomenon of decreased mobility and motor initiation should be called akinesia rather than catatonia (30). This behavior was fully reversed by naloxone, a specific antagonist for opiate, L-DOPA with a peripheral decarboxylase inhibitor, or apomorphine. L-DOPA or apomorphine did not reverse the analgesia, whereas naloxone at least partially reversed both analgesia and akinesia. Indeed, apomorphine (20 mg/kg) fully reversed the akinesia induced by β-endorphin and produced its characteristic stereotyped behavioral effect 7 min following drug injection. The complete akinesia-reversal effect of apomorphine lasted for about 17 min, then its efficacy decreased gradually. This observed time course in the action of apomorphine seems to be parallel to the time course of accumulation and disappearance of the drug in the rat brain (14). As seen in Fig. 3, L- and D-amphetamine (15 mg/kg) can also reverse the endorphin-induced akinesia. These findings, together with the recent report that dopamine release from a rat striatal slice is inhibited by β-endorphin and that enkephalins stimulate dopamine synthesis in the caudate nucleus (13), indicate that the peptide acts preferentially on dopaminergic neurons, probably at presynaptic sites. It is also of great interest that evidence for a long leu-enkephalin striopallidal pathway in rat brain has been advanced (19).

The observation that naloxone could reverse the akinesia-catatonia signs produced in animals by the intraventricular injection of β-endorphin prompted studies of the use of this compound in human Parkinson's disease. With R. Labrecque (unpublished studies) we investigated the effect of a single i.v. naloxone injection (0.4 mg of naloxone chlorhydrate) on a battery of motor performance tests in 20 akinetic parkinsonian patients and 10 age-matched normal controls. There were no significant changes in tremor, rigidity, akinesia, or total motor performance scores at 30, 60, or 90 min post-injection. The parkinsonian state did not improve objectively, but subjectively most patients stated that some of the tests (particularly the puzzle) were carried out with less difficulty. We subsequently pursued this

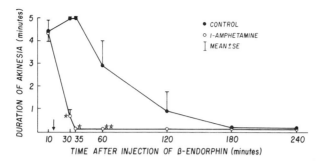

FIG. 3. Effects of L-amphetamine (15 mg/kg) on a β-endorphin-induced akinesia. Test rats received L-amphetamine (15 mg/kg) intraperitoneally 15 min after the intraventricular administration of β-endorphin (13 nmoles). Control rats received 0.85% saline 15 min after the peptide injection. The arrow indicates the time of injection of L-amphetamine or 0.85% saline. The cut-off time was determined to be 5 min. Each value represents a mean ± SE of 3 control or 4 test rats. Significant difference between duration of akinesia in test and control rats is shown by *p < 0.01 and **p < 0.05. (Unpublished data of C. Viallet, K. Izumi, M. Lis, N. Seidah, M. Chrétien, T. T. Ngo, and A. Barbeau, 1978.)

observation by studying the performance of a color and of a black and white puzzle (both representing an identical duck and consisting of 10 pieces) by 10 parkinsonian patients, 10 subjects with essential tremor, and 10 normal controls. The puzzle test was carried out at 0, 30, and 90 min. In normal subjects and essential tremor patients, there is a significant *apprentissage* from the first to the third test with the color puzzle test but not with the black and white puzzle. Parkinsonian patients are unable to improve this score with either puzzles. However, this last group of patients, alone, significantly improved their performance with the color puzzle after the i.v. injection of naloxone (0.4 mg). We are investigating further this interesting improvement in *apprentissage* with naloxone.

Thus the above evidence indicates that many peptides derived from the prohormone β-LPH could be involved in the production of some of the symptoms of Parkinson's disease, particularly tremor and akinesia.

THE PRO-LEU-GLY-NH₂ STORY

In 1971 Nair, Kastin, and Schally (35) synthesized a tripeptide, L-prolyl-L-leucyl-glycine amide (Pro-Leu-Gly-NH₂; PLG) which they claimed had MSH release-inhibitory (MIF) properties. They called this peptide MIF-I, but we would now prefer to use the initials PLG because subsequent studies by some authors have failed to confirm the hormonal activity. However, animal experiments soon revealed that this substance was neurologically active, in that it potentiated the actions of L-DOPA and oxotremorine in both intact and hypophysectomized animals (37).

Based on these premises, Kastin and Barbeau (31) carried out a number of experiments in Montreal. The first set of studies consisted in the slow intravenous infusion of 20 to 40 mg of PLG in 100 ml of saline over a 30-min period in 8 patients. Rigidity was improved by an average 20%, whereas tremor was markedly reduced in 4 of the 8 patients. To our surprise this benefit persisted some 2 or 3 days after the infusion. One week later the same 8 patients were given 30 mg/day of oral PLG for 2 days. Motor performance tests, objectively measured, improved by an average 19% and justified longer trials in 3 patients. The latter received 50 mg/day of oral PLG for a minimum of 2 months. Again the objective motor performance tests were improved, by 30% at the end of the observation period. A further 5 patients who were taking L-DOPA but presented with oscillations in performance and dyskinesias were given, on a single occasion, 50 mg of PLG orally. Although a slight decrease in the dyskinesias was noted, no clear-cut potentiation of performance could be observed.

These results were soon partially confirmed by Chase et al. (16) who found some antiparkinsonian activity with small infusions of the drug, but could not confirm the decrease in dyskinesias. The same year Fischer and collaborators (23) in Germany made similar positive observations in 10 patients. They observed simultaneous mood brightening and thought that the effect of PLG was mostly on mood and motivation. Our own studies were followed by a 4-month double-blind experiment with gradually increasing oral doses of PLG in 20 parkinsonian patients, followed by 6 months of open observation (12). Unfortunately, objective measurements of various parameters did not reveal important differences when the initial and final results were compared. Functional impairment and finger dexterity, to all intents and purposes, remained identical. However, there was a significant downward trend in rigidity and tremor scores for the patients receiving PLG. This corresponded to 20 and 44% decreases, respectively, figures of the same order of magnitude as seen in the initial study.

A further study, this time using the intravenous approach already shown to be effective, again demonstrated the efficacy of a single bolus injection of 200 mg PLG in 8 parkinsonian patients (10). This effect persisted for nearly 6 hr.

Animal studies quoted above had shown that PLG potentiates the L-DOPA-induced effect on motility. In a further set of experiments (4), we were able to show the same type of potentiation in human parkinsonian subjects (Fig. 4). Six of our patients who had been treated with L-DOPA for an average of a little over 4 years were chosen for evaluation. After this period of time the average motor performance score was still significantly improved over the pre-DOPA period. On the first day of the experiment, at 10 A.M., the patients were given their usual 500 mg dose of oral L-DOPA. At the same time they received an intravenous injection of 10 ml of NaCl. Performance scores were measured before and hourly after the injection. L-DOPA produced an average 21% further improvement. On the second day, 200 mg of intravenous PLG was substituted for the NaCl. This pro-

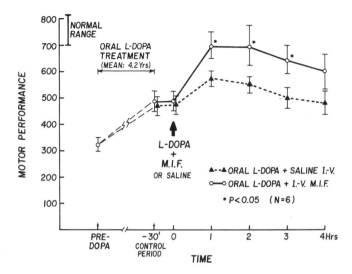

FIG. 4. Potentiation of motor performance by L-DOPA + PLG (MIF) in Parkinson's disease (see text for description).

duced an improvement in performance scores of 44% which lasted for at least 4 hr. In 4 of the 6 patients, and for the first time since the onset of treatment with L-DOPA, performance scores within the normal range were obtained. All patients also noted a marked amelioration in the clarity of their thinking. Similar results were recently obtained by Gerstenbrand and collaborators (25) and by our group over more chronic periods (26).

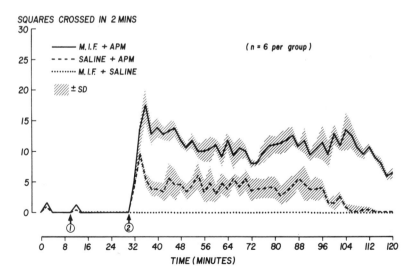

FIG. 5. Potentiation of apomorphine (5 mg/kg) by PLG (MIF, 2 mg/kg) in rats with a bilateral hypothalamic lesion induced by 6-OH-dopamine and producing severe hypokinesia.

PLG was ineffective, in our studies (10), in modifying brain levels, turnover, or distribution of catecholamines. Neither could we demonstrate inhibition of monoamine oxidase or catecholamine-O-methyl transferase activity by PLG. Furthermore, there was no evidence that PLG acted on the reuptake mechanism or facilitated the release of catecholamines in an amphetamine-like fashion. Therefore a presynaptic or metabolic mode of action is unlikely. PLG is still active in animals after hypophysectomy, indicating that the effect on the brain is probably not through peripheral hormones. Finally, we have demonstrated (10) that PLG potentiates the action of apomorphine in reversing the akinesia produced by bilateral hypothalamic lesions with 6-hydroxydopamine in the rat (Fig. 5). This would favor a postsynaptic site of action for PLG, probably through modulation of the receptor.

Recently we have begun studying in animals and man some analogs of PLG which, in rats at least, appear to be as effective as PLG but less subject to biological degradation. It is hoped that these new products will prove to be useful against the symptoms of Parkinson's disease.

SUMMARY

Peptides have found a progressively more important role in the biochemistry and physiology of the brain in recent years. Many possess neurological and behavioral actions in addition to their function in endocrinology. This chapter reviewed the formation and distribution, as well as the neurological action, of peptides probably involved in Parkinson's disease: β-LPH and its derivatives (MSH, ACTH$_{4-10}$, β-endorphin). It also recounted the experience of many authors with prolyl-leucyl-glycine amide (PLG) in that disease and new data on naloxone in parkinsonism. Finally, we proposed a new theory of the etiology of Parkinson's disease, based on a postulated deficiency in the important trophic function on catecholaminergic neurons, of fibers originating from some A.P.U.D. cells.

ACKNOWLEDGMENTS

The studies from the author's laboratory quoted in the chapter were supported in part through grants from the Medical Research Council of Canada (MT-4938) and the United Parkinson Foundation. Thanks are due to Drs. R. F. Butterworth, M. Gonce, C. Viallet, M. Lis, K. Izumi, M. Chrétien, and A. J. Kastin for collaboration in these studies

REFERENCES

1. Barbeau, A. (1962): The pathogenesis of Parkinson's disease: A new hypothesis. *Can. Med. Assoc. J.,* 87:802–807.

2. Barbeau, A. (1969): L-DOPA therapy in Parkinson's disease: A critical review of nine years' experience. *Can. Med. Assoc. J.,* 101:791–800.
3. Barbeau, A. (1973): Aging and the extrapyramidal system. *J. Am. Geriatr. Soc.,* 21:145–149.
4. Barbeau, A. (1975): Potentiation of L-DOPA effect by intravenous L-prolyl-L-leucyl-glycine amide in man. *Lancet,* 2:683.
5. Barbeau, A. (1976): Parkinson's disease: Etiological considerations. In: *The Basal Ganglia,* edited by M. D. Yahr, pp. 281–292. Raven Press, New York.
6. Barbeau, A. (1976): Six years of high level Levodopa therapy in severely akinetic parkinsonian patients. *Arch. Neurol.,* 33:333–338.
7. Barbeau, A., Campanella, G., Butterworth, R. F., and Yamada, K. (1975): Uptake and efflux of ^{14}C-dopamine in platelets: Evidence for a generalized defect in Parkinson's disease. *Neurology (Minneap.),* 25:1–9.
8. Barbeau, A., and Donaldson, J. (1974): Zinc, taurine and epilepsy. *Arch. Neurol.,* 30:52–58.
9. Barbeau, A., Inoue, N., and Cloutier, T. (1976): The role of manganese in dystonia. In: *Advances in Neurology,* Vol. 14, edited by F. McDowell and A. Barbeau, pp. 339–351. Raven Press, New York.
10. Barbeau, A., and Kastin, A. J. (1976): Polypeptide therapy in Parkinson's disease— A new approach. In: *Advances in Parkinsonism,* edited by W. Birkmayer and O. Hornykiewicz, pp. 483–487. Editiones Roche, Basel.
11. Barbeau, A., Rojo-Ortega, J. M., Brecht, H. M., Donaldson, J., Minnich, J. L., and Genest, J. (1972): Effect of a magnesium-deficient diet on the striatal content of amines in the dog. *Experientia,* 28:289–291.
12. Barbeau, A., Roy, M., and Kastin, A. J. (1976): Double-blind evaluation of oral L-prolyl-L-leucyl-glycine amide in Parkinson's disease. *Can. Med. Assoc. J.,* 114:120–122.
13. Biggio, G., Casis, M., Corda, M. G., Di Bello, C., and Gessa, G. L. (1978): Stimulation of dopamine synthesis in caudate nucleus by intrastriatal enkephalins and antagonism by naloxone. *Science,* 200:552–554.
14. Butterworth, R. F., and Barbeau, A. (1975): Apomorphine: Stereotyped behaviour and regional distribution in rat brain. *Can. J. Biochem.,* 53:308–311.
15. Celis, M. E., Taleisnik, S., and Walter, R. (1971): Regulation of formation and proposed structure of the factor inhibiting the release of melanocyte-stimulating hormone. *Proc. Natl. Acad. Sci. USA,* 68:1428–1433.
16. Chase, T. N., Woods, A. C., Lipton, M. A., and Morris, C. E. (1974): Hypothalamic releasing factors and Parkinson's disease. *Arch. Neurol.* 31:55–56
17. Chrétien, M., and Li, C. H. (1967): Isolation, purification and characterization of gammalipotropic hormone from sheep and pituitary glands. *Can. J. Biochem.,* 45:1163–1174.
18. Cotzias, G. C., Van Woert, M. H., and Schiffer, L. M. (1967): Aromatic amino acids and modifications of parkinsonism. *N. Engl. J. Med.,* 276:374–379.
19. Cuello, A. C., and Paxinos, G. (1978): Evidence for a long Leu-enkephalin striopallidal pathway in rat brain. *Nature,* 271:178–180.
20. De Wied, D., Witter, A., and Lande, S. (1970): Anterior pituitary peptides and avoidance acquisition of hypophysectomized rats. *Prog. Brain Res.,* 32:213–230.
21. Elizan, T. S., Schwartz, Yahr, M. D., and Casals, J. (1978): Antibodies against arboviruses in postencephalitic and idiopathic Parkinson's disease. *Arch. Neurol.,* 35:257–260.
22. Finch, C. E. (1973): Catecholamine metabolism in the brains of aging male mice. *Brain Res.,* 52:261–276.
23. Fischer, P. A., Schneider, E., Jacobi, P., and Maxion, H. (1974): Effect of melanocyte-stimulating hormone-release inhibiting factor (MIF) in Parkinson's syndrome. *Eur. Neurol.,* 12:360–368.
24. Gamboa, E. T., Wolf, A., Yahr, M. D., Harter, D. H., Duffy, P. E., Barden, H., and Hsu, K. C. (1974): Influenza virus antigen in post-encephalitic parkinsonism brain. *Arch. Neurol.,* 31:228–232.
25. Gerstenbrand, F., Binder, H., Grünberger, J., Kozma, C., Push, S., and Reisner, T.

(1976): Infusion therapy with MIF (melanocyte inhibiting factor) in Parkinson. In: *Advances in Parkinsonism,* edited by W. Birkmayer and O. Hornykiewicz, pp. 456–461. Editiones Roche, Basel.

26. Gonce, M., and Barbeau, A. (1978): Expériences thérapeutiques avec le Propyl-Leucyl-Glycine amide dans la maladie de Parkinson. *Rev. Neurol. (Paris),* 139: 141–150.

27. Hökfelt, T., Elde, R., Fuxe, K., Johansson, O., Ljungdahl, A., Goldstein, M., Luft, R., Efendic, S., Nilsson, G., Terenuis, L., Ganten, D., Jeffcoate, S. L., Rehfeld, J., Said, S., Perez, de la Mora, M., Possani, L., Tapia, R., Teran, L., and Palacios, R. (1978): Aminergic and peptidergic pathways in the nervous system with special reference to the hypothalamus. In: *The Hypothalamus,* edited by S. Reichlin, B. J. Baldessarini, and J. B. Martin, pp. 69–135. Raven Press, New York.

28. Hughes, J., Smith, T. W., Kosterlitz, H. W., Fothergill, L. A., Morgan, B. A., and Morris, H. R. (1975): Identification of two related pentapeptides from the brain with potent opiate agonist activity. *Nature,* 258:577–579.

29. Izumi, K., Donaldson, J., and Barbeau, A. (1973): Yawning and stretching in rats induced by intraventricularly administered zinc. *Life Sci.,* 12:203–210.

30. Izumi, K., Motomatsu, T., Chrétien, M., Butterworth, R. F., Lis, M., Seidah, N., and Barbeau, A. (1977): β-Endorphin induced akinesia in rats: Effect of apomorphine and α-methyl-p-tyrosine and related modifications of dopamine turnover in the basal ganglia. *Life Sci.,* 20:1149–1156.

31. Kastin, A. J., and Barbeau, A. (1972): Preliminary clinical studies with L-prolyl-L-leucyl-glycine amide in Parkinson's disease. *Can. Med. Assoc. J.,* 107:1079–1081.

32. Lycke, E., and Roos, B. E. (1969): Some virological and biochemical aspects of the pathogenesis of Parkinson's disease. In: *Third Symposium on Parkinson's Disease,* edited by F. J. Gillingham and I. M. C. Donaldson, pp. 16–21. E. and S. Livingstone, Ltd., Edinburgh.

33. Mobley, W. C., Server, A. C., Ishii, D. N., Riopelle, R. J., and Shooter, E. M. (1977): Nerve growth factor. Parts 1, 2, and 3. *N. Engl. J. Med.,* 297:1096–1104; 1149–1158; 1211–1218.

34. Moskowitz, M. A., and Wurtman, R. J. (1975): Catecholamines and neurologic diseases. Parts 1 and 2. *N. Engl. J. Med.,* 293:274–280, 332–338.

35. Nair, R. M. G., Kastin, A. J., and Schally, A. V. (1971): Isolation and structure of hypothalamic MSH release-inhibiting hormone. *Biochem. Biophys. Res. Commun.,* 43:1376–1381.

36. Pearse, A. G. E. (1969): The cytochemistry and ultrastructure of polypeptide hormone-producing cells of the APUD series and the embryologic, physiologic and pathologic implications of the concept. *J. Histochem. Cytochem.,* 17:303–313.

37. Plotnikoff, N. P., and Kastin, A. J. (1974): Pharmacological studies with a tripeptide, prolyl-leucyl-glycine amide. *Arch. Int. Pharmocodyn. Ther.,* 211:211–224.

38. Shuster, S., Thody, A. Y., Goolamali, S. K., Burton, J. L., Plummer, N., and Bates, D. (1973): Melanocyte-stimulating hormone and parkinsonism. *Lancet,* 1:463–464.

39. Steiner, D. F., and Oyer, P. E. (1967): The biosynthesis of insulin and a probable precursor of insulin by a human islet cell adenoma. *Proc. Natl. Acad. Sci. USA,* 57:473–480.

Central Nervous System Effects of Hypothalamic Hormones and Other Peptides, edited by Collu et al. Raven Press, New York © 1979.

Clinical Utilization of MIF-I

F. Gerstenbrand, W. Poewe, F. Aichner, and C. Kozma

Clinic of Neurology, University of Innsbruck, Innsbruck, Austria

After 15 years of clinical experience with levodopa substitution therapy for Parkinson syndrome, the implications and problems of this form of therapy require some fundamental reorientation in the management of this disease entity. The possible role of the tripeptide L-prolyl-L-leucyl-glycine amide (PLG), which has melanocyte-inhibiting factor (MIF) activity, is one of the items being discussed among neuropharmacologists (10,11) and clinicians (3,5,7,9).

Kastin and Barbeau (9) in 1972 were the first to use PLG in patients with Parkinson's syndrome. In their first set of studies they supplied the substance by i.v. infusion. Although rather low doses of 20 to 40 mg were used, clinical improvement of up to 20% was observed. However, when the same authors gave PLG orally in gradually increasing amounts up to 1.5 g daily, results were disappointing on a long-term basis, although initial improvement could be detected (4). Barbeau (1) then continued to use PLG intravenously with very good results when given as a potentiating agent with levodopa therapy. Although his patients had been under levodopa therapy for a mean of 4 years, additional PLG injection still produced improvement in motor performance of up to 44% (1). Concerning the different clinical manifestations of parkinsonism, no differentiation was done (3). According to Barbeau (2), akinesia and rigidity are more affected than tremor by PLG.

PLG was available to our own group in Vienna for clinical utilization first in 1975. Under the impression that the doses for infusion therapy used by Kastin and Barbeau in 1972 had been too low, we raised the PLG dosage to 400 mg daily and administered it as a 24-hr continuous i.v. infusion over 10 days. In total, 10 patients were treated, and PLG was given as sole therapeutic agent with no other antiparkinsonian therapy. After the 10-day period of clinical observation, the patients were controlled during a follow-up period of 4 weeks at weekly intervals (7,8).

As can be seen from Table 1, all 9 patients in whom MIF infusion therapy was completed—1 patient declined further treatment after the first day— showed global clinical improvement. In 5 patients this improvement averaged 75%, in 2 it was 50%, and 2 patients with severe clinical manifestations at

TABLE 1. Evaluation of treatment with MIF-I (400 mg daily) i.v. in 10 patients with Parkinson syndrome

No. of patient	Initials	Age	Sex	Diagnosis[a]	Degree[b] Pre- A R T	Degree[b] Post- A R T	Global clinical improvement (%)	Psychological state Pre-	Psychological state Post-	Depot effect	Remarks
1	F.R.	47	M	P.a.	3 3 0	1 1 0	75	D	N	+	—
2	J.F.	67	M	P.a.	3 3 3	1 2 2	50	D	N	±	—
3	J.K.	61	M	P.a./T	1 1 3	0 0 2	75	D	Hm	±	A second course of treatment produced the same effect
4	E.W.	70	M	P.a.	1 3 2	0 2 1	50	N	N	+	An i.v. injection course produced the same effect
5	J.D.	66	M	P.a.	4 4 1	3 3 1	25	D	N	—	—
6	P.K.	62	F	P.a.	3 3 0	1 2 0	75	N	N	+	—
7	M.S.	67	F	P.a./T	2 2 3	2 2 3	0	D	D	—	Interruption of study; patient declined further treatment
8	L.H.	64	M	P.a.	1 2 1	0 1 0	75	N	N	+	—
9	Th.Z.	60	M	P.a.	2 2 1	1 1 1	75	D	N	+	—
10	B.S.	68	F	P.a./T	2 1 4	1 1 3	25	D	D	±	Rapid deterioration of tremor after cessation of treatment

[a] P.a., paralysis agitans.
[b] A, akinesia; R, rigidity; T, tremor.
[c] Psychological state: D > depressed; N, normal; Hm, hypermanic.

the onset showed mild improvement of 25%. Regarding the cardinal symptoms, there was improvement of akinesia (Fig. 1) in all patients—significant in 3, moderate in 4, and mild in 2 patients. Rigidity (Fig. 2) was also improved in all patients, significantly in 1, moderately in 3, and mildly in 4 cases. Tremor (Fig. 3) was least affected.

The improvement in motor performance correlated with a remarkable improvement in handwriting, which is demonstrated in Figs. 4 and 5. The motor performance was controlled by a test battery consisting of six single test units in a fixed combination.

We paid particular attention to the time course of the PLG effect. In our first study, evaluation of the different rating systems had revealed a first positive effect after 48 hr with the maximum effect becoming evident on the 7th day. Remarkable was a depot effect, which could be observed in 8 patients and lasted for about 3 weeks after PLG treatment had been stopped, then a gradual deterioration of all symptoms became visible. Four weeks after maximum improvement had been reached, the therapeutic effect had disappeared. However, it was possible to restore the original clinical improvement by single i.v. injections of 200 mg PLG twice daily for 3 days. Again a depot effect was reached lasting shorter than after the infusion period. Like Barbeau (2) we could observe no significant side effects, apart from a positive influence on the patient's mood. Out of 7 patients with depression at the onset of treatment period, 4 achieved a normal psychological state, 1 showed hypomanic features, and 2 remained in an unchanged depressive mood (see Table 1).

Based on these encouraging results and Barbeau's clinical experience (1) about the DOPA-potentiating effect of PLG, we started another set of PLG studies in Innsbruck (6). In a group of 7 patients, consisting of 5 men and 2 women, with a mean age of 61 years and a Parkinson syndrome of grades 2 through 4, we applied PLG intravenously additional to oral levodopa

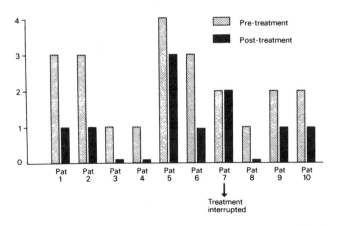

FIG. 1. Effect of MIF i.v. (400 mg daily through 10 days) on akinesia of 10 patients with Parkinson syndrome.

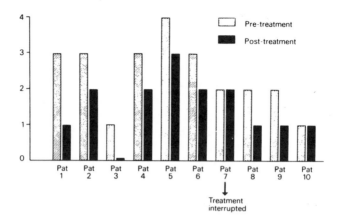

FIG. 2. Effect of MIF i.v. (400 mg daily through 10 days) on rigidity of 10 patients with Parkinson syndrome.

medication. All patients had been under levodopa for at least 6 months prior to the study, the mean duration of previous DOPA therapy being 3½ years. Levodopa had been given in a dosage from 400 to 750 mg either with benserazide (Madopar) or carbidopa (Sinemet). In 3 of the 7 patients PLG was given twice daily (as a 200-mg i.v. injection) over a period of 10 days. Four patients received PLG over 15 days. In this group we gave the substance in a crossover manner every second day for the first 6 days, alternating with placebo. In the crossover phase PLG was injected as a single 400-mg bolus, the following 9 days the administration was as in the first group. Another 2 patients had been under previous therapy with Budipine, a diphenylpiperidine derivative with anticholinergic and hypothetic dopaminergic properties. Additional PLG (200 mg i.v.) was given twice daily for 10 days.

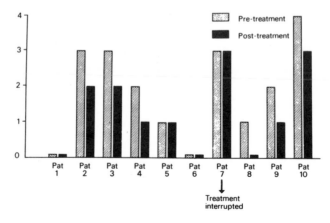

FIG. 3. Effect of MIF i.v. (400 mg daily through 10 days) on tremor of 10 patients with Parkinson syndrome.

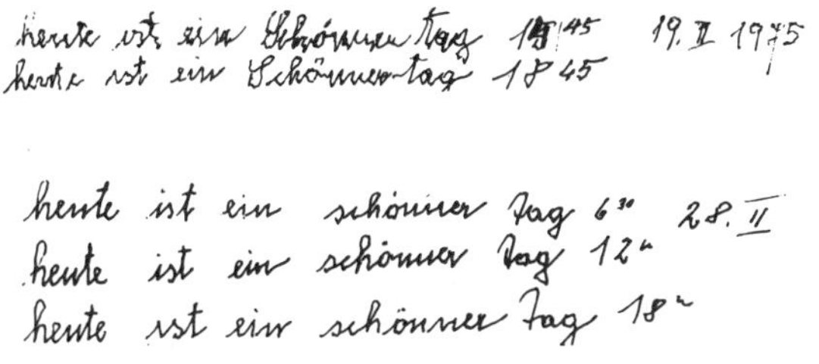

[handwriting samples]

FIG. 4. Pattern of handwriting of a 61-year-old male patient, J. K., with paralysis agitans. Comparison before treatment and 9 days after infusion therapy (400 mg daily).

In 2 patients with a Parkinson syndrome of mild degree who had been without previous antiparkinson therapy, PLG was administered twice daily (200 mg i.v.) as sole therapy over 10 days. Finally, we administered PLG to 2 patients with Parkinson symptoms following a traumatic apallic syndrome.

Table 2 gives a synopsis of all patients studied. In the first group, all 3 patients had Parkinson's syndrome of grade 3, and in all of them akinesia and rigidity were more prominent than tremor. Their cumulative score in our test battery ranged from 226 to 480, the maximal score being 1,000. We also used the peg-board test, prosupination recording, button press test, and the motor performance test of Grünberger. In addition, each patient had to perform drawing and handwriting tests. Finally the patients were rated by doctors and nurses.

In all 3 patients there was global improvement of 25% to 50%. The additional improvement became evident already on the first day of treatment, improvement having reached the maximum after the 4th or 5th day. As in our first group, improvement was more prominent for akinesia and rigidity than for tremor. The motor performance score proved to be a particularly sensitive indicator of the PLG-induced effect. A depot effect was evident in our first set of studies, lasting between 10 days and 3 weeks. Again, restoring of the original improvement could be achieved with a second 3-day PLG period. Remarkable side effects were the influence on

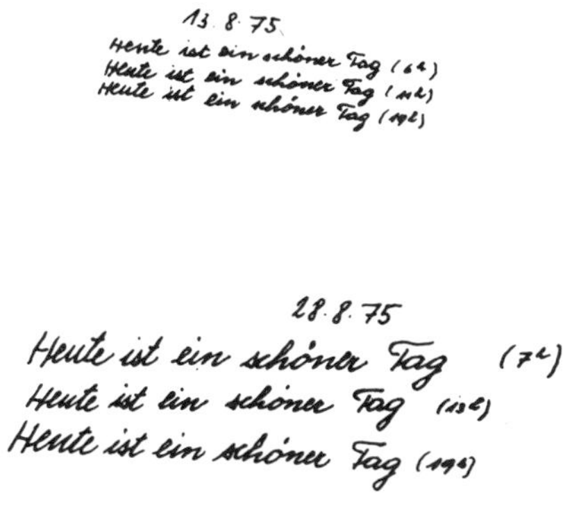

[handwriting samples]

FIG. 5. Pattern of handwriting of a 67-year-old male patient, J. F., with paralysis agitans. Comparison before treatment and 5 days after infusion therapy with MIF (400 mg daily through 10 days).

TABLE 2. Results of PLG studies (second series)[a]

Name	Age	Sex	Diagnosis[b]	Levodopa	Other AP therapy	Degree[a] Pre-ART	Degree[a] Post-ART	Motor performance Pre-	Motor performance Post-	Clinical improvement (%)	Psychological State Pre-	Psychological State Post-	Remarks
F.H.	63	M	PS/3	625 mg/S	—	432	221	226	488	50	D	N	Dyskinesia
J.W.	61	M	PS/3	750 mg/S	—	332	221	480	650	25	D	D	Dyskinesia
M.K.	61	F	PS/3	400 mg/M	—	331	221	420	532	25	N	Hm	—
H.R.	64	M	PS/3	750 mg/S	—	333	112	395	615	75	N	N	Dyskinesia
R.H.	58	M	PS/2	500 mg/S	—	220	110	526	730	50	D	N	—
F.B.	61	M	PS/2	400 mg/M	—	122	112	473	586	25	D	N	—
M.P.	72	F	PS/4	600 mg/M	—	441	220	160	356	50	N	Hm	—
G.W.	65	F	PS/3	—	Budipine	333	112	235	480	50	D	Hm	—
R.M.	59	F	PS/2	—	Budipine	220	120	368	475	25	N	N	—
S.J.	61	M	PS/2	—	—	221	121	375	492	25	N	N	—
J.M.	56	F	PS/2	—	—	220	110	486	640	50	D	N	—
H.Z.	30	M	TAS + PS/2	—	—	210	110	380	540	25	N	N	Cerebellar
M.S.	24	M	TAS + PS/2	—	—	310	210	245	456	25	N	N	Cerebellar

[a] Abbreviations as in Table 1.
[b] PS, Parkinson's syndrome; TAS, traumatic apallic syndrome.

preexisting dyskinesias which showed transient exacerbation in 2 patients during this series. This observation is in accordance with previously published studies (13). The effect on the psychological state was the same as reported earlier (7).

Four patients in whom the 9-day period was preceded by a crossover application of PLG and placebo during 6 days showed globally similar results, as can be seen in Table 2. The improvement ranged from 25 to 75%. There was no correlation between the severity of symptoms at onset and final improvement. The same effects on dyskinesia and mood could be observed. Figure 6 shows a patient before the study had started and at the end of the 15-day period.

Figure 7 summarizes the results of the clinical ratings of akinesia, rigidity, and tremor in all 7 patients treated with the combination of levodopa and PLG. Again, it is visible that tremor is less influenced than akinesia and rigidity.

The crossover trial in the second group revealed another remarkable aspect of the PLG effect. As can be seen from Fig. 8 there is an overhanging effect of PLG demonstrable during the placebo days. The graph represents the rigidity scores of all four extremities of one of the patients (case 4) of this group in a continuous 15-day rating period with 6 daily ratings during the first 7 days and 3 daily ratings thereafter. A daily profile with a minimum at 2 P.M. was evident on DOPA when placebo was added. A 400-mg bolus in the morning accentuated this profile. This PLG effect not only was maintained during the following placebo days but was still accentuated. Up to the 6th

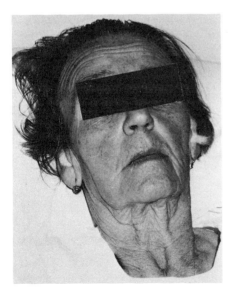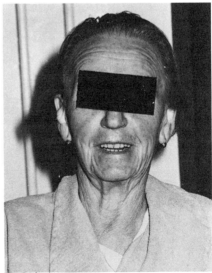

FIG. 6. Left: patient before the start of the study. Right: patient at the end of 15-day treatment period.

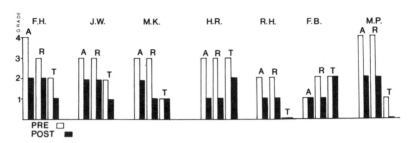

FIG. 7. Effect of treatment with PLG (200 mg) twice daily in addition to previous levadopa treatment on akinesia rigidity and tremor in 7 patients with Parkinson syndrome.

day an additional and cumulative effect became evident. In the permanent application period (with application of 200 mg PLG twice daily) only a slight further decrease in rigidity was reached, whereas the circadian profile was progressively lost.

In order to find out more details about the immediate effect of PLG and its time course as already examined by Barbeau and Kastin (3), we followed motor performance in one of the patients out of group 1 (case 3) in a continuous 24-hr rating after a single 200-mg dose of PLG i.v. It can be seen from Fig. 9 that a marked increase is reached after 1 hr, becoming maximal 3 to 4 hr after the injection, with a gradual decrease in the following 20 hr. After 24 hr performance score was still 20% higher than the control value.

Two patients who had been treated with an anticholinergic agent (Budipine) for 3 months received additional PLG 200 mg i.v. twice daily for 10 days. Potentiation of the Budipine effect could be demonstrated on a long-term basis as well as during an 8-hr rating period. Table 2 shows a global improvement of 25% in one patient (case 9) and of 50% in case 8. Figure 10 shows the result of 8-hr rating in such a patient.

With the fifth group, it was possible to confirm our previous results on the effect of PLG on Parkinson symptoms when used without any other antiparkinson therapy.

Based on the experience that PLG as the sole agent is effective in relieving Parkinson symptoms, we administered the substance to 2 patients in a deficiency state after a traumatic apallic syndrome with prominent Parkinson signs as well as cerebellar symptoms. Both showed mild clinical improvement approximating 25%. The drawing and writing performance of 1 of the 2 patients showed significant improvement under PLG. This effect was in part due to a diminution of the cerebellar symptoms.

In summarizing the results of our second set of studies with PLG, we confirm Barbeau's clinical observation of potentiation of levodopa effect by MIF (1). Although our first set of studies showed a dependence of PLG-induced improvement on the severity of parkinsonian symptoms, this correlation was not confirmed by the results of our second series.

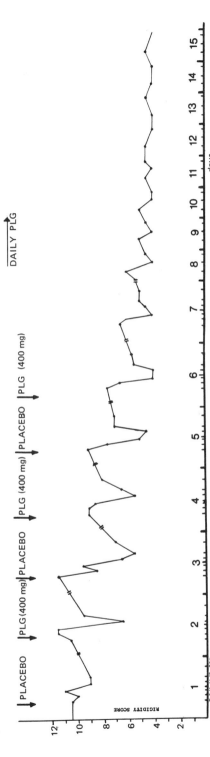

FIG. 8. Hans R., a 64-year-old male with Parkinson syndrome of grade 3. Oral levodopa therapy (Sinemet, $6 \times \frac{1}{2}$, 1 year). Additional PLG treatment for 15 days. During first 6 days every second day 400 mg PLG i.v. as a bolus and from the 7th day 400 mg PLG i.v. daily. Rigidity, total score for all four extremities.

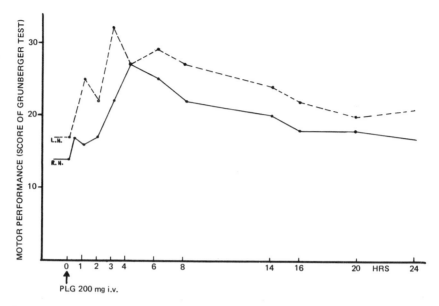

FIG. 9. Maria K., a 61-year-old female with Parkinson syndrome of grade 3. Oral levodopa therapy (Maldopar, 125 mg 4 × 1, 1½ years). Motor performance profile over 24 hours. Period after bolus injection of 200 mg PLG i.v. (L.H. = left hand; R.H. = right hand.)

In analyzing the clinical effect of PLG, it seems that the bolus injection of 200 or 400 mg is superior to the slow infusion. Whereas in the first series there was a delay of 3 days before the effects were visible, the bolus administration of the substance led to first effects after 10 to 15 min, with a maximum reached after 3 hr. When we used the bolus injection alternating with a placebo, a cumulative effect was discovered. From current experimental data, it thus seems that PLG acts as a receptor-activating substance at the postsynaptic site. From our clinical experience, we would suggest that this activation is dependent on dosage as well as on the factor of time. According to our experience, a dose of 200 mg PLG as a bolus (i.v.) is necessary for rapid clinical effects. Lower doses seem to be less effective. On the other hand, we could not increase the clinical improvement or its rapidity of onset with daily doses higher than 400 mg. It is our impression that a slow intravenous infusion needs the cumulative property of PLG to become clinically effective, and therefore onset of improvement is delayed.

The question whether PLG can cause dyskinesias or worsen preexisting levodopa dyskinesias is still unanswered. From our experience transient activation of dyskinesias seems possible. We could not find that PLG reduced the dyskinesias in our patients.

Cerebellar symptoms in one of our patients with a deficiency state from a traumatic apallic syndrome were diminished under PLG. The influence of

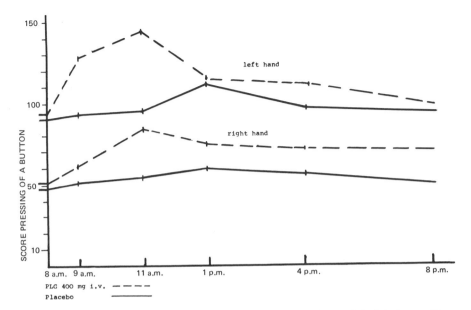

FIG. 10. Gertraud W., a 65-year-old female with Parkinson syndrome (Postenc.). Budipin therapy 80 mg (3 months). Motor performance (pressing a button) after PLG 200 mg i.v. as bolus (----) as compared to placebo (—).

PLG on the depressive state was reconfirmed, which suggests further clinical investigation in endogenous depression.

In closing, we would again like to emphasize that PLG is opening a new way in therapy for Parkinson's syndrome.

REFERENCES

1. Barbeau, A. (1975): Potentiation of L-Dopa effect by intravenous L-prolyl-L-leucyl-glycine amide in man. *Lancet,* 2:683.
2. Barbeau, A. (1977): Peptides and extrapyramidal disease. Delivered at the 11th World Congress of Neurology, Amsterdam.
3. Barbeau, A., and Kastin, A. J. (1976): Polypeptide therapy in Parkinson's disease —A new approach. In: *Advances in Parkinsonism,* edited by W. Birkmayer and O. Hornykiewicz, pp. 483–487. Editiones Roche, Basel.
4. Barbeau, A., Roy, M., and Kastin, A. J. (1976): Double-blind evaluation of oral L-prolyl-L-leucyl-glycine amide in Parkinson's disease. *Can. Med. Assoc. J.,* 114: 120–122.
5. Fischer, P. A., Schneider, E., Jacobi, P., and Maxion, H. (1974): Effect of melano-cyte-stimulation hormone-release inhibiting factor (MIF) in Parkinson's syndrome. *Eur. Neurol.,* 12:360.
6. Gerstenbrand, F. (1977): Discussion of peptides and extrapyramidal disease. Delivered at the 11th World Congress of Neurology, Amsterdam.
7. Gerstenbrand, F., Binder, H., Kozma, C., Pusch, S., and Reisner, T. (1975): Infusionstherapie mit MIF (melanocyte inhibiting factor) beim Parkinson-Syndrom. *Wien. Klin. Wochenschr.,* 87:822–823.

8. Gerstenbrand, F., Binder, H., Grünberger, J., Kozma, C., Pusch, S., and Reisner, T. (1976): Infusion therapy with MIF (melanocyte inhibiting factor) in Parkinson's disease. In: *Advances in Parkinsonism,* edited by W. Birkmayer and O. Hornykiewicz, pp. 456–461. Editiones Roche, Basel.
9. Kastin, A. J., and Barbeau, A. (1972): Preliminary clinical studies with L-prolyl-L-leucyl-glycine amide in Parkinson's disease. *Can. Med. Assoc. J.,* 107:1079.
10. Plotnikoff, N. P., and Kastin, A. J. (1974): Oxotremorine antagonism by prolyl-leucyl-glycine amide administered by different routes and with several anticholinergics. *Pharmacol. Biochem. Behav.,* 2:417.
11. Plotnikoff, N. P., Minard, F. N., and Kastin, A. J. (1974): Dopa potentiation in ablated animals and brain levels of biogenic amines in intact animals after prolyl-leucyl-glycine amide. *Neuroendocrinology,* 14:271.
12. Shuster, S., Burton, J. L., Thody, A. J., Plummer, N., Goolamali, S. K., and Bates, D. (1973): Melanocyte-stimulating hormone and parkinsonism. *Lancet,* 1:463.
13. Woods, A. C., and Chase, T. N. (1973): M.I.F.: Effect on levodopa dyskinesias in man. *Lancet,* 2(9):513.

Subject Index